# Progress in Inflammation Research

## Series Editor

Prof. Dr. Michael J. Parnham
PLIVA
Research Institute
Prilaz baruna Filipovica 25
10000 Zagreb
Croatia

T Cells in Arthritis, P. Miossec, W. van den Berg, G. Firestein (Editors), 1998
Chemokines and Skin, E. Kownatzki, J. Norgauer (Editors), 1998
Medicinal Fatty Acids, J. Kremer (Editor), 1998
Inducible Enzymes in the Inflammatory Response, D. A. Willoughby, A. Tomlinson (Editors), 1999
Cytokines in Severe Sepsis and Septic Shock, H. Redl, G. Schlag (Editors), 1999
Fatty Acids and Inflammatory Skin Diseases, J.-M. Schröder (Editor), 1999
Immunomodulatory Agents from Plants, H. Wagner (Editor), 1999
Cytokines and Pain, L. Watkins, S. Maier, (Editors), 1999
In vivo Models of Inflammation, D. Morgan, L. Marshall, (Editors), 1999
Pain and Neurogenic Inflammation, S. D. Brain, P. Moore (Editors), 1999

## Forthcoming titles:

Apoptosis and Inflammation, James D. Winkler (Editor), 1999
Novel Inhibitors of Leukotrienes, G. Folco, B. Samuelsson, R.C. Murphy (Editors), 1999
Vascular Adhesion Molecules and Inflammation, J. D. Pearson (Editor), 1999
Metalloproteinases as Targets for Anti-Inflammatory Drugs, K.M.K. Bottomley, D. Bradshaw, J.S. Nixon (Editors), 1999
Free Radicals and Inflammation, P. Winyard, D. Blake, Ch. Evans, (Editors), 1999
Gene therapy in Inflammatory Diseases, Ch. Evans, P. Robbins (Editors), 1999

# Anti-Inflammatory Drugs in Asthma

Anthony P. Sampson
Martin K. Church

Editors

Birkhäuser Verlag
Basel · Boston · Berlin

1999

Editors

Dr. Anthony P. Sampson
Prof. Martin K. Church
Immunopharmacology Group
Southampton General Hospital
Tremona Road
Southampton, SO16 6YD
UK

A CIP catalogue record for this book is available from the Library of Congress, Washington D.C., USA


Deutsche Bibliothek Cataloging-in-Publication Data
**Anti-inflammatory drugs in asthma** / Anthony B. Sampson ;
Martin K. Church (ed.). - Basel ; Boston ; Berlin : Birkhäuser, 1999
  (Progress in inflammation research)
  ISBN 3-7643-5873-4 (Basel...)
  ISBN 0-8176-5873-4 (Boston)

© 1999 Birkhäuser Verlag, P.O. Box 133, CH-4010 Basel, Switzerland
Printed on acid-free paper produced from chlorine-free pulp. TCF ∞
Cover design: Markus Etterich, Basel
Printed in Germany
ISBN 3-7643-5873-4
ISBN 0-8176-5873-4

9 8 7 6 5 4 3 2 1

# Contents

# List of contributors

Neil C Barnes, Department of Respiratory Medicine, The London Chest Hospital, Bonner Road, London E2 9X, UK

Peter J. Barnes, Department of Thoracic Medicine, National Heart and Lung Institute, Dovehause St., London SW3 6 LY, UK; e-mail: p.j.barnes@ic.ac.uk

Li Chee Loh, Department of Respiratory Medicine, The London Chest Hospital, Bonner Road, London E2 9JX, UK

Steven J. Compton, Immunopharmacology Group, University of Southampton, Southampton General Hospital, Southampton, SO16 6YD, UK;
e-mail: sjc1@soton.ac.uk

Zuzana Diamant, Erasmus University Medical Centre Rotterdam, Department of Respiratory Diseases, Dr Molewaterplein 40, NL-3015 GD Rotterdam, The Netherlands; e-mail: z.diamant@gems.demon.nl

Ratko Djukanović, University Medicine (810), Level D, Centre Block, Southampton General Hospital, Tremona Road, Southampton, SO16 6YD, UK

Paul S. Foster, Division of Biochemistry and Molecular Biology, John Curtin School of Medical Research, Australian National University, Acton ACT 0200;
e-mail: Paul.Foster@anu.edu.au

Simon P. Hogan, Division of Biochemistry and Molecular Biology, John Curtin School of Medical Research, Australian National University, Acton ACT 0200;
e-mail: Simon.Hogan@anu.edu.au

Guy F. Joos, Department of Respiratory Diseases, University Hospital Ghent, De Pintelaan 185, B-9000 Ghent, Belgium; e-mail: guy.joos@rug.ac.be

James L. Lordan, University Medicine (810), Level D, Centre Block, Southampton General Hospital, Tremona Road, Southampton, SO16 6YD, UK; e-mail: jll1@soton.ac.uk

Francesco Patalano, SkyePharma AG, Eptingerstr. 51, CH-4132 Muttenz, Switzerland; e-mail: f.patalano@skyepharma.ch

Romaine A. Pauwels, Department of Respiratory Diseases, University Hospital Ghent, De Pintelaan 185, B-9000 Ghent, Belgium

Renaat A. Peleman, Department of Respiratory Diseases, University Hospital Ghent, De Pintelaan 185, B-9000 Ghent, Belgium

Anthony P. Sampson, Immunopharmacology Group, Level F, Centre Block (825), Southampton General Hospital, Tremona Road, Southampton, SO16 6YD, UK; e-mail: aps@soton.ac.uk

Christian Schudt, Byk Gulden Lomberg, Chemische Fabrik GmbH. Byk Gulden Strasse 2, D-78467 Konstanz, Germany; e-mail: Christian.Schudt@byk.de

Anne E. Tattersfield, Division of Respiratory Medicine, ity Hospital, Mucknall Road, Nottingham, NG 1PB, UK

Hermann Tenor, Byk Gulden Lomberg, Chemische Fabrik GmbH, Byk Gulden Strasse 2, D-78467 Konstanz, Germany; e-mail: Hermann.Tenor@byk.de

Joanna S. Thompson Coon, Division of Respiratory Medicine, City Hospital, Hucknall Road Nottingham, NG5 1PB, UK; e-mail: mfzjtc@unix.ccc.nottingham.ac.uk

Andrew F. Walls, Immunopharmacology Group, University of Southampton, Mailpoint 837, Southampton General Hospital, Southampton, SO16 6YD, UK; e-mail: afw1@soton.ac.uk

# Anti-inflammatory drugs in asthma: The pathophysiology of asthma

*James L. Lordan and Ratko Djukanović*

University Medicine (810), Level D, Centre Block, Southampton General Hospital, Tremona Road, Southhampton, SO16 6YD, UK

## Introduction

Asthma is a chronic condition characterised by widespread, variable and reversible airflow obstruction which is either spontaneous or pharmacologically induced. The underlying pathophysiological feature of asthma is increased airway responsiveness which develops on a basis of diffuse bronchial inflammation. The prevalence of asthma is increasing worldwide despite improved treatment which has resulted from a more comprehensive understanding of its pathogenesis [1]. In most countries asthma affects between 4 and 8% of the population, with a trend towards an increase in morbidity as judged by increased hospital admissions [2]. The reasons for this are unclear, but environmental factors such as indoor and outdoor air pollution and changes in lifestyle are considered to be amongst the contributing factors.

Asthma is clearly a complex process mediated by inflammatory cells and the formed and structural elements of the airway, involving numerous cytokines, chemokines, and costimulatory and adhesion molecules that interact in a complex network (Fig. 1). There is accumulating evidence establishing a link between chronic inflammation and remodelling of the airways in asthma. The present evidence of relatively permanent, irreversible structural changes found at an early stage in asthma supports the recommendations of current asthma management guidelines that effective anti-inflammatory treatment be introduced at an early stage in the management of asthma.

Asthma has been closely associated with atopy, the ability to generate an IgE response to environmental allergens which is detected by positive skin tests to one or more allergens, although it is interesting to note that only one-fifth of atopic individuals actually develop asthma. Whilst the presence of allergen specific IgE has been considered to be central to allergic responses in human allergic disease, studies using IgE-deficient mice have demonstrated that bronchial eosinophilic inflammation and airway hyperresponsiveness (AHR) can occur in the absence of IgE [3]. To what extent these observations are relevant to human disease remains to be elucidated. Clinical studies using a humanised monoclonal antibody to IgE show that

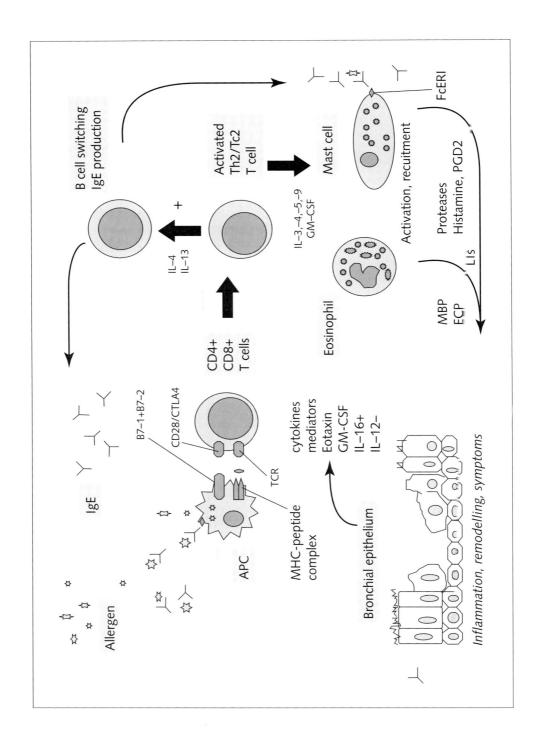

despite a dramatic depletion of IgE from the circulation with the prevention of the early and late phase response to allergen challenge, the clinical response in allergic asthmatics is quite poor [4, 5]. These studies suggest that while IgE is likely to be contributing to the inflammatory process in asthma, other immune mechanisms must be operating in parallel [6].

## The genetic basis of asthma

There is evidence from family aggregation studies to support an important role for genetic contributionfactors into the development of atopy and asthma. The prevalence of asthma in first-order relatives of asthmatics is 20–25% compared with 4–5% in the general population [1]. The relative contribution of genetic factors to the onset of allergy and asthma is estimated at 40–60% [7]. Twin studies, including a large study of 7000 same-sex twins by Edfors-Lubs, provide evidence for the genetic contribution to the onset of asthma, with concordance for asthma in monozygotic twins being 19%, and only 4.8% for dizygotic twins, who share less common genetic material [8]. Asthma is a complex genetic disorder, with studies suggesting a polygenic inheritance pattern which interacts with environmental factors to express the full clinical and pathophysiological phenotype [1].

Genetic studies are being used to characterise and map the genes responsible for the asthmatic phenotype. Studies in British families by Cookson and colleagues were the first to provide evidence of linkage of atopy to a marker (D11S97) on chromosome 11q13 in the vicinity of genes for CD20 (a B cell marker) and FcεRI-β, the β component of the high affinity IgE receptor [9–12]. An iso-leucine to leucine polymorphism at position 181 was identified in the FcεRI-β gene and was found in 15% of individuals, being associated with the phenotype of high total serum IgE [13]. A polymorphism (Glu 237-Gly) was found in 5.3% of the population in a study by Hill and colleagues and this was associated with AHR and atopy [5014]. There is

*Figure 1*
*The inflammatory process in asthma involves the activation of Th2 type T cells by antigen presenting cells (APCs) resident in the airway wall (i.e. dendritic cells). T cell derived cytokines, including Interleukin-4 and IL-13 promote the switching of B cells to the synthesis of IgE. Cytokines are involved in the activation and differentiation of eosinophils and mast cells with release of pro-inflammatory mediators, leading to epithelial damage, bronchoconstriction and symptoms of asthma. The bronchial epithelium plays an active role by the release of mediators and cytokines. MHC, major histocompatibility complex class II; TCR, T cell receptor; FcεRI, high affinity IgE receptor; MBP, major basic protein; ECP, eosinophil cationic protein; LT, leukotrienes; $PGD_2$, Prostaglandin $D_2$.*

also evidence for linkage of atopy and AHR to chromosome 5q31–33, which contains the genes for many cytokines considered to play an important role in asthma (interleukins- (IL-) 3, 4, 5, 9, and 13 and GM-CSF) [15]. In a study of Amish families involving 349 affected sib pairs, Marsh and colleagues provided evidence of linkage of total serum IgE with markers located at 5q31 [16]. A study in Dutch families, using affected sib pair analysis and linkage analysis, has also provideds evidence of linkage of total serum IgE and AHR to markers on chromosome 5q [17, 18]. Asthma and elevated serum IgE levels have further been linked to markers on chromosome 12q which contains candidate asthma genes including IFNγ, mast cell growth factor (MGF), insulin-like growth factor-1 (IGF-1), and the constitutive form of nitric oxide synthase (NOS-1) [19, 20].

In agreement with the complex nature of asthma pathogenesis, tThere is evidence that the human leucocyte antigen (HLA) and T cell receptor (TCR) genes may genetically also contribute to determine antigen- specific IgE responses. Studies have shown associations between HLA alleles (HLA DRB1) and specific IgE responses [21]. HLA-DQw2 is more prevalent in Chinese children with asthma and house dust mite (HDM) allergy [22]. An association is found with certain alleles (HLA-DQB1*0503 and HLA-DQB1*0201/0301) and the onset of isocyanate-induced asthma in exposed individuals, while other alleles (HLA-DQB1*0501 and DQA1*0101-DQB1*0501-DR1) appeared to be protective (HLA-DQB1*0501 and DQA1*0101-DQB1*0501-DR1 [23]. The alpha chain of the T cell receptor (TCR), located on chromosome 114, has been linked to specific IgE responses in a population of atopic asthmatics [24]. On chromosome 5q31–33 the β2 adrenoreceptor gene has been linked with a phenotype based on elevated IgE and bronchial hyperreactivity. Of significant relevance to treatment of asthma are the genes which might determine response to anti-inflammatory drugs, and one such plausible candidate for corticosteroid resistance is the glucocorticoid receptor gene [2, 25].

## Prenatal origin of asthma and allergy

A familial tendency is seen in allergic patients, with 50% of children with one parent and 80% of those with two allergic parents becoming atopic [26]. Significantly more infants of an atopic mother develop allergy than those with an allergic father [27]. It is hypothesized that factors which determine allergic responses may cross the placenta and activate the process of initial sensitization of the fetal immune system. Thus, IL-10, a cytokine known believed to deviate the immune response to a Th2 type immune response, thus favouring the development of atopy in the foetus of an atopic mother [28], is detectable in amniotic fluid with at higher levels seen in atopic mothers than non-atopic mothers [29]. The maternal antigen presenting cells (APC) of the mother may pre-process antigen to peptides capable of crossing the placenta, allowing the foetal APCs to present this specific peptide to foetal T cells [76]. There is also evidence to suggest that house dust mite antigens are present in cord blood, enabling foetal exposure to allergen to occur *in utero*. Infants who subsequently develop allergy during later childhood demonstrate an altered immune response at birth, with raised proliferative responses of T cells from cord blood and defective IFNγ production of IFNγ (a cytokine which downregulates allergic responses) to specific allergic stimulation [30]. Circulating allergen-specific T cells can be demonstrated as early as 15 weeks of gestation, and increased proliferative responses to antigen can be seen from 22 weeks, suggesting that the second trimester may be vital for initial sensitisation [30]. Circulating allergen-specific T cells are detectable at birth and these cells are thought to migrate over the following 6 to 12 months to tissue sites where disease will be expressed [31–33]. The early origin of atopy therefore appears to be central to a strategy aimed at early intervention. In keeping with this notion, studies are under way to assess whether allergen avoidance during the second trimester of pregnancy and the first year of life is effective in preventing the sensitization and subsequent development of atopy and allergy.

## Pathological features of asthma

Asthma is characterised by variable damage to the epithelium with and increased numbers of mucosal and submucosal inflammatory cells, including eosinophils, mast cells and lymphocytes [34, 35]. Other prominent features of asthma are hypertrophy of airway smooth muscle, thickening of the basement membrane, mucosal oedema and excessive secretion of mucus, all of which contribute to airways narrowing. In severe exacerbations both large and small airways show gross damage and shedding of the epithelium, and the airways may become occluded by inspissated mucus and cellular debris which form tenacious plugs [34, 35]. Studies suggest differences in the type of inflammation depending on the time-course of asthma exacerbation, with infiltration of eosinophils being noted in slow-onset fatal asthma and an excess of neutrophils being seen the prominent feature of sudden acute asthma deaths [36].

## Cellular mechanisms in asthma

The ability to obtain representative samples of the lower respiratory tract and technological improvements in analysing samples hasve revolutionised our understanding of the cellular and molecular basis of asthma. The advent of flexible bronchoscopy as a research tool, and the ability to safely obtain and analyse bronchial biopsies, bronchial brushings and bronchoalveolar lavage (BAL) fluid in asthmatic individuals, together with the recent validation of induced sputum techniques, have provided essential samples for research purposes.

Traditionally asthma has been viewed as a condition characterised by airway infiltration with activated mast cells and eosinophils, orchestrated by specific Th2 polarised T lymphocytes [37]. It is increasingly evident that other structures, including the bronchial epithelium, endothelium, fibroblasts and the extracellular matrix are involved in the recruitment of inflammatory cells, tissue damage and the subsequent repair and remodelling process that is characteristic of asthma.

## Antigen presentation and co-stimulation

Environmental allergens and antigen presentation play an important role in the initiation and maintenance of airway inflammation. As with any immune response, antigen presentation of allergens to the immune system is central to subsequent responses. On exposure to antigen, T cells require the assistance of antigen-presenting cells (APC), such as dendritic cells, tissue macrophages, or in the case of secondary presentation, B cells, for optimal activation [38]. Antigen presentation involves the intracellular processing of allergen to peptides which are presented to the T cell receptor (TCR) in the context of major histocompatibility complex (MHC) class II molecules on the surface of APCs. For this process to be effective at eliciting a T cell response, ligation of costimulatory molecules on the surface of T cells and APC is required, resulting in optimal T cell clonal expansion and activation (Fig. 2).

The dendritic cells (DC), which form an intricate network within the bronchial epithelium, are believed to be the main APC in the airways. They develop from monocytes in the presence of IL-3, stem cell factor (SCF) and GM-CSF, having a unique capacity to stimulate naïve T cells. In rats, dendritic cells can be shown to migrate to regional (peribronchial, and mediastinal) lymph nodes for presentation of antigen to the immune system [39]. Of relevance to antigen presentation in asthma is the finding that dendritic cell numbers are elevated in the mucosa of asthmatic individuals and are reduced by treatment with inhaled corticosteroids in association with improved disease control [40, 41]. Although the mechanisms responsible for this increase in DC numbers are largely unknown, local T cell-mediated inflammation is enhanced by increased production of granulocyte macrophage-colony stimulating factor (GM-CSF) which enhances the ability of DC to differentiate and present antigen effectively [39]. Other cells, such as macrophages or B cells, may be involved in antigen presentation, but their role in asthma is poorly understood. Macrophages recovered by BAL are generally poor antigen presenting cells and have predominantly an immuno-suppressive role in the lungs, despite the fact that tissue macrophages promote inflammation through the production of pro-inflammatory mediators, such as $PGE_2$, hydrogen peroxide, leukotrienes, and cytokines such as IL-1, GM-CSF and MCP-1 [42–46]. Alveolar macrophages have a reduced capacity to bind with T cells, which may be due to reduced density of LFA-1 expression on their

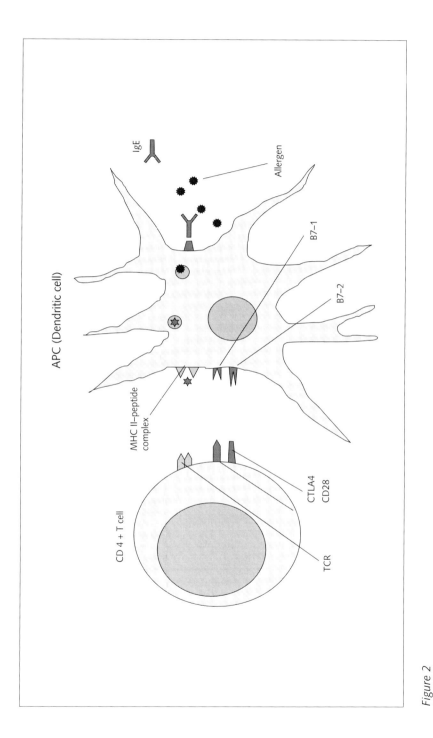

*Figure 2*

*Activation of T cells by antigen presenting cells (APCs) involves the processing of allergen by APCs and presentation of peptide to the T cell receptor via the major histocompatibility complex (MHC) class II molecules. Optimum T cell activation requires a costimulatory signal delivered via the CD28/CTLA4-CD80 (B7-1)/CD86 (B7-2) pathway. Antigen uptake by APCs is potentiated by IgE-facilitated mechanisms involving the high affinity IgE receptor (FcεRI).*

cell surface AM [47, 48]. Defective expression of B7-1 and B7-2 expression has previously been shown on AMs which would reduce the ability to present antigen efficiently [49], although a recent study by Agea and coworkers has shown elevated expression of B7-2 on AM in BAL fluid from atopic asthmatics compared with normal control subjects [50].

## Costimulation via the CD28:B7 pathway

There is considerable evidence to support an important role for costimulatory molecules in regulating the proliferation and activation of T cells in the immune response. Of particular relevance are the interaction between CD28 and B7, and the CD40 binding with CD40 ligand (CD40L) [51, 52].

Following interaction between the T cell receptor (TCR) on the T cell membrane and the major histocompatibility (MHC) antigen-peptide complex on the APC, CD28 molecules expressed on the surface of T cells interact with B7-1 (CD80) and B7-2 (CD86) ligands expressed on the surface of APCs to provide a powerful augmenting stimulus to T cell activation. Studies have suggested that binding of another molecule present on activated T cells, CTLA-4, to B7-1 and B7-2 delivers a negative signal and functions to downregulate T cell activity [53, 54]. However, the role of CTLA4 remains uncertain, with recent studies suggesting that CTLA-4 might also deliver a positive signal to T cell activation [55, 56]. The development of CTLA4-Ig, a fusion protein consisting of the extracellular domain of CTLA4 and the Fc portion of a human immunoglobulin $G_1$ (Ig$G_1$), has provided a useful tool to study the role of CD28/B7 interactions in immune responses. A number of studies have shown that interference with interaction by CTLA4-Ig is able to switch off T cell activation [57]. Recent studies using an ovalbumin sensitive murine model of asthma showed that systemic or intra-nasal CTLA4-Ig treatment suppresses the response to inhaled allergen (increased AHR, IgE production, irecruitment of eosinophils into the lungs, production of IL-4, IL-5, and IL-10 and increased IFNγ production from CD3-TCR-activated T cells) [31, 54, 58–60]. Anti B7-2 treatment was has been shown seen to have effects similiar in magnitude on eosinophil infiltration, cytokine production, IgE production and to reduce bronchial hyperresponsiveness, suggesting that interaction of B7-2 with CD28 is important in the development of a Th-2 type inflammatory response in mice.

This observation has recently been shown to be of relevance to human allergic disease. *In vitro* studies have shown that exposure of naïve cord blood mononuclear cells to Der P allergen or Th-2 type cytokines, IL-4 or GM-CSF, results in increased expression of B7-2 and to a lesser extent B7-1. Blockade of CD28-B7 signalling by CTLA4-Ig or anti-B7-2 antibody has been shown to inhibit allergen-induced proliferation and cytokine mRNA production by PBMC from both atopic and non-atopic subjects [61]. A recent study by Spinozzi and colleagues has also shown increased expression of B7-2 on BAL fluid alveolar macrophages from atopic asthmatics compared to normal controls, and to patients with pulmonary sarcoidosis or extrinsic allergic alveolitis [50].

The role of co-stimulation was recently studied in a human bronchial explant model of asthma. Bronchial biopsies obtained at bronchoscopy from house dust mite (HDM) sensitive atopic asthmatics were cultured for 24 h in the presence of house dust mite allergen extract. In this bronchial explant model, allergen was shown to stimulate the production of the cytokines IL-5 and IL-13 [62]. Addition of CTLA4-Ig fusion protein to the culture medium effectively blocked production of both IL-5 and IL-13 found on stimulation *ex vivo* with house dust mite antigen [62]. These studies confirm the requirement for interaction between co-stimulatory molecules in cytokine production and allergic inflammation, and point to the CD28-B7 pathway as being important to the allergen-induced AHR in asthma. Studies of organ transplantation in primates suggest that CTLA4-Ig is extremely effective in preventing organ rejection. While Phase I clinical trials have shown CTLA-4-Ig treatment of patients with psoriasis vulgaris to be well tolerated and to result in clinical improvement, its role in asthma management merits further investigation [63].

## The role of CD40-CD40L interaction

There is considerable recent interest in the role of CD40 and its ligand CD40L in inflammation. CD40 is expressed on a number of cells, including B cells, T cells, monocytes, dendritic cells, eosinophils, and endothelial cells [64]. Ligation of CD40 ligation on monocytes and dendritic cells results in the secretion of cytokines IL-1, -6, -8, -10, -12, TNFα, MIP1α and up-regulation of costimulatory molecule expression such as CD54 (ICAM-1), CD58 (LFA-3), B7-1 and B7-2 on the cell surface. In co-cultures of dendritic cells and T cells, the interruption of CD40 signalling with an anti-CD40L monoclonal antibody results in reduced T cell proliferation. Ligation of CD40L on human activated T cells by specific monoclonal antibodies or with CD40 transfected T cells considerably enhances their cytokine production [65]. The interruption of CD40-CD40L interactions appears to improve the disease state in murine models of many conditions (e.g. collagen arthritis, lupus nephritis, experimental allergic encephalomyelitis and Leishmania infection) [64]. However, while its effects on B cell function and IgE production in allergy have been well studied, the role in T cell function is less clear.

## Facilitated antigen presentation

Emerging evidence suggests that IgE may potentiate allergen-specific responses by binding to high- and low- affinity IgE receptors (FcεRI and FcεRII) on the surface

9

of antigen presenting cells and facilitating the capture and internalization of antigen which can subsequently be processed and presented to T cells. It has recently been demonstrated that IgE/FcɛRI-mediated antigen uptake results in 100–1000-fold increased effectiveness in antigen presentation by APCs [66]. A recent study of bronchial biopsies has shown that pulmonary DCs and mast cells stain positively for the α sub-unit of FcɛRI [67]. This suggests a possible role for IgE and facilitated antigen presentation in the induction and mainteanance of chronic inflammation in asthma.

## Transcription factors

There is increasing research interest in the role of transcription factors in the expression of cytokine genes involved in asthma. Transcription factors are intra-cellular proteins that bind to regulatory sequences of target genes, activating gene transcription, and subsequent cytokine mRNA and protein production. It is also increasingly recognised that therapies for asthma, such as corticosteroids and cyclosporin A, may function through interaction with transcription factors. Many stimuli including cytokines, activators of protein kinase C, viruses, and oxidants activate transcription factors including NFκB [68]. Cytokines act by binding to receptors on target cells with increased intracellular production of various protein kinases and phosphorylation of nuclear factor kappa B (NFκB) and activator pro-tein (AP)-1. NFκB is present in the cytoplasm in an inactive form complexed to an inhibitory protein IκB. Various protein kinase molecules phosphorylate IκB to release free NFκB which then localises to the nucleus and binds to a specific κB recognition element on the promoter region of several genes. NFκB is an important regulator of several inducible genes, such as inducible nitric oxide synthase (iNOS), TNFα, GM-CSF, MIP-1α, MCP-1, eotaxin, ICAM-1 and VCAM-1 [68, 69]. TNFα stimulates the activation of NFκB and AP-1 in the lung, and treatment with corti-costeroids inhibits activation of these transcription factors via a direct interaction between activated glucocorticosteroid receptor (GR), and the p65 subunit of NFκB [70].

## The cytokine mediators of asthma

A number of cytokines have been implicated in controlling and perpetuating the chronic inflammation in asthma [71]. While studies of BAL and bronchial biopsies using *in situ* hybridisation show T cells to be a major source of cytokines in asthma, it is clear that other cells including eosinophils, mast cells, bronchial epithelial cells and the structural elements of the airways contribute to the production of cytokines (Table 1).

Table 1 - The cellular origin of cytokines and chemokines in asthma

| Cell type | Cytokines and chemokines produced |
|---|---|
| T lymphocytes | IL-2, -3, -4, -5, -10, -12, -13, -16 |
| | GM-CSF, TNFα, IFNγ, RANTES, MIP-1α, MCP-3 |
| Eosinophil | IL-1α, -2, -3, -4, -6, -8, -10, -16, |
| | GM-CSF, TNFα, IFNγ, TGFα, TGFβ1, MIP-1α, IGF-II |
| Mast cell | IL-3, -4, -5, -6, -8, -10, -13, -16, |
| | GM-CSF, SCF, TNFα |
| Bronchial epithelium | IL-5 [72], -6, -8, -16, GM-CSF, TNFα, PDGF, |
| | IL-18, IDGF, MIP-1α, MCP-3, RANTES, Eotaxin |
| Alveolar macrophages | IL-1, -10, -12, -13, -18, |
| | GM-CSF, TNFα, MCP-1 |

Cytokines derived from T cells and mast cells, such as IL-4, IL-5, and IL-10 play central roles in the pathogenesis of asthma by their ability to promote recruitment, activation, terminal differentiation, and prolonged survival of eosinophils in the airways, and, in the case of IL-4, to promote B cell switching to IgE production [73]. IL-4 enhances eosinophil recruitment to the airways by increasing VCAM-1 expression on endothelial cells to promote adherence of eosinophils bearing VLA-4 [74, 75, 121]. IL-3 and GM-CSF also contribute to eosinophilic inflammation by promoting eosinophil survival and mast cell and basophil development. GM-CSF is also involved in priming neutrophils and eosinophils [7Barnes PJ 941]. Although T cells and mast cells are likely to initiate the production of eosinophilotactic cytokines, eosinophils are also capable of enhancing eosinophilic inflammation by producingtion of IL-4, IL-5, GM-CSF and TNFα [76]. A number of studies have confirmed increased expression of the Th2-type cytokines which promote the allergic response (IL-4 and IL-5), but not the Th1-type cytokine IFNγ, in BAL and bronchial biopsies from asthmatics [77, 78].

While there is a considerable body of evidence to support the role of cytokines such as IL-3, IL-4, IL-5, IL-6 and GM-CSF in asthma, a number of studies have recently focussed on IL-10, IL-12, IL-13, IL-16 and IL-18. IL-10 inhibits T cell proliferation and cytokine production [79, 80]. *In vivo* studies in murine models of allergic disease show that IL-10 treatment can reduce the airway eosinophilic response to allergen inhalation by preventing the release of pro-inflammatory cytokines IL-3, IL-5, GM-CSF and TNFα [76]. It has been suggested that IL-10 is produced as a late event after T cell activation in asthma [Robinson DS 9680], with IL-10 mRNA expression being increased after allergen challenge and localised predominantly to CD3+ T cells, but also to CD68+ alveolar macrophages. It has thus been suggested This suggests that IL-10 may be useful as a potential therapeutic agent in asthma by controlling Th2-mediated inflammatory processes and preventing eosinophil accumulation [76, 80].

*In vitro* studies show that IL-12 promotes IFNγ production, suppresses IgE production, and promotes development of a Th1 phenotype [81, 82, 77]. For In sensitised mice, IL-12 treatment has been shown to abrogate airway hyperresponsiveness, eosinophilia and the production of Th-2 type cytokines after allergen inhalation [Gavett 9583]. Studies using anti-IFNγ antibodies show that the action of IL-12, at least in mice, is partially mediated by IFNγ production. The expression of IL-12 in bronchial biopsies is lower in asthmatics than normal controls, with mRNA for IL-12 being localised to alveolar macrophages and T cells [77]. A recent observation that treatment with prednisolone results in a significant increase in IL-12 mRNA positive cells in bronchial biopsies from steroid sensitive (SS) asthmatics but not steroid resistant (SR) asthmatic patients [77]. IL-12 provides further insight into the mechanisms of severe asthma that does not respond readily to corticosteroids. In addition, it suggests that treatment with IL-12 may prove useful in the management of asthma.

IL-13 is produced mainly by activated T cells and has a potentially important role in regulating allergic inflammation in asthma by promoting B cell proliferation, differentiation and immunoglobulin secretion via enhancement of class switching from IgG to IgE. This cytokine upregulates MHC class II and FcεRII (low affinity IgE receptor) molecules and can promote dendritic cell development [84, 85]. IL-13 also upregulates VCAM-1 expression on vascular endothelial cells, which togetheor with IL-4 and TNFα promotes eosinophil accumulation [86, 87]. Segmental allergen challenge in asthmatics has conclusively shown elevated expression of cells expressing BAL IL-13 mRNA and IL-13 levels in BAL [85, 88]. As noted for IL-2 and IL-4, treatment with prednisolone results in improvement in lung function which is associated with a significant downregulation in IL-13 mRNA cellular expression in glucorticosteroid sensitive (GS) asthmatics, but not in glucocorticosteroid resistant (GR) asthmatics who showed little clinical improvement after treatment [77, 86]. These observations support the hypothesis that corticosteroid action is mediated partly by influencing IL-12 and IL-13 expression [77].

IL-16 is a newly characterised cytokine which has been shown to be produced by CD4+ and CD8+ T cells, epithelial cells, mast cells and eosinophils [89, 92, 113]. It uses the surface molecule CD4 as its ligand and thus activates cells that are CD4+, namely monocytes and CD4+ T cells [90]. Bronchial biopsy studies using ISH show expression of IL-16 mRNA on epithelial cells from asthmatics but not normal or atopic controls. The epithelial and subepithelial IL-16 mRNA expression was significantly associated with airways hyperresponsiveness and CD4+ T cell infiltration in the bronchial mucosa [91]. IL-16 has been detected early in BAL post endobronchial allergen challenge in asthmatics but not in control subjects [92]. This suggests a role for early IL-16 release in the selective recruitment of CD4+ T cells and eosinophils to the inflammmed bronchial mucosa in asthma.

IL-18 is a recently characterised cytokine synthesised by activated macrophages and bronchial epithelial cells [93]. In association with IL-12, IL-18 acts on Th1 type T cells to produce IFNγ, and *in vivo* and *in vitro* studies in mice show that IL-12 and IL-18 strongly activate B cells to produce IFNγ [94]. Further studies are necessary to characterise the function of IL-18 in asthma.

TNFα is produced by many cells including mast cells, T cells, neutrophils, epithelial cells and monocytes [95–97]. Bronchial biopsy studies confirm mast cells to be a major source of TNFα in the human airways, with increased expression seen in asthmatics [96]. TNFγ levels in BAL are also raised in asthmatics in comparison to controls with higher levels seen in more symptomatic subjects [98]. TNFα may cause increased AHR via induction of pro-inflammatory mediators or by acting directly on bronchial smooth muscle [Kips JC 17,9299]. It is a chemoattractant for neutrophils and monocytes, and enhances eosinophil and mast cell cytotoxicity. Furthermore, TNFα increases vascular permeability [100–102]. TNFα also acts indirectly on eosinophils by stimulating myofibroblasts to produce GM-CSF which prolongs their survival. TNFα upregulates adhesion molecules, including VCAM-1, E-selectin and ICAM-1 involved in the recruitment of eosinophils, T cells and neutrophils to the site of inflammation [103–105]. Finally, TNFα appears to play an important role in airways remodelling by promoting fibroblast activity [106].

## The orchestrating role of T lymphocytes in the inflammation of asthma

There is considerable evidence to support the view that the fine balance between Th1 and Th2 cytokines that exists in disease is dysfunctional, leading to a predominant Th2 type pattern in asthma. The asthmatic process is driven by the persistence of chronically activated memory T cells sensitised to specific allergens which localise to the airways after appropriate antigen exposure, or as some evidence suggests, after viral infection. This hypothesis is supported by observations in studies using BAL and bronchial biopsies from asthmatic subjects, including those studying treatment effects. Elevated numbers of activated CD4+, CD25+ cells are seen in blood in acute severe asthma, with a direct correlation being evident between activated peripheral blood T cells and airflow obstruction [107, 202]. Using immunohistochemistry, an increased number of activated (CD25+, CD3+) T cells can be demonstrated in the lamina propria and submucosa of bronchial biopsies from symptomatic asthmatics [108, 109]. Flow cytometry of BAL cells from asthmatics shows a correlation between CD4+, CD25+ lymphocytes and eosinophils, and the majority of CD4+ T cells are of the memory (CD45RO+) phenotype [110].

Using techniques such as double ISH , immunohistochemistry and semi-quantitative PCR, T cells have been shown to be the major source of mRNA encoding IL-4 and IL-5 in bronchial biopsies from both atopic and non-atopic asthmatics [111,

112]. Furthermore, CD4+ lymphocytes expressing mRNA for IL-4, IL-5 and GM-CSF, but not IL-2, IL-3 or IFNγ, are increased in the peripheral blood of asthmatics. The percentage of CD4+ T lymphocytes expressing IL-5 mRNA correlates with disease severity and the number of eosinophils in bronchial biopsy specimens. Glucocorticoid treatment improves lung function and reduces the percentage of CD4+ T cells expressing mRNA encoding IL-3, IL-5 and GM-CSF but not IL-2, IL-4 or IFNγ [115]. An elevated number of IL-5 mRNA expressing cells are seen in mucosal biopsies of asthmatics in comparison to controls, and these correlate with the number of CD25+ and EG2+ cells and total eosinophil counts suggesting that T cell products regulate eosinophil accumulation and function [116]. BAL from atopic asthmatics shows an increased number of cells expressing mRNA for IL-3, IL-4, IL-5 and GM-CSF, with IL-4 and IL-5 being localised to T cells, suggesting activation of, and cytokine production by, Th2 type T cells [78]. Prednisolone treatment of asthmatics results in clinical improvement and reduced AHR, accompanied by reduced eosinophil counts and reduced expression of mRNA for IL-4 and IL-5 and increased expression of IFNγ by cells in BAL [117, 118].

*In situ* hybridisation (ISH) techniques demonstrate significant associations between IL-4, IL-5 and GM-CSF expression by BAL cells and airflow obstruction, bronchial hyper-responsiveness and asthma symptom scores [119]. IL-5 is significantly higher in asthmatics than atopic non-asthmatic controls while IL-4 is elevated in both atopic groups compared to normal non-atopic controls [111, 112]. This suggests that IL-5 may be more closely related to the asthmatic phenotype while IL-4 may be associated with the overproduction of IgE [120]. The combined use of immunohistochemistry and *in situ* hybridisation localises mRNA for IL-4 and IL-5 predominantly to CD4+, but also to CD8+ T cells [121].

## T cells – determinants of asthma severity

The notion that asthma is not a single disease entity but a spectrum of what is best referred to as the asthma syndrome is well accepted. Since the natural history of asthma has not been a subject of scrutiny in large studies, it is unclear what proportion of asthmatics are predisposed to develop severe disease early in their life as opposed to progressing gradually from mild, through moderate, to severe disease. Severe asthma is characterised by decreased responsiveness, both in clinical and pathological terms, to corticosteroid treatment. A minority of these patients can be shown to be truly resistant irrespective of the dose of corticosteroids used.

Peripheral blood mononuclear cells (PBMCs) from patients with glucocorticosteroid resistant (GR) asthma are seen to proliferate in response to the mitogen, phytohaemagglutinin (PHA), despite the presence of high doses of dexamethasone

[120]. A clear relationship can be shown between clinical responsiveness to steroids and *in vitro* effects of steroids on PHA induced T cell proliferation [1201ref??]. After treatment with oral prednisolone, glucorticosteroid sensitive (GS) asthmatics experience a significant decrease in the number of cells in BAL expressing mRNA for IL-4 and IL-5 with an increase in IFNγ expression. GR asthmatics show no change in the number of cells expressing IL-4 or IL-5, but display a significant reduction in the number of IFNγ positive cells [122]. These findings are compatible with reports of a defect in glucocorticosteroid receptor binding affinity in GR asthmatics which can be maintained *in vitro* by the addition of IL-2 and IL-4 together, but not individually [123, 124]. It has been suggested that steroid resistance may be due to altered expression of genes regulating T cell cytokine production [125]. Studies suggest that corticosteroid resistance results from an altered ability of the cellular glucocorticosteroid receptor (GCR) to bind to glucocorticoid response elements (GREs) in the promoter region of the glucocorticoid responsive genes in GR patients [125]. Another hypothesis is that a dysregulation of transcription factors, with increased expression of the pro-inflammatory molecule AP-1 in GR asthmatics, may be involved in steroid resistance by interfering with steroid action by binding to the glucocorticosteroid receptor preventing GCR DNA binding [125, 126]. Leung et al. have identified GRC abnormalities using a [$^3$H]-dexamethasone radio ligand-binding assay of PBMCs, categorising GR asthmatics as Type 1 when a decrease in GCR binding affinity restricted to T cells was present, and Type 2 when the GCR binding affinity was normal but the numbers of GCR binding sites per cell were found to be abnormally low in both T cells and non-T cells.

Unfortunately, effective and safe agents enabling suppression of corticosteroid-resistant components of airway inflammation are not available. A number of drugs used to inhibit organ rejection in transplanted patients (cyclosporin) and so-called corticosteroid sparing agents (methotrexate, azathioprine) have been used in severe asthma. Cyclosporin inhibits T cell activation by blocking calcium dependent transcription of mRNA encoding a number of cytokines. In a group of GR asthmatics it is seen to improve lung function, reduce the number of exacerbations and have a cortico-steroid- sparing effect [126–128, 201]. Cyclosporin reduces the magnitude of the late allergic response (LAR) to allergen challenge, suggesting cyclosporin action through inhibition of T cell function in this model of asthma [129, 201]. However, the clinical efficacy of cyclosporin remains to be fully established. For this reason, a number of novel therapeutic agents are being considered for the treatment of severe asthma, including :immuno-suppressive agents (e.g. FK506, mycophenolate mofetil and rapamycin), ;anti-CD4 antibodies, ;cytokine receptor antagonists (e.g. IL-1 receptor antagonist), anti-cytokine antibodies (e.g. anti-IL-4 and anti-IL-5 antibodies), IL-12 modulation of the Th2 response, and agents that may block the co-stimulatory pathways required for T cell activation (e.g. CTLA4Ig fusion protein and anti-B7-2 antibody) [130].

## The effector role of eosinophils

Eosinophils are considered to be responsible for much of the mucosal inflammation and resulting epithelial damage in asthma. A number of proteins are released by eosinophils on activation , including major basic protein (MBP), eosinophil cationic protein (ECP), eosinophil-derived neurotoxin and eosinophil peroxidase, which have been shown to damage epithelial integrity by disruption of epithelial desmosomes and tight junctions [6]. Eosinophil counts are consistently shown to be increased in the lumen and in sub-mucosa and epithelium of bronchial biopsies both in unchallenged airways and after segmental allergen challenge [131, 132].

Whilst a correlation between disease severity and eosinophils can be demonstrated using cell counts in the lumen and mucosa, the strength of correlation is best when luminal eosinophils, counted in sputum, are investigated [133]. In addition to producing vaso- and bronchoactive mediators, eosinophils have been shown to synthesise a number of pro-inflammatory cytokines including IL-3, IL-4, IL-5, IL-6, TNFα, GM-CSF and transforming growth factors (TGFα and TGFβ) [134]. In addition, using recombinant polymerase chain reaction (RT-PCR), mRNA for IL-4 has been detected in blood eosinophils of asthmatic patients [135]. IL-3, IL-5 and GM-CSF are thought to prime eosinophil mediator release and prolong eosinophil survival by inhibiting apoptyosis [118].

## Mast cells

Mast cells have long been viewed as pivotal to the development of anaphylactic or immediate type reactions .They produce a number of inflammatory mediators including histamine, heparin, tryptase, prostaglandins ($PGD_2$), leukotriene $C_4$ ($LTC_4$) and thromboxane $A_2$ ($TXA_2$) which possess potent broncho- and vasoactive properties [6]. Mast cells containing tryptase alone ($MC_T$) are found in increased numbers in the airway biopsies of asthma patients and correlated inversely with $PC_{20}$ (i.e.the cumulative dose of spasmiogen, such as histamine, required to cause a 20% fall in $FEV_1$ from baseline) [37]. Mast cell activation markers have also been shown to correlate positively with markers of vascular permeability and negatively with $FEV_1$, suggesting an association with disease activity. Studies have shown an increased release of mast cell mediators in the BAL fluid of asthmatics [6].

In the presence of specific allergen, cross linkage of IgE molecules bound to high affinity IgE receptors(Fcε R1) on the mast cell surface causes cellular activation and release of mediators resulting in acute bronchoconstriction. Mast cells can be activated by stimuli such as airway fluid osmolar changes as in exercise-induced asthma, and by drugs such as non-steroidal anti-inflammatory drugs (NSAIDS) in susceptible individuals [136].

It is now fully appreciated that mast cells have the capacity to produce a number of cytokines which have previously been attributed to T cells, including IL-4, IL-5, IL-6, IL-8, GM-CSF and TNFα [137]. IL-4 has been shown to bind to glycosaminoglycan (GAG) side-chains of heparin produced by mast cells and stored in their granules, which is likely to mediate local cytokine signalling. The production of cytokines such as TNFα and IL-5 and the release of the neutral protease tryptase by mast cells, in association with the later recruitment and activation of Th-2 type T cells, are likely to contribute significantly to the LAR [138, 139]. To what extent the cytokines secreted by mast cells contribute to allergic inflammation is unclear. Using a combination of immunohistochemistry and *in situ* hybridisation, studies have shown that the greatest proportion of cells producing IL-3, IL-4 and IL-5 are T cells [121]. However, in view of the relatively low frequency of allergen specific T cells in the airways of asthmatics [115] it is uncertain what the trigger factors for the synthesis of these cytokines may be. The relative contribution of mast cells and T cells is further complicated by the fact that probably all of the mast cells in the airways possess specific IgE which enables them to respond in an allergen specific manner.

## The bronchial epithelium as a source of pro-inflammatory cytokines

The bronchial epithelium was previously thought to be a passive barrier that was damaged by inflammation in asthma. It is now known to be an important source of mediators including arachidonic acid products, nitric oxide, endothelins, cytokines and molecules involved in repair, demonstrating an active role for the epithelium in regulating the inflammation, repair and remodelling processes of asthma. The epithelium can be activated by mediators such as histamine, cytokines, leukotrienes, by IgE dependent mechanisms or by stimuli including, occupational chemicals, pollutants, viruses, or the shifts in epithelial lining fluid osmolarity that may occur in exercise induced asthma [140–144]. The epithelium is a major source of 15-HETE, $PGE_2$, nitric oxide (NO) and endothelin-1 [6]. The arachidonic acid metabolite, 15-HETE induces chemotaxis of inflammatory cells, increases mucus production and enhances the EAR. $PGE_2$ has vasodilator and bronchodilator properties. Increased $PGE_2$ production by the epithelium inhibits IL-12 production by dendritic cells promoting Th2 differentiation by T cells [97, 145].

The bronchial epithelium is capable of storing and releasing cytokines (IL-1β, IL-6, IL-11, GM-CSF, IL-16 and IL-18) and chemokines (IL-8, MIP-1α, MCP-3, RANTES and eotaxin) [146–149]. Cytokine release is controlled by inducible genes activated by pro-inflammatory cytokines (TNFα, IL-1α and IFNγ), by growth factors (TGFα, HB-EGF and amphiregulin) and by epithelial detachment and deformation [68, 150, 151]. The transcription factors, NF-κB and STATS, control inducible genes that regulate mediator release. Immuno-histochemical studies show increased expression of NF-κB and STATS in asthmatic bronchial epithelium [152]. Asthmatic bronchial epithelium expresses the adhesion molecules ICAM-1, α3β1 and αvβ6 [153]. ICAM-1 is the binding receptor for rhinovirus and increased ICAM-1 expression may contribute to virus-induced exacerbations in asthma [154]. α3β1 is a ligand for fibronectin, laminins and collagens, the extracellular matrix proteins involved in repair and remodelling [155]. αvβ6 is a ligand for fibronectin and tenascin, the structural proteins deposited in increased amounts beneath the epithelial basement membrane.

Nitric oxide (NO) is a highly soluble free radical with a short half-life, involved in cellular signalling and is produced by constitutive and inducible forms of NO synthase (iNOS). Increased levels of NO are found in the exhaled air of patients with active asthma or rhinitis. In severe asthma, the epithelium is likely to be a major source of NO [156–158]. Bronchial biopsy studies show that iNOS immune activity localises to the bronchial epithelium in asthmatics but is rarely seen in airway biopsies of normal controls [6]. Bronchial epithelial iNOS activity is downregulated in corticosteroid sensitive asthma and is associated with a reduction in exhaled NO levels. It may be a useful marker of disease activity in asthma [159, 160].

Human endothelins include three polypeptides (ET-1, ET-2 and ET-3). ET-1 is a potent vasoconstrictor, contractor of smooth muscle, mitogen for airway smooth muscle and fibroblasts and is capable of activating collagen synthesis [161]. ET-1 is produced by bronchial epithelial cells [162], vascular endothelial cells [163], mast cells and macrophages and ET-1 expression is increased in bronchial epithelial biopsies of asthmatics [164]. Studies show that ET-1 levels in BALF of asthmatics are increased in proportion to the level of resting airflow obstruction in asthma [165]. ET-1 levels in BALF and bronchial biopsy epithelial expression of ET-1 have been shown to fall to normal levels in asthmatics treated with effective doses of corticosteroids [165]. This suggests a role for endothelins in asthma , particularly in the late allergic reaction (LAR) but also possibly in the remodelling process.

Inhaled anti-inflammatory drugs such as corticosteroids have a dramatic effect in improving asthma symptoms, lung function and airway reactivity. These agents have powerful inhibitory effects on mediator release and cytokine production by the asthmatic epithelium [166, 167]. Inhaled corticosteroids promote a reduction in bronchial eosinophilic infiltration and downregulate the expression of transcription factors such as NF-κB known to be important in inflammation [168].

## The process of airway remodelling in asthma

A number of studies indicate that irreversible airway obstruction can occur in asthma, which suggests that structural changes consistent with a remodelling process occurs in the airways of asthmatics [169]. In patients who died from severe asthma, prominent airway wall thickening is noted. The bronchi of wall diameter greater than 2 mm in thickness demonstrate increased thickness of the total wall, sub-epithelial layer and muscle layer with associated hypertrophy and hyperplasia of the airway smooth muscle layer [170, 171]. A recent three-dimensional morphometric study of asthmatic airways suggests that smooth muscle hyperplasia is more prominent in large airways whereas hypertrophy is more prominent in the affected smaller airways [171]. Studies have demonstrated prominent hyperplasia of mucus glands in the airway wall in cases of fatal asthma [172]. Increased angiogenesis and airway smooth muscle hypertrophy is also a feature of the remodelling process of asthma [173, 174]. Computerised tomography studies of asthmatics demonstrated abnormalities in airway wall thickness in 90% of the cases studied; these were related to both the duration and severity of asthma in cases with an irreversible component of airways disease [175, 176]. Thickened basement membrane zone abnormalities noted at postmortem of asthmatics have been confirmed in bronchial biopsy studies using fibreoptic bronchoscopy. Electron microscopy studies localise the increased basement membrane thickness to the lamina reticularis layer. Immunohistochemistry studies confirm that this thickened layer is composed of collagen types III, V, I and fibronectin [177]. Myofibroblast numbers are increased in the airway walls of asthmatics and are considered to be responsible for this collagen deposition [178]. A recent study has shown that the submucosa, as well as the reticular basement membrane, contains significantly more collagen than normal controls, suggesting that airway scar formation may have more significant effects than were previously considered [179]. *In vitro* studies suggest that this remodelling process involves a number of growth factors and cytokines including TGF$\beta_1$, platelet-derived growth factor, basic fibroblast growth factor, TNF$\alpha$, IL-4, endothelin and other molecules including tryptase and histamine suggesting a role for mast cells in tissue remodelling in asthma [180, 181]. A number of extra-cellular matrix proteins contribute to the inflammation and remodelling of asthma. Eosinophils express integrins such as VLA-4, VLA-6 and LFA-1 which are known to adhere to matrix proteins such as laminin, fibronectin and fibrinogen [182, 183].This is thought to encourage the accumulation, increase the activation and prolong the survival of eosinophils locally in the bronchial tissue [184]. Studies of asthmatic bronchial biopsies, using *in situ* hybridisation and immunohistochemistry techniques have shown activated eosinophils in the reticular lamina to be a major source of TGF$\beta_1$ mRNA and immunoreactivity which is associated with the degree of airway fibrosis, linking chronic allergic inflammation with the structural remodelling and decline in FEV$_1$ seen in asthma [185]. Mast cells also express integrins and *in vitro* studies have shown that fibronectin adherence encourages both IgE mediated mast cell degranulation, chemotaxis and proliferation. In asthmatics, matrix protein interaction is capable of altering IgE mediated cytokine release by basophils [184]. Elevated levels of glycosaminoglycan (GAG) side-chains, particularly chondroitin and dermatan sulphate have been noted in the urine of asthmatics during a severe asthmatic attack [186].It is considered that these are produced by the breakdown of extracellular matrix proteoglycan in the bronchi of asthmatics. Tryptase is known to cleave certain components of the extracellular matrix (e.g.fibronectin, collagen VI) and activate matrix metalloproteases (stromolysin). Tryptase can also enhance proliferation of fibroblasts, smooth muscle and epithelial cells. Asthmatic airways have an increased expression of these mediators which are thought to promote mitogenesis of myofibroblasts and airway smooth muscle and synthesis of collagen [187].

Studies in children and occupational asthma indicate that airway changes of remodelling occur at an early stage of the disease [188]. The majority of studies in asthmatics treated with inhaled corticosteroids show no significant reversibility of airway collagen deposition despite relieving symptoms, improving lung function and modifying bronchial hyperreactivity [189, 190]. This supports the recommendation of early introduction of effective anti-inflammatory treatment in an attempt to prevent the development of irreversible structural changes.

## Mechanisms of asthma severity and chronicity

Despite the considerable improvement in the understanding of asthma pathogenesis, the mechanisms which determine disease severity remain poorly understood. The degree of sputum, BALF and blood eosinophilia and, to a lesser extent, levels of ECP detected in clotted blood have been found to broadly relate to disease severity. T cell activation and expression of Th2 type cytokines are found in all degrees of asthma but, as discussed above, it is most prominent in severe disease, which is poorly controlled by corticosteroids [191]. Physiological indices of asthma severity such as methacholine responsiveness are related to the number and activity of eosinophils and activated CD4+ T cells in BALF from atopic asthmatics [192, 193]. AHR but not symptom scores have been shown to be inversely related to the number of activated eosinophils and mast cells in bronchial biopsies from asthmatics not treated with corticosteroids [194]. In asthmatics treated with inhaled corticosteroids, AHR, but not symptom score or lung function, is inversely related to the number of infiltrating mast cells, activated eosinophils, CD8+, and CD45RO+ T cells in bronchial biopsies from these patients [193].

Studies involving *post mortem* examination of patients with sudden asthma related deaths, and sputum analysis of patients in *status asthmaticus* support the role of neutrophils in severe asthma [195, 196]. A recent bronchoscopy study showed that whilst eosinophil numbers may or may not be raised in the mucosa, a significantly higher neutrophil count is seen in bronchial and transbronchial biopsies of severe, high-dose oral corticosteroid dependent asthmatics compared with moderate asthmatics and normal controls. Lipid-derived and mast cell derived mediators remained elevated in the severe patients despite treatment with high dose corticosteroids [197]. Interestingly, a lower percentage of macrophages was seen in the severe asthmatics compared to moderate asthmatics. Some studies have shown that corticosteroids can enhance neutrophil function through increased leukotriene and superoxide production and inhibition of apoptosis [198]. It is possible that corticosteroids could reduce the lymphocyte and eosinophil mediated inflammation but exacerbate neutrophil mediated inflammation in severe asthmatics [199].

## Concluding remarks

The last few years have seen a dramatic improvement in our understanding of asthma which has probably surpassed that of other respiratory diseases. We have learned about the orchestrating role of Th2-type cytokines which dominate inflammatory responses in asthma and are beginning to understand the regulation of their production at the gene level. Detailed morphological studies have led to the concept of airways remodellling as a consequence of chronic inflammation which is most likely fixed. This has contributed to better management of asthma. However, many issues remain unresolved, the most important being the inability to completely abrogate the inflammatory response in more severe disease, which is not only becoming more prevalent but is also draining a major proportion of funds dedicated to asthma amanagement [200]. The identification of several cytokines as participating in airways inflammaamtion has meant that targetting individual cytokines is unlikely to lead to major improvements in disease management. Future efforts will have to be directed at elucidating the relative contribution of individual cell types and mediators in the hope that the wide syndrome of asthma may eventually be broken down into subtypes, hopefully with distinct patterns of mediators that are involved in their pathogenesis.

## References

1    Davies RJ, Tang J, Abdelaziz MM et al (1997) New insights into the understanding of asthma. *Chest* 111: 2–10
2    Sandford A, Weir T, Pare Ph (1996) The genetics of asthma. *Am J Respir Crit Care Med* 153: 1749–1765
3    Mehlhop PD, Van de Rijn M, Goldberg AB et al (1997) Allergen-induced bronchial reactivity and eosinophilic inflammation occur in the absence of IgE in a mouse model of asthma. *Proc Natl Acad Sci USA* 94: 1344–1349
4    Fahy JV, Fleming E , Wong HH et al (1997) The effect of an anti-IgE monoclonal antibody on the early- and late responses to allergen inhalation. *Am J Respir Crit Care Med* 155: 1828–1834
5    Corne J, Djukanovic R, Lynette T, Holgate ST et al (1997) The effect of intravenous administration of a chimeric anti-IgE antibody on serum IgE levels in atopic subjects: Efficacy, safety and pharmacokinetics. *J Clin Invest* 99: 879–887

6     Holgate ST (1997) Asthma: A dynamic disease of inflammation and repair. The rising trends in asthma. *The Ciba Foundation Bulletin* 206: 5–34

7     Morton NE (1996) Statistical consideration for genetic analysis of atopy and asthma, In: DA Meyers, SB Liggett (eds): *The genetics of asthma*. Marcel Dekker, New York, 367–378

8     Edfors-Lubs M (1971) Allergy in 7,000 twin pairs. *Acta Allergol* 26: 249–285

9     Cookson W, Sharp PA, Faux JA et al (1989) Linkage between IgE responses underlying asthma and rhinitis and chromosome 11q13. *Lancet* 1: 1292–1295

10    Young RP, Lynch J, Sharp PA et al (1992) Confirmation of genetic linkage between atopic IgE responses and chromosome 11q13. *J Med Genetics* 29: 236–238

11    Sandford AJ, Shirakawa T, Moffatt MF (1993) Localisation of atopy and the β subunit of the high affinity IgE receptor(FcεRI) on chromosome 11q13. *Lancet* 341: 332–334

12    Manian P (1997) Genetics of asthma: A review. *Chest* 112: 1397–1408

13    ShirakawaT, Li A, Dubowitz M et al (1994) Association between atopy and variants of the β subunit of the high affinity IgE receptor. *Nat Genetics* 7: 125–130

14    Hill MR, Cookson W (1996) A new variant of the β subunit of the high affinity receptor for IgE (FcεRI-β E237G): associations with measures of atopy and bronchial hyper-reponsiveness. *Hum Mol Genet* 5: 959–962

15    Chandrashekharappa SC, Rebelesky MS, Firak TA et al (1990) A long range restriction map of the interleukin-4 and IL-5 linkage group on chromosome 5. *Genomics* 6: 94–99

16    Marsh DG, Neely JD, Breazeale DR et al (1994) Linkage analysis of IL-4 and other chromosome 5q31.1 markers and total serum IgE concentrations. *Science* 264: 1152–1156

17    Meyers DA, Postma DS, Panhuysen CIM et al (1994) Evidence for a locus regulating total serum IgE mapping to chromosom 5. *Genomics* 23: 464–470

18    Postma DS, Bleecker ER, Amelung PJ et al (1995) Genetic susceptibility to asthma-bronchial hyperresponsiveness co-inherited with a major gene for atopy. *N Engl J Med* 333: 894–900

19    Barnes KC, Neely JD, Duffy DL et al (1996) Linkage of asthma and total IgE concentration to markers on chromosome 12q: evidence from Afro-Carribean and Caucasian populations. *Genomics* 37: 41–50

20    Wilkinson J, Thomas S, Loi P et al (1996) Evidence for linkage for atopy and asthma to markers on chromosome 12q. *Eur Respir J* 9: 435s

21    Howell WM, Holgate ST (1995) HLA genetics and allergic disease. *Thorax* 50: S15–18

22    Hsieh K, Shieh C, Hsieh R et al (1991). Association of HLA-DQw2 with Chinese childhood asthma. *Tissue antigens* 38: 181–182

23    Bignon JS, Yolande A, Ju L et al (1994) HLA class II alleles in isocyanate-induced asthma. *Am J Respir Crit Care Med* 149: 71–75

24    Moffatt MF, Hill MR, Cornelis F et al (1994) Genetic kinkage of T cell receptor α/δ complex to specific IgE responses. *Lancet* 343: 1597–1600

25    Rosenwasser LJ (1997) Genetics of atopy and asthma: promoter-based candidate gene studies for IL-4. *Int Arch Allergy Immunol* 113: 61–64

26  Cooke RA, Vander Veer A (1916) Human sensitisation. *J Immunol* 1: 201–305

27  Ruiz RGG, Richards D, Kemeny DM et al (1991) Neonatal IgE: A poor screen for atopic disease. *Clin Exp Allergy* 21 : 467–472

28  D'Andrea A, Aste-Amezaga M, Valianta NM et al (1993) IL-10 inhibits human lymphocyte IFNγ production by suppressing natural killer cell stimulatory factor/IL-12 synthesis in accessory cells. *J Exp Med* 178: 1041–1048

29  Warner J, Jones AC, Miles EA et al (1997) Prenatal origins of allergy and asthma. The rising trends in asthma. *Ciba Foundation Symposium* 206: 220–232

30  Warner JA, Miles EA, Jones AC et al (1994) Is deficiency of interferon gamma production by allergen triggered blood cells a predictor of atopic eczema. *Clin Exp Allergy* 24: 423–430

31  Nicod LP (1996) Role of antigen-presenting cells in lung immunity. *Eur Respir Rev* 6: 142–150

32  Sporik R, Holgate ST, Platts-Mills TAE et al (1990) Exposure to house dust mite allergen (Der P1) and the development of allergy in childhood: A prospective study. *N Eng J Med* 323: 502–507

33  Warner JA, Jones AC, Miles EA et al (1996) Materno-fetal interaction and allergy. *Allergy* 51: 447–451

34  Azzawi M, Johnston PW, Majumdar S et al (1992) T lymphocytes and activated eosinophils in asthma and cystic fibrosis. *Am Rev Respir Dis* 145: 1477–1482

35  Kay AB (1996) Pathology of mild, severe and fatal asthma. *Am J Respir Crit Care Med* 154: S66–S69

36  Sur S, Crotty TB, Kephart GM et al (1993) Sudden onset fatal asthma – A distinct entity with few eosinophils and relatively more neutrophils in the airway submucosa? *Am Rev Respir Dis* 148: 713–719

37  Koshino T, Arai Y Miyamoto Y et al (1996) Airway basophil and mast cell density in patients with bronchial asthma relationship to bronchial hyperresponsiveness. *J Asthma* 33 (2): 89–95

38  Linsley PS, Ledbetter JA (1993) The role of CD28 receptor during T cell responses to antigen. *Annu Rev Immunol* 11: 191–212

39  Holt FG (1996) Current concepts in pulmonary immunology: regulation of primary and secondary responses to inhaled antigen. *Eur Respir Rev* 6 (36): 128–135

40  Semper AE, Hartley JA (1996) Dendritic cells in the lung-what is their relevance to asthma. *C in Exp Allergy* 26(5): 485–490

41  Moller GM, Overbeek SE, Van-HeldenMeeuwsen CG et al (1996) Increased numbers of dendritic cells in the bronchial mucosa of atopic asthmatic patients: downregulation by inhaled corticosteroids. *Clin Exp Allergy* 26(5): 517–524

42  Holt FG (1986) Downregulation of immune responses in the lower respiratory tract: The role of alveolar macrophages. *Clin Exp Immunol* 63: 261–270

43  Sousa AR, Trigg CJ, Lane SJ et al (1997) Effect of inhaled glucocorticosteroids on IL-1β and IL-1 receptor antagonist (IL-lra) expression in asthmatic bronchial epithelium. *Thorax* 52 407–410

44 Aubas P, Cosso B, Godard P et al (1984) Decreased suppressor cell activity of alveolar macrophages in bronchial asthma. *Am Rev Respir Dis* 130: 875–878

45 Gosset P, Lassalle P, Tonnel AB et al (1988) Production of an interleukin 1 inhibitory factor by human alveolar macrophages from normals and allergic asthmatic patients. *Am Rev Respir Dis* 138: 40–46

46 Metzger ZWI, Hoffeld JT, Oppenheim JJ (1980) Macrophage mediated suppression. *J Immunol* 124: 983–988

47 Lyons CR, Ball EJ, Toews GB et al (1986) Inability of human alveolar macrophages to stimulate resting T-cells correlates with decreased antigen-specific T-cell macrophage binding. *J Immunol* 137: 1173–1180

48 Van Kooyk Y, Van de Wiel-Van Kemenade P et al (1989) Enhancement of LFA-1 mediated cell adhesion by triggering through CD2 or CD3 on T-lymphocytes. *Nature* 342: 811–813

49 Chelen CJ, Fang Y, Freeman GJ et al (1995) Human alveolar antigens present antigen ineffectively due to defective expression of B-7 co-stimulatory cell surface molecules. *J Clin Invest* 95: 1415–1421

50 Agea E, Spinozzi F et al (1998) Expression of B7 costimulatory molecules and CD1a antigen by alveolar macrophages in bronchial asthma. *Clin Exp Allergy* 28: 1359–1367

51 van Gool S, Vandenberghe P, De Boer M, Ceuppens JL (1996) CD80, CD86 and CD40 provide accessory signals in a multiple-step T-cell activation model. *Immunol Rev* 153: 111: 129–155

52 Bluestone JA (1997) Is CTLA-4 a master switch for peripheral T cell tolerance? *J Immunol* 58: 1989–1993

53 Krummel MF, Allison JP (1995) CD28 and CTLA-4 have opposing effects on the response of T cells to stimulation. *J Exp Med* 182: 459–465

54 Klinzman SJ, DeSanctis GT, Cemades M et al (1996) Inhibition of T cell costimulation abrogates airway hyperresponsiveness in a murine model. *J Clin Invest* 98: 2693–2699

55 Wu Y, Guo Y, Huang A et al (1997) CTLA-4-B-7 interaction is sufficient to costimulate T cell clonal expansion. *J Exp Med* 185(7): 1327–1335

56 Liu Y (1997) Is CTLA-4 a negative regulator for T cell activation? *Immunology Today* 18(12): 569–572

57 Lenschow DJ, Walunas TL, Bluestone JA (1996) CD28/B7 system of cell costimulation. *Annu Rev Immunol* 14: 233–258

58 Tsuyuki S, Tsuyuki J, Einsle K et al (1997) Co-stimulation through B7-2(CD86) is required for the induction of a lung mucosal T helper cell 2(TH2)immune response and altered airway hyperresponsiveness. *J Exp Med* 185(9): 1671–1679

59 Keane-Myers A, Gause WC, Linsley PS et al (1997) B7-CD28/CTLA4 costimulatory pathways are required for the development of T helper cell 2-mediated allergic airway responses to inhaled antigens. *J Immunol* 158: 2042–2049

60 Keane-Myers A, Gause WC, Finkelman FD et al (1998) Development of murine allergic asthma is dependent upon B7-2 costimulation. *J Immunol* 160: 1036–1043

61 van Neerven RJ, van de Pol MM, van der Zee JS et al (1998) Inhibition of allergen-spe-

cific proliferation and cytokine production of human T lymphocytes by blocking the CD28-CD86 costimulatory pathway. *Clin Exp Allergy* 28 (7): 808–816

62 Jaffer Z, Roberts K, Pandit A et al (1997) B7 costimulation is required for IL-5 and IL-13 expression by T cells resident in bronchial biopsy tissue of asthmatics after allergen stimulation. *Immunology* 92(S1): 45–A12.15

63 Lebwohl MJ, Kang S, Guzzo C et al (1997) CTLA4-Ig (BMS-188667)-mediated blockade of T cell co-stimulation in patients with psoriasis vulgaris. *J Inv Dermatology* 108: 570, A198

64 Cees van Cooten, Banchereau J (1997) Functions of CD40 on B cells, dendritic cells and other cells. *Current Opinions in Immunology* 9: 330–337

65 Boussiotis VA, Freeman GJ, Gribben JG, Nadler LM (1996) The role of B7-1/B7-2: CD28/CTLA4 pathways in the prevention of anergy, induction of productive immunity and downregulation of the immune response. *Immunological Reviews* 153: 5–25

66 Maurer D, Ebner C, Reininger B et al (1995) The high affinity IgE receptor (FcεRI) mediates IgE-dependent allergen presentation. *J Immunol* 154: 6285–6290

67 Tuncn-de-lara JM, Redington AE, Bradding P, Holgate ST et al (1996) Dendritic cells in normal and asthmatic airways: expression of the alpha subunit of the high affinity IgE receptor (FcERI-a). *Clin Exp Allergy* 26: 648–655

68 Barnes PJ, Karin M (1997) Nuclear factor-KB – A pivotal transcription factor in chronic inflammatory diseases. *N Engl J Med* 336 (15): 1066–1071

69 Muegge K, Durum SK (1990) Cytokines and transcription factors. *Cytokine* 2: 1–8

70 Adcock IM, Gelder CM, Shirasaki H et al (1992) Effects of steroids on transcription factors n human lung. *Am Rev Respir Dis* 145: A834

71 Barnes PJ, Adcock IM (1995) Transcription factors. *Clin Exp Allergy* 25 (S2): 46–49

72 Salvi SS, Semper AE, Papi A et al (1998) Human lung epithelial cells express IL-5 mRNA. *J Allergy Clin Immunol* 101(1): S19

73 Romagniani S (1990) Regulation and deregulation of human IgE synthesis. *Immunol Today* 11: 316–321

74 Schleimer RP, Sterbinsky CA, Kaiser CA et al (1992) Interleukin 4 induces adherence of human eosinophils and basophils but not neutrophils to endothelium: association with expression of VCAM-1. *J Immunology* 148: 1086–1092

75 Walsh GM, Mermod JJ, Hartnell A et al (1991) Human eosinophil, but not neutrophil, adherence to IL-1 stimulated HWEC is α4β1 (VLA-4) dependent. *J Immunol* 146: 3419

76 Pretolani M, Goldman M (1997) IL-10: A potential therapy for allergic inflammation *Immunol Today* 277–280

77 Naseer T, Minshall EM, Leung DYM et al (1997) Expression of IL-12 and IL-13 mRNA in asthma and their modulation in response to steroid therapy. *Am J Respir Crit Care Med* 155: 845–851

78 Robinson DS, Hamid Q, Ying S et al (1992) Predominant Th2-type bronchoalveolar lavage T lymphocyte population in atopic asthma. *N Eng J Med* 326: 298–304

79 Del Prete G, de Carli M, Almerigogna F et al (1993) Human IL-10 is produced by Th1

and Th2 T cell clones and inhibits their antigen specific proliferation and cytokine production. *J Immunol* 150: 353–360

80    Robinson DS, Tsicopoulos A, Meng Q et al (1996) Increased IL-10 mRNA expression in atopic allergy and asthma. *Am J Respir Cell Mol Biol* 14: 113–117

81    Hseih CS, Macatonia SE, Tripp CS et al (1993) Development of Th1 CD4+ T cells through IL-12 produced by Listeria induced macrophages. *Science* 260: 547–549

82    Manetti R, Parronchi P, Guidizi MG et al (1993) Natural killer stimulatory factor(IL-12) induces Th1-specific immune responses and inhibits the development of IL-4 producing Th cells. *J Exp Med* 177: 1199–1204

83    Gavett SH, O'Hearn DJ, Li Z et al(1995) Interleukin-12 inhibits antigen-induced airway hyperresponsiveness, inflammation and Th2 cytokine expression in mice. *J Exp Med* 182 (5): 1527–1536

84    Defrance T, Carayon P, Billian G et al (1994) Interleukin 13 is a B-cell stimulating factor. *J Exp Med* 179: 135–143

85    Kroegel C, Julius P, Matthys H et al (1996) Endobronchial secretion of IL-13 following local allergen challenge in atopic asthma: relationship to IL-4 and eosinophil counts. *Eur Respir J* 9: 899–904

86    Humbert M, Durham SR, Kimmitt P et al (1997) Elevated expression of mRNA encoding IL-13 in the bronchial mucosa of atopic and nonatopic subjects with asthma. *J Allergy Clin Immunol* 99: 657–665

87    Bochner BS, Klunk DA, Sterbinsky SA et al (1995) IL-13 selectively induces vascular cell adhesion molecule-1expression in human endothelial cells. *J Immunol* 154: 799–803

88    Shau-Ku Huang, Hui-Qing Xiao, Jorg Kleine-Tebbe et al (1995) IL-13 expression at the sites of allergen challenge in patients with asthma. *J Immunol* 155: 2688–2694

89    Cruikshank WW, Long A, Tarpy RE et al (1995) Early identification of IL-16 (Lymphocyte chemoattractant factor) and macrophage inflammatory protein 1α(MIP1α) in BALF of antigen-challenged asthmatics. *Am J Respir Cell Mol Biol* 13: 738–747

90    Cruikshank WW, Berman JS, Theodore AC et al (1987) Lymphokine activation of T4+ lymphocytes and monocytes. *J Immunol* 138: 3817–3825

91    Laberge S, Ernest P, Ghaffar O et al (1997) Increased expression of IL-16 in bronchial mucosa of subjects with atopic asthma. *Am J Respir Cell Mol Biol* 17 (2): 193–202

92    Bellini A, Yoshimura H, Vitori E et al (1993) Bronchial epithelial cells of patients with asthma release chemoattractant factors for T lymphocytes. *J Allerg Clin Immunol* 92: 412–424

93    Okamura H, Tsutsui H, Komatsu T et al (1995) *Nature* 378: 88–91

94    Yoshimoto T, Okamura H, Tagawa Y et al (1997) Interleukin 18 togethor with interleukin 12 inhibits IgE production by induction of IFNγ production from activated B cells. *Proc Natl Acad Sci USA* 94 (8): 3948–3953

95    Bradding P (1996) Human mast cell cytokines. *Clin Exp Allergy* 26: 13–19

96    Bradding P, Roberts JA, Britten KM et al (1994) Interleukin-4, -5, and -6 and tumor necrosis factor-α in normal and asthmatic airways: Evidence for the human mast cell as a source of these cytokines. *Am J Respir Cell Mol Biol* 10: 471–480

97  Andersson U, Matsuda T (1989) Human interleukin 6 and tumor necrosis factor-α production studied at a single cell level. *Eur J Immunol* 19: 1157–1160

98  Broide DH, Lotz M, Cuomo AJ et al (1992) Cytokines in symptomatic asthma airways. *J Allerg Clin Immunol* 89: 958–967

99  Kips JC, Tavernier J, Pauwels RA (1992) Tumor necrosis factor (TNF) causes bronchial hyperresponsiveness in rats. *Am Rev Respir Dis* 145: 2–336

100  Ming WJ, Bersani L, Mantovani A (1987) Tumor necrosis factor is chemotactic for monocytes and polymorphonuclear leucocytes. *Immunol* 138: 1469–1474

101  Silberstein DS, Davis JR (1986) Tumor necrosis factor enhances eosinophil toxicity to *Schistosoma Mansoni* larvae. *Proc Natl Acad Sci USA* 83: 1055–1059

102  Slungaard A, Vercellotte GM, Walker G et al (1990) Tumor necrosis factor/cachectin stimulates eosinophil oxidant production and toxicity towards human endothelium. *J Exp Med* 171: 2025–2031

103  Bevilacqua MP, Stengelin S, Gimbrone MA et al (1989) Endothelial leucocyte adhesion molecule-1: An inducible receptor for neutrophils related to complement regulatory proteins and lectins. *Science* 243: 1160–1165

104  Osborn L, Hession R, Tizard R et al (1989) Direct expression and cloning of vascular cell adhesion molecule-1, a cytokine -endothelial protein that binds to lymphocytes. *Cell* 59: 1203–1211

105  Pober JS, Gimbrone MA, Lapierre LA et al (1986) Overlapping pattern of activation of human endothelial cells by interleukin 1, Tumor necrosis factor, and immune interferon. *Immunol* 137: 1893–1896

106  Shah A, Church MK, Holgate ST (1995) Tumor necrosis factor-α: a potential mediator of asthma. *Clin Exp Allergy* 25: 1038–1044

107  Corrigan CJ, Hartnell A, Kay AB (1988) T lymphocyte activation in acute severe asthma. *Lancet* I: 1129–1132

108  Azzawi M, Bradley B, Jeffery PK et al (1990) Identification of activated T lymphocytes and eosinophils in bronchial biopsies in stable atopic asthmatics. *Am Rev Respir Dis* 142: 1407–1413

109  Hamd Q, Barkans J, Robinson DS et al (1992) Co-expression of CD25 and CD3 in atopic allergy and asthma. *Immunol* 75: 659–663

110  Robinson DS, Bentley AM, Hartnell A et al (1993) Activated memory T helper cells in bronchoalveolar lavage from atopic asthmatics. Relationship to asthma symptoms, lung function and bronchial responsiveness. *Thorax* 48: 26–32

111  Ying S, Durham SR, Corrigan CJ et al (1995) Phenotype of cells expressing mRNA for Th2-type (IL-4 and IL-5) and Th1-type (IL-2 and interferon gamma) cytokines in bronchoalveolar lavage and bronchial biopsies from atopic asthmatics and normal control subjects. *Am J Respir Cell Mol Biol* 12: 477–487

112  Humbert M, Durham SR, Ying S et al (1996) IL-4 and IL-5 mRNA and protein in bronchial biopsies from atopic and non-atopic asthmatics: evidence against intrinsic asthma being a distinct immunopathological entity. *Am J Respir Crit Care Med* 154: 1497–1504

113 Center DM, Kornfeld H, Cruikshank WW (1996) Interleukin 16 and its function as a CD4 ligand. *Immunol Today* 476–481

114 Gause WC, Mitro V, Via C et al (1997) Do effector and memory T helper cells also need B7 ligand costimulatory signals? *J Immunol* 159: 1055–1058

115 Corrigan CJ, Hamid Q, North J et al (1995) Peripheral blood CD4 but not CD8 T-lymphocytes in patients with exacerbation of asthma transcribe and translate mRNA encoding cytokines which prolong eosinop~hil survival in the context of a Th2-type pattern: effect of glucocorticosteroid therapy. *Am J Respir Cell Mol Biol* 12: 567–578

116 Hamid Q, Azzawi M, Ying S et al (1991) Expression of mRNA for interleukin-5 in mucosal bronchial biopsies from asthmatics. *J Clin Invest* 87: 1541–1546

117 Robinson DS, Hamid Q, Ying S (1993) Prednisolone treatment in asthma is associated with modulation of broncho-alveolar lavage cell IL-4, IL-5 and interferon-γ cytokine gene expression. *Am Rev Respir Dis* 148: 401–406

118 Bentley AM, Hamid Q, Robinson DS et al (1996) Prednisolone treatment in asthma. Reduction in the number of eosinophils, T-cells, tryptase-only positive mast cells, and modulation of IL-4, IL-5 and interferon gamma cytokine gene expression within the bronchial mucosa. *Am J Respir Crit Care Med* 153: 551–556

119 Robinson DS, Ying S, Bentley AM et al (1993) Relationship among numbers of bronchoalveolar lavage cells expressing mRNA for cytokines, asthma symptoms and airway methacholine responsiveness in atopic asthma. *Allergy Clin Immunol* 92: 397–403

120 Kay AB (1997) T cells as orchestrators of the asthmatic response. The rising trends in asthma. *Ciba Foundation Symposium* 206: 56–70

121 Sun Ying, Humbert M, Barkans J et al (1997) Expression of IL-4 and IL-5 mRNA and protein product by CD4+ and CD8+ T-cells, eosinophils and mast cells in bronchial biopsies obtained from atopic and non-atopic asthmatics. *J Immunol* 158: 3539–3544

122 Leung DYM, Martin RJ, Szefler SJ et al (1995) Dysregulation of IL-4, IL-5 and IFNγ gene expression in steroid-resistant asthma. *J Exp Med* 181: 33–40

123 Sher E, Leung DYM, Surs W et al (1994) Steroid resistant asthma. Cellular mechanisms contributing to inadequate response to glucocorticosteroid therapy. *J Clin Invest* 93: 33–39

124 Szefler SJ, Leung DYM (1997) Glucorticoid-resistant asthma: pathogenesis and clinical implications for management. *Eur Respir J* 10: 1640–1647

125 Lane SJ, Lee TH (1997) Mechanisms and detection of glucocorticoid insensitivity in asthma. *ACI International* 9/6

126 Adcock IM, Lane SJ, Brown CR et al (1995) Abnormal glucocorticosteroid receptor-activator protein 1 interaction in steroid resistant asthma. *J Exp Med* 182: 1951–1958

127 Alexander AG, Barnes NC, Kay AB (1992) Trial of cyclosporin A in corticosteroid-dependent chronic severe asthma. *Lancet* 339: 324–328

128 Lock SH, Kay AB, Barnes NC (1996) Double-blind placebo-controlled study of cyclosporin A as a corticosteroid-sparing agent in corticosteroid-dependant asthma. *Am J Respir Crit Care Med* 153: 509–514

129 Sihra BS, Durham SR, Walker S et al (1997) Effect of Cyclosporin A on the allergen-induced late asthmatic response. *Thorax* 52: 447–452

130 Kay AB, Frew AJ, Corrigan CJ et al (1998) The T cell hypothesis of chronic asthma. In: AB Kay (ed): *Allergy and allergic diseases*. Blackwell Science, Oxford

131 Teran LM, Carroll M, Frew AJ (1996) Leucocyte recruitment after local endobronchial allergy challenge in asthma: relationship to procedure and to airway IL-8 release. *Am J Respir Crit Care Med* 154: 469–476

132 Holgate ST (1993) Mediators and cytokine mechanisms in asthma. Altyounan address. *Thorax* 48: 103–109

133 Louis R, Shute J, Biagi S et al (1997) Cell infiltration, ICAM-1 expression, and eosinophil chemotactic activity in asthmatic sputum. *Am J Respir Crit Care Med* 155: 466–472

134 Weller PF(1997) Updates on cells and cytokines. Human eosinophils. *J Allergy Clin Immunol* 100: 283–287

135 Mochel R, Ying S, Barkans J et al (1995) Identification of mRNA for IL-4 in human eosinophils with granule localisation and release of the translated product. *J Immunol* 155 10): 4939–4947

136 Makker HK, Holgate ST (1994) Mechanisms of exercise-induced asthma. Eur J Clin Inv 24: 571–585

137 Bradding P, Feather IH, Wilson S et al (1993) Immunolocalisation of cytokines in the nasal mucosa of normal and perennial rhinitic subjects: the mast cell as a source of IL-4, IL-5 and IL-6 in human allergic mucosal inflammation. *J Immunol* 151: 3853–3865

138 Okayama Y, Lau LC-K, Church MK (1996) TNFα production by human lung mast cells in response to stimulation by stem cell factor and FcER1 cross-linkage. *J Immunol; in press*

139 Montefort S, Gratziou C, Goulding D (1994) Bronchial biopsy evidence for leucocyte infiltration and upregulation of leucocyte endothelial cell adhesion molecules 6 hours after local allergen challenge of sensitised asthmatic airway. *J Clin Inv* 93: 1411–1421

140 Campbell AM (1997) Bronchial epithelial cells in asthma. *Allergy* 52: 483–489

141 Devalia JL, Campbell AM, Sapeford RJ et al (1993) Effects of nitrogen dioxide on synthesis of inflammatory cytokines expressed by human bronchial epithelial cells *in vitro*. *Am J Respir Cell Mol Biol* 9: 271–278

142 Vignola AM, Campbell AM, Chanez P et al (1993) Activation by histamine of bronchial epithelial cells from nonasthmatic subjects. *Am J Respir Cell Mol Biol* 9: 411–417

143 Altman LC, Ayars GH, Baker C et al (1993) Cytokines and eosinophil-derived cationic proteins upregulate ICAM-1 on human nasal epithelial cells. *J Allergy Clin Immunol* 92: 527

144 Souques F, Crampette L, Mondain M et al (1995) Stimulation of dispersed nasal polyp cells by hyperosmolar solutions. *J Allergy Clin Immunol* 96: 980–985

145 Kalinski P, Hilkens CMU, Snijders A et al (1997) IL-12 deficient dendritic cells, generated in the presence of $PGE_2$ promote type 2 cytokine production in maturing human naive T helper cells. *J Immunol* 159: 28–35

146 Campbell AM, Vignola AM, Chanez P et al (1994) Low affinity receptors for IgE on human bronchial epithelial cells. *Immunol* 82: 506–508

147 Marini M, Vittori E, Hollemborg J et al (1992) Expression of the potent inflammatory cytokines, GM-CSF and IL-6 and IL-8, in bronchial epithelial cells of patients with asthma. *J Allergy Clin Immunol* 89: 1001–1009

148 Cromwell O, Hamid Q, Corrigan CJ et al (1992) Expression and generation of IL-8, IL-6 and GM-CSF by bronchial epithelial cells and enhancement by IL-1β and TNFα. *Immunol* 77: 330–337

149 Wang DH, Devalia JL, Xia C et al (1996) Expression of RANTES by human bronchial epithelial cells *in vitro* and *in vivo* and the effect of corticosteroids. *Am J Respir Cell Mol Biol* 14: 27–35

150 Barnes PJ (1997) NFκB. *N Engl J Med* 336: 1066–1071

151 Asano K, Nakamura H, Lilly CM et al (1997) IFNγ induces prostaglandin GIH synthase-2 through an autocrine loop via the epidermal growth factor receptor in human bronchial epithelial cells. *J Clin Inv* 99: 1057–63

151 Shibata Y, Nakamura H, Kato S et al (1996) Cellular detachment and deformation induce IL-8 gene expression in human bronchial epithelial cells. *J Immunol* 156: 772–777

152 Wilson SJ, Leone BA, Anderson D, Manning A, Holgate ST (1999) Immunohistochemical analysis of the activation of NF-κB and expression of associated cytokines and adhesion molecules in human models of allergic inflammation. *J Pathology; submitted for publication*

153 Manolitsas ND, Trigg CJ, McAulay AE et al (1994) The expression of intercellular adhesion molecule-1 and the β1-integrins in asthma. *Eur Respir J* 7: 1439–1444

154 Corne J, Holgate ST (1997) Mechanisms of virus induced exacerbations of asthma. *Thorax* 52: 380–389

155 Vignola AM, Merendino AM, Chiapparo G et al (1999) Heterogeneous effects of TGFβ, EGF, IL-4 and IL-5 on ICAM-1 and α3β1 expression on fibronectin release by human pulmonary epithelial cells. *Thorax; in press*

156 Alving K, Weitzberg E, Lundberg JM (1993) Increased amounts of nitric oxide in exhaled air. *Eur Resp J* 6: 1268–1270

157 Kharitonov SA, Yates D, Robbins RA, Logan-Sinclair R et al (1994) Increased nitric oxide in exhaled air of asthmatic patients. *Lancet* 343: 133–135

158 Nijkamp FP, Folkerts G (1997) Nitric oxide: Initiator and modulator. *Clin Exp Allergy* 27: 347–350

159 Holgate ST (1996) The inflammation-repair cycle in asthma: possible new biomarkers of disease activity. *Eur Respir Rev* 6: 4–10

160 Barnes PJ (1995) Nitric oxide and airway disease. *Ann Int Med* 27: 91–97

161 Redington AE, Springall DR, Holgate S et al (1997) Airway endothelin levels in asthma: influence of allergen challenge and maintenance corticosteroid therapy. *Eur Resp J* 10: 1026–1032

162 Mattoli S, Mezzetti M, Riva G et al (1990) Specific binding of endothelin on human

bronchial smooth muscle cells in culture and secretion of endothelin-like material from bronchial epithelial cells. *Am J Resp Cell Mol Biol* 3: 145–151

163 Yanagisawa M, Kurihara H, Kimura S et al (1988) A novel potent vasoconstrictor peptide produced by vascular endothelial cells. *Nature* 332: 411–415

164 Springall DR, Howarth PH, Counihan H et al (1991) Endothelin immunoreactivity of airway epithelium in asthmatic patients. *Lancet* 337: 697–701

165 Redngton AE, Springall DR, Ghatei MA et al (1995) Endothelin in BALF and its relationship to airflow obstruction in asthma. *Am Rev Resp Crit Care Med* 151: 1034–1039

166 Newton R, Kuitert LM, Slater DM et al (1997) Cytokine induction of cytosolic phospholipase A2 and cyclooxygenase-2 mRNA is suppressed by glucocorticosteroids in human epithelial cells. *Life Science* 60: 67–78

167 Souza A, Trigg CJ, Lane SJ et al (1997) Effect of inhaled glucocorticosteroids on IL-1β and IL-1ra expression in asthmatic bronchial epithelium. *Thorax* 52: 407–410

168 Wilson S, Wallin A, Sandstrom T et al (1997) Effects of budesonide treatment on expression of NF-κB and NF-κB regulated cytokines and adhesion molecules in bronchial mucosa of mild asthmatics. *Am J Respir Crit Care Med* 155(2): A698

169 Brown PJ, Greville HW, Finucane KE (1980) Asthma and irreversible airflow obstruction *Thorax* 35: 298–302

170 Huber HL, Koessler KK (1922) The pathology of bronchial asthma. *Arch Int Med* 30: 689–760

171 Ebira M, Takahashi T, Chiba T et al (1993) Cellular hypertrophy and hyperplasia of airway smooth muscles underlying bronchial asthma: a 3-D morphometric study. *Am Rev Resp Dis* 148: 720–726

172 Takizawa T, Thurlbeck WM (1971) Muscle and mucus gland size in the major bronchi of patients with chronic bronchitis, asthma and asthmatic bronchitis. *Am Rev Resp Dis* 104 331–336

173 Li X, Wilson JW (1997) Increased vascularity of the bronchial mucosa in mild asthma. *Am J Respir Crit Care Med* 156: 229–233

174 Hirst SJ (1996) Airway smooth muscle cell culture: Application to studies of airway wall remodelling and phenotype plasticity in asthma. *Eur Respir J* 9: 808–820

175 Lynch DA, Newell JD, Tschomper BA et al (1993) Uncomplicated asthma in adults: comparison of CT appearances of the lungs in asthmatic and healthy subjects. *Radiology* 188: 829–833

176 Paganin F, Seneterre E, Chanez P et al (1996) Computerised tomography of the lungs in asthma: influence of disease severity and aetiology. *Am J Respir Crit Care Med* 153: 110–114

177 Roche WR, Beasley R, Williams JH et al (1989) Subepithelial fibrosis in the bronchi of asthmatics. *Lancet* i: 520–524

178 Brewster CEP, Howarth PH, Djukanovic R et al (1990) Myofibroblasts and subepithelial fibrosis in bronchial asthma. *Am J Respir Cell Mol Biol* 3: 507–511

179 Wilson JW, Li X (1997) The measurement of reticular basement membrane and submucosal collagen in the asthmatic airway. *Clin Exp Allergy* 27: 363–371

180 Redington AE, Howarth PH (1997) Airway wall remodelling in asthma. *Thorax* 52: 310–312

181 Redington AE, Madden J, Frew AJ et al (1997) Transforming growth factor β1 in asthma-measurement in bronchoalveolar lavage fluid. *Am J Respir Crit Care Med* 156: 642–647

182 Anwar AR, Moqbel R, Walsh GM et al (1993) Adhesion to fibroneetin prolongs eosinophil survival. *J Exp Med* 177: 839–843

183 Georas SN, McIntyre WB, Ebisawa M (1993) Expression of a functional laminin receptor a6bl (VLA-6) on human eosinophil. *Blood* 82: 2872–2879

184 Goldring K, Warner JA (1997) Cell matrix interactions in asthma. *Clin Exp Allergy* 27: 22–27

185 Minshall EM, Leung DYM, Martin RJ et al (1997) Eosinophil-associated TGF-β1 mRNA expression and airways fibrosis in bronchial asthma. *Am J Respir Cell Mol Biol* 17: 326–333

186 Shute J, Parmar J, Holgate ST (1997) Urinary glyeosaminoglyean levels are increased in acute severe asthma – a role for eosinophil-derived gelatinase B? *Int Arch Allergy Immunol* 113: 366–367

187 Ruoss SJ, Hartmann T, Caughey GH (1991) Mast cell tryptase is a mitogen for cultured fibroblasts. *J Clin Inv* 88: 493–499

188 Cutz E, Levison H, Cooper DM (1978) Ultrastructure of airways in children with asthma. *Histopathology* 2: 407–421

189 Djukanovic R, Wilson JW, Britten KM et al (1992) Effect of inhaled corticosteroids on airway inflammation and symptoms in asthma. *Am Rev Respir Dis* 145: 669–674

190 Laitinen LA, Laitinen A (1996) Remodelling of asthmatic airways by glucocorticosteroids. *J Allergy Clin Immunol* 97: 153–158

191 Djukanovic R, Howarth PH, Vrugt B et al (1995) Determinants of asthma severity. *Int Arch Allergy Immunol* 107: 389

192 Walker, C, Kaegi MK, Braun P et al (1991) Activated T cells and eosinophilia in bronchoalveolar lavages from subjects with asthma correlated with disease severity. *J Allergy Clin Immunol* 88: 935–942

193 Sont JK, Han J, van Krieken JM et al (1996) Relationship between the inflammatory infiltrate in bronchial biopsy specimens and clinical severity of asthma in patients treated with inhaled steroids. *Thorax* 51: 496–502

194 Bradley BL, Azzawi M, Jacobson M et al (1991). Eosinophils, T-lymphocytes, mast cells, neutrophils, and macrophages in bronchial biopsy specimens from atopic subjects with asthma: comparison with biopsy specimens from atopic subjects without asthma and normal control subjects and relationship to bronchial hyperresponsiveness. *J Allergy Clin Immunol* 889: 661–74

195 Sur S, Crotty TB, Kephart GM et al (1993) Sudden onset fatal asthma – A distinct entity with few eosinophils and relatively more neutrophils in the airway submueosa? *Am Rev Respir Dis* 148: 713–719

196 Fahy JV, Kim KW, Liu J et al (1995) Respiratory pathophysiological responses-promi-

nent neutrophilic inflammation in sputum from subjects with asthma exacerbations. *J Allergy Clin Immunol* 95 (4): 843–852

197 Wenzel SE, Szefler SJ, Leung DYM et al (1997) Bronchoscopic evaluation of severe asthma, persistent inflammation associated with high dose glucocorticosteroids. *Am J Respir Crit Care Med* 156: 737–743

198 Cox G (1995) Glucocorticosteroid treatment inhibits apoptosis in human neutrophils. *J Immunol* 154: 4719–4725

199 Chanez P, Paradis A, Vignola M et al (1996) Changes in bronchial epithelium of steroid (GCs) dependent asthmatics. *Am J Respir Crit Care Med* 153: 212

200 Weiss KB, Gergen PJ, Hodgson TA (1992) An economic evaluation of asthma in the United States. *N Engl J Med* 326: 862–866

201 Nizankowska E, Soja J, Pinis G et al (1995) Treatment of steroid-dependant bronchial asthma with cyclosporin. *Eur Respir J* 8: 1091–1099

202 Corrigan CJ, Kay AB (1990) CD4+ T lymphocyte activation in acute severe asthma: relationship to disease severity. *Am Rev Respir Dis* 140: 970–977

# Corticosteroids

*Peter J Barnes*

Department of Thoracic Medicine, National Heart and Lung Institute, Imperial College School of Medicine, Dovehouse St., London SW3 6LY, UK

## Introduction

Corticosteroids are the most effective therapy currently available for asthma and improvement with corticosteroids is one of the hallmarks of asthma. Inhaled glucocorticoids have revolutionised asthma treatment and have now become the mainstay of therapy for patients with chronic disease [1]. There has recently been an enormous increase in our understanding of the molecular mechanisms whereby glucocorticoids suppress inflammation in asthma and this has led to changes in the way corticosteroids are used and may point the way to the development of more specific therapies in the future [2, 3].

## Molelcular mechanisms

Glucocorticoids are very effective antiinflammatory therapy in asthma and the molecular mechanisms involved in suppression of inflammation in asthma have recently become clarified. It is evident that corticosteroids are so effective because they block may of the inflammatory pathways that are abnormally activated in asthma.

### Glucocorticoid receptors

Glucocorticoids exert their effects by binding to glucocorticoid receptors (GR) which are localised to the cytoplasm of target cells. The affinity of cortisol binding to GR is approximately 30 nM, which falls within the normal range for plasma concentrations of free hormone. There is a single class of GR that binds glucocorticoids, with no evidence for subtypes of differing affinity in different tissues. Recently a splice variant of GR, termed GR-β, has been identified that does not bind glucocorticoids, but binds to DNA and may therefore interfere with the action of corticosteroids [6]. However, it is unlikely that there is sufficient GR-β present in cells to

Anti-Inflammatory Drugs in Asthma, edited by A.P. Sampson and M.K. Church

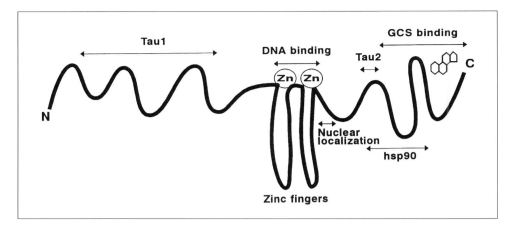

*Figure 1*
*Domains of the glucocorticoid receptor.*

functionally inhibit glucocorticoid action. The structure of GR has been elucidated using site-directed mutagenesis, which has revealed distinct domains [7, 8]. The glucocorticoid binding domain is at the C-terminal end of the molecule and in the middle of the molecule are two finger-like projections that interact with DNA. Each of these "zinc fingers" is formed by a zinc atom bound to four cysteine residues (Fig. 1). An N-terminal domain ($\tau$1) that is involved in transcriptional trans-activation of genes once binding to DNA has occurred and this region may also be involved in binding to other transcription factors [9]. Another trans-activating domain ($\tau$2) is adjacent to the steroid-binding domain and is also important for the nuclear translocation of the receptor. The inactivated GR is bound to a protein complex (~300 kDa) that includes two molecules of 90 kDa heat shock protein (hsp90) and various other inhibitory proteins. The hsp 90 molecules act as a "molecular chaperone" preventing the unoccupied GR localising to the nuclear compartment. Once the glucocorticoid binds to GR hsp90 dissociates, thus exposing two nuclear localisation signals and allowing the nuclear localisation of the activated GR-corticosteroid complex and its binding to DNA (Fig. 2).

## Effects on gene transcription

Glucocorticoids produce their effect on responsive cells by activating GR to directly or indirectly regulate the transcription of certain target genes [10, 11]. The number of genes per cell directly regulated by corticosteroids is estimated to be between 10 and 100, but many genes are indirectly regulated through an interaction with

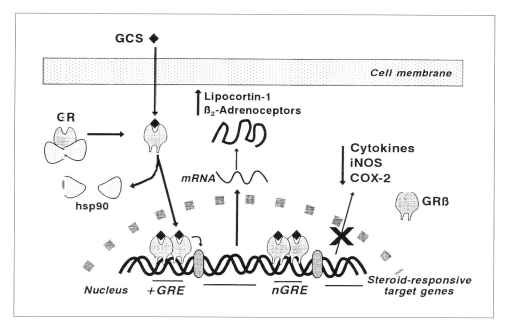

*Figure 2*
*Classical model of glucocorticoid action. The glucocorticoid enters the cell and binds to a cytoplasmic glucocorticoid receptor (GR) that is complexed with two molecules of a 90 kDa heat shock protein (hsp90). GR translocates to the nucleus where, as a dimer, it binds to a glucocorticoid recognition sequence (GRE) on the 5'-upstream promoter sequence of corticosteroid responsive genes. GREs may increase transcription and nGREs may decrease transcription, resulting in increased or decreased messenger RNA (mRNA) and protein synthesis.*

other transcription factors, as discussed below. Upon activation GR forms a homodimer which binds to DNA at consensus sites termed glucocorticoid response elements (GREs) in the 5'-upstream promoter region of corticosteroid-responsive genes. This interaction changes the rate of transcription, resulting in either induction or repression of the gene. The consensus sequence for GRE binding is the palindromic 15-base pair sequence *GGTACAnnnTGTTCT* (where n is any nucleotide), although for repression of transcription the putative negative GRE (nGRE) has a more variable sequence (*ATYACnnTnTGATCn*). Crystallographic studies indicate that the zinc finger binding to DNA occurs within the major groove of DNA with one finger of each receptor in the homodimer interacting with one-half of the DNA palindrome. Interaction with other transcription factors may also be important in determining differential corticosteroid responsiveness in different cell types. Other transcription factors binding in the vicinity of GRE may influence the transactivat-

37

ing efficiency of GRE binding and the relative abundance of different transcription factors may contribute to the corticosteroid responsiveness of a particular cell type. GR may also inhibit protein synthesis by reducing the stability of mRNA via enhanced transcription of specific ribonucleases that break down mRNA containing constitutive AU-rich sequences in the untranslated 3'-region, thus shortening the turnover time of mRNA.

## Interaction with transcription factors

Activated GR may bind directly with other activated transcription factors as a protein-protein interaction. This could be an important determinant of corticosteroid responsiveness and is a key mechanism whereby glucocorticoids exert their anti-inflammatory actions [4]. This interaction was first demonstrated for the collagenase gene which is induced by the transcription factor activator protein-1 (AP-1), which is a heterodimer of Fos and Jun oncoproteins. AP-1, activated by phorbol esters or tumour necrosis factor-$\alpha$ (TNF$\alpha$), forms a protein-protein complex with activated GR, and this prevents GR interacting with DNA and thereby reduces corticosteroid responsiveness [12]. In human lung TNF$\alpha$ and phorbol esters increase AP-1 binding to DNA and this is inhibited by glucocorticoids [13, 14]. GR also interacts with other transcription factors that are activated by inflammatory signals, including nuclear factor-$\kappa$B (NF-$\kappa$B) in a similar manner [13–17] (Fig. 3). There is also evidence that $\beta_2$-agonists, via cyclic AMP formation and activation of protein kinase A, result in the activation of the transcription factor CREB that binds to a cyclic AMP responsive element (CRE) on genes. A direct interaction between CREB and GR has been demonstrated [18]. These interactions between activated GR and transcription factors occur within the nucleus, but recent observations suggest that these protein-protein interactions may also occur in the cytoplasm [19].

## Effects on chromatin structure

There has recently been increasing evidence that glucocorticoids may have effects on the chromatin structure. DNA in chromosomes is wound around histone molecules in the form of nucleosomes. Several transcription factors interact with large co-activator molecules, such as CREB binding protein (CBP) and the related p300, which bind to the basal transcription factor apparatus [20]. Several transcription factors have now been shown to bind directly to CBP, including AP-1, NF-$\kappa$B and STATs [21]. Since binding sites on this molecule may be limited, this may result in competition between transcription factors for the limited binding sites available, so that there is an indirect rather than a direct protein-protein interaction (Fig. 4). CBP also interacts with nuclear hormone receptors, such as GR. These nuclear hormone

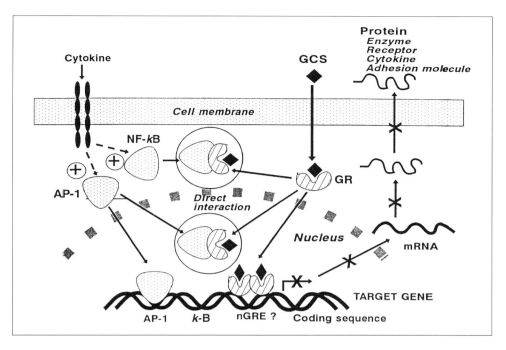

*Figure 3*
*Direct interaction between the transcription factors activator protein-1 (AP-1) and nuclear factor-kappa B (NF-κB) and the glucocorticoid receptor (GR) may result in mutual repression. In this way corticosteroids may counteract the chronic inflammatory effects of cytokines that activate these transcription factors.*

receptors may interact with CBP and the basal transcriptional apparatus through binding to other nuclear coactivator proteins, including corticosteroid receptor coactivator-1 (SRC-1) [22, 23], transcription factor intermediary factor-2 (TIF2) or glucocorticoid receptor interacting protein-1 [24]. DNA is wound around histone proteins to form nucleosomes and the chromatin fibre in chromosomes. At a microscopic level that chromatin may become dense or opaque due to the winding or unwinding of DNA around the histone core. CBP and p300 have histone acetylation activity which is activated by the binding of transcription factors, such as AP-1 and NF-κB [25]. Acetylation of histone residues results in unwinding of DNA coiled around the histone core, thus opening up the chromatin structure, which allows transcription factors to bind more readily, thereby increasing transcription (Fig. 4). Repression of genes reverses this process by histone deacetylation [26]. The process of deacetylation involves the binding of hormone or vitamin receptors to co-repressor molecules, such as nuclear receptor co-repressor (N-CoR) which forms a

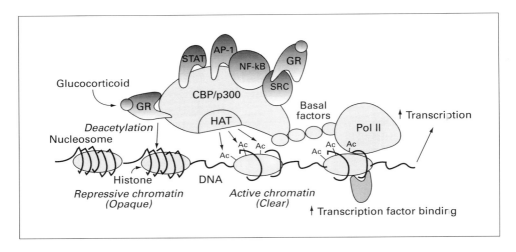

*Figure 4*

*Effect of glucocorticoids on chromatin structure. Transcription factors, such as STATs, AP-1 and NF-κB bind to co-activator molecules, such as CREB binding protein (CBP) or p300, which have intrinsic histone acetyltransferase (HAT) activity, resulting in acetylation (-Ac) of histone residues. This leads to unwinding of DNA and this allows increased binding of transcription factors resulting in increased gene transcription. Glucocorticoid receptors (GR) after activation by glucocorticoids bind to a glucocorticoid receptor co-activator which is bound to CBP. This results in deacetylation of histone, with increased coiling of DNA around histone, thus preventing transcription factor binding leading to gene repression.*

complex with another repressor molecule Sin3 and a histone deacetylase [27, 28]. Deacetylation of histone increases the winding of DNA round histone residues, resulting in dense chromatin structure and reduced access of transcription factors to their binding sites, thereby leading to repressed transcription of inflammatory genes. Activated GR may bind to several transcription co-repressor molecules that associate with proteins that have histone deacetylase activity, resulting in deacetylation of histone, increased winding of DNA round histone residues and thus reduced access of transcription factors to their binding sites and therefore repression of inflammatory genes [26] (Fig. 4).

## Target genes in inflammation control

Glucocorticoids may control inflammation by inhibiting many aspects of the inflammatory process through increasing the transcription of anti-inflammatory genes and decreasing the transcription of inflammatory genes [2, 4] (Tab. 1).

*Table 1 - Effect of corticosteroids on gene transcription*

**Increased transcription**

Lipocortin-1 (phospholipase $A_2$ inhibitor)
$\beta_2$-Adrenoceptor
Secretory leukocyte inhibitory protein
Clara cell protein (CC10)
IL-1 receptor antagonist
IL-1R2 (decoy receptor)
I$\kappa$B-$\alpha$ (inhibitor of NF-$\kappa$B)

**Decreased transcription**

Cytokines        (IL-1, IL-2, IL-3, IL-4, IL-5, IL-6, IL-11, IL-12, IL-13, TNF$\alpha$, GM-CSF, SCF)
Chemokines       (IL-8, RANTES, MIP-1$\alpha$, MCP-1, MCP-3, MCP-4, eotaxin)
Inducible nitric oxide synthase (iNOS)
Inducible cyclooxygenase (COX-2)
Cytoplasmic phospholipase $A_2$ (cPLA$_2$)
Endothelin-1
NK$_1$-receptors, NK$_2$-receptors
Adhesion molecules (ICAM-1, E-selectin)

## Antiinflammatory proteins

Glucocorticoids may suppress inflammation by increasing the synthesis of anti-inflammatory proteins. Corticosteroids increase the synthesis of lipocortin-1, a 37 kDa protein that has an inhibitory effect on phospholipase $A_2$ (PLA$_2$), and therefore may inhibit the production of lipid mediators. Corticosteroids induce the formation of lipocortin-1 in several cells and recombinant lipocortin-1 has acute anti-inflammatory properties [29]. However, glucocorticoids do not induce lipocortin-1 expression in all cells and this may be only one of many genes regulated by glucocorticoids. Glucocorticoids also increase the synthesis of secretory leukocyte protease inhibitor (SLPI) in human airway epithelial cells by increasing gene transcription [30]. SLPI is the predominant antiprotease in conducting airways and may be important in reducing airway inflammation by counteracting inflammatory enzymes, such as tryptase.

Interleukin (IL)-1 receptor antagonist (IL-1ra) is a cytokine that blocks the binding of IL-1 to its receptors. Its synthesis is increased by glucocorticoids, thus counteracting the effect of the proinflammatory cytokine IL-1. Thus, treatment of asthmatic patients with inhaled glucocorticoids results in an increased expression of IL-1ra in airway epithelial cells *in vitro* and *in vivo* [31, 32]. IL-1 interacts with two types of surface receptor, designated IL-1R1 and IL-1R2. The inflammatory effects of IL-1β are mediated exclusively via IL-1R1, whereas IL-1R2 has no signalling activity, but binds IL-1 and therefore acts as a "molecular decoy" that interferes with the actions of IL-1. Glucocorticoids are potent inducers of this decoy IL-1 receptor and result in release of a soluble form of the receptor, thus reducing the functional activity of IL-1 [33].

IL-10 is another antiinflammatory cytokine secreted predominantly by macrophages in the lung which inhibits the transcription of many proinflammatory cytokines and chemokines and this appears to be mediated via an inhibitory effect on NF-κB [34]. IL-10 secretion by alveolar macrophages may be impaired in asthmatic patients, resulting in increased macrophage cytokine secretion [35, 36]. Glucocorticoid treatment in asthmatic patients increases IL-10 secretion by these cells, although this appears to be an indirect effect, since treatment of alveolar macrophages *in vitro* with glucocorticoids tends to decrease IL-10 secretion [36].

NF-κB is regulated by the inhibitory protein IκB to which it is bound in the cytoplasm [37]. There is some evidence that glucocorticoids increase the synthesis and transcription of the predominant form of IκB, IκB-α, in mononuclear cells and T lymphocytes, thus terminating the activation of NF-κB [38, 39], but this has not been seen in other cell types [40–42]. The IκB-α gene does not appear to have any GRE consensus sequence, so any effect of glucocorticoids is probably mediated via other transcription factors.

In epithelial cells glucocorticoids also increase the expression of the enzyme neutral endopeptidase (NEP), which degrades inflammatory peptides such as substance P, bradykinin and endothelin-1 [43]. Asthmatic patients treated with inhaled glucocorticoids have a higher level of NEP expression that untreated patients [44].

## $\beta_2$-Adrenoceptors

Corticosteroids increase the expression of $\beta_2$-adrenoceptors by increasing the rate of transcription and the human $\beta_2$-receptor gene has three potential GREs [45]. Corticosteroids double the rate of $\beta_2$-receptor gene transcription in human lung *in vitro*, resulting in increased expression of $\beta_2$-receptors [46]. Using autoradiographic mapping and *in situ* hybridisation in animals to localise the increase in $\beta_2$-receptor expression, there appears to be an increase in all cell types, including airway epithelial cells and airway smooth muscle, after chronic glucocorticoid treatment [47]. This may be relevant in asthma as it may prevent down-regulation in response to prolonged treatment with $\beta_2$-agonists. In rats glucocorticoids prevent the down-regulation and reduced transcription of $\beta_2$-receptors in response to chronic β-agonist exposure [47].

## Cytokines

Although it is not yet possible to be certain of the most critical aspects of corticosteroid action in asthma, it is likely that their inhibitory effects on cytokine synthesis are of particular relevance. Corticosteroids inhibit the transcription of several cytokines that are relevant in asthma, including IL-1β, TNFα, granulocyte-macrophage colony-stimulating factor (GM-CSF), IL-2, IL-3, IL-4, IL-5, IL-6, IL-11 and the chemokines IL-8, RANTES, macrophage chemotactic protein (MCP)-1, MCP-3, MCP-4, macrophage inflammatory protein (MIP)-1α and eotaxin. These inhibitory effects were at one time thought to be mediated directly via interaction of GR with a nGRE in the upstream promoter sequence of the cytokine gene, resulting in reduced gene transcription. Surprisingly, there is no apparent nGRE consensus sequence in the upstream promoter region of these cytokines, suggesting that glucocorticoids inhibit transcription indirectly. Thus, the 5'-promoter sequence of the human IL-2 gene has no GRE consensus sequences, yet glucocorticoids are potent inhibitors of IL-2 gene transcription in T-lymphocytes. Transcription of the IL-2 gene is predominantly regulated by a cell-specific transcription factor nuclear factor of activated T-cells (NF-AT), which is activated in the cytoplasm on T-cell receptor stimulation via calcineurin. A nuclear factor is also necessary for increased activation and this factor appears to be AP-1, which binds directly to NF-AT to form a transcriptional complex [48]. Glucocorticoids therefore inhibit IL-2 gene transcription indirectly by binding to AP-1, thus preventing increased transcription due to NF-AT [49]. There may be marked differences in the response of different cells and of different cytokines to the inhibitory action of glucocorticoids and this may be dependent on the relative abundance of transcription factors. Thus in alveolar macrophages and peripheral blood monocytes GM-CSF secretion is more potently inhibited by glucocorticoids than IL-1β or IL-6 secretion [50].

## Inflammatory enzymes

Nitric oxide (NO) synthase may be induced by proinflammatory cytokines, resulting in increased NO production. NO may amplify asthmatic inflammation and contribute to epithelial shedding and airway hyperresponsiveness through the formation of peroxynitrite. The induction of the inducible form of NOS (iNOS) is potently inhibited by glucocorticoids. In cultured human pulmonary epithelial cells pro-inflammatory cytokines result in increased expression of iNOS and increased NO formation, due to increased transcription of the iNOS gene, and this is inhibited by glucocorticoids [51]. There is no nGRE in the promoter sequence of the iNOS gene, but NF-κB appears to be an important transcription factor in regulating iNOS gene transcription [52]. Glucocorticoids may therefore prevent induction of iNOS by inactivating NF-κB, thereby inhibiting transcription.

Glucocorticoids inhibit the synthesis of several inflammatory mediators implicated in asthma through an inhibitory effect on enzyme induction. Glucocorticoids inhibit the induction of the gene coding for inducible cyclooxygenase (COX-2) in monocytes and epithelial cells and this also appears to be via NF-κB activation [53-55]. Glucocorticoids also inhibit the gene transcription of a form of $PLA_2$ ($cPLA_2$) induced by cytokines [56].

Corticosteroids also inhibit the synthesis of endothelin-1 in lung and airway epithelial cells and this effect may also be via inhibition of transcription factors that regulate its expression [57].

## Inflammatory receptors

Glucocorticoids also decrease the transcription of genes coding for certain receptors. Thus the NK1-receptor which mediates the inflammatory effects of substance P in the airways may show increased gene expression in asthma [58]. This may be inhibited by corticosteroids through an interaction with AP-1 as the $NK_1$ receptor gene promoter region has no GRE, but has an AP-1 response element [59]. Glucocorticoids also inhibit the transcription of the $NK_2$-receptor which mediates the bronchoconstrictor effects of tachykinins [60].

## Apoptosis

Corticosteroids markedly reduce the survival of certain inflammatory cells, such as eosinophils. Eosinophil survival is dependent on the presence of certain cytokines such as IL-5 and GM-CSF. Exposure to corticosteroids blocks the effects of these cytokines and leads to programmed cell death or apoptosis [61].

## Adhesion molecules

Adhesion molecules play a key role in the trafficking of inflammatory cells to sites of inflammation. The expression of many adhesion molecules on endothelial cells is induced by cytokines and corticosteroids may lead indirectly to a reduced expression via their inhibitory effects on cytokines, such as IL-1β and TNFα. Corticosteroids may also have a direct inhibitory effect on the expression of adhesion molecules, such as ICAM-1 and E-selectin at the level of gene transcription [62]. ICAM-1 expression in bronchial epithelial cell lines and monocytes is inhibited by glucocorticoids [63].

# Effects on cell function

Corticosteroids may have direct inhibitory actions on several inflammatory cells implicated in pulmonary and airway diseases (Fig. 5).

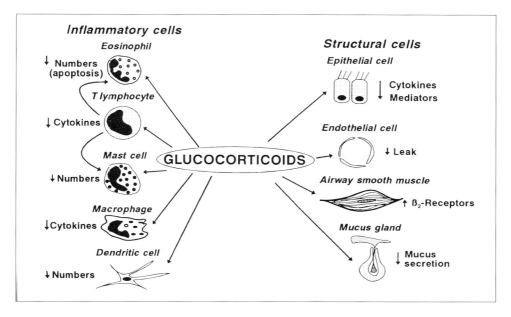

*Figure 5*
*Cellular effect of glucocorticoids.*

## Macrophages

Corticosteroids inhibit the release of inflammatory mediators and cytokines from alveolar macrophages *in vitro* [50], although their effect after inhalation *in vivo* is modest [64]. Corticosteroids may be more effective in inhibiting cytokine release from alveolar macrophages than in inhibition of lipid mediators and reactive oxygen species *in vitro* [65]. Inhaled corticosteroids reduce the secretion of chemokines and proinflammatory cytokines from alveolar macrophages from asthmatic patients, whereas the secretion of IL-10 is increased [36]. Oral prednisone inhibits the increased gene expression of IL-1β in alveolar macrophages obtained by bronchoalveolar lavage from asthmatic patients [66].

## Eosinophils

Corticosteroids have a direct inhibitory effect on mediator release from eosinophils, although they are only weakly effective in inhibiting secretion of reactive oxygen species and eosinophil basic proteins [67]. Corticosteroids inhibit the permissive action of cytokines such as GM-CSF and IL-5 on eosinophil survival [68, 69] and this contributes to the reduction in airway eosinophils seen with corticosteroid therapy. One of the best described actions of corticosteroids in asthma is a reduction in circulating eosinophils, which may reflect an action on eosinophil production in the bone marrow. Inhaled corticosteroids inhibit the increase in circulating eosinophil count at night in patients with nocturnal asthma and also reduce plasma concentrations of eosinophil cationic protein [70]. After inhaled corticosteroids (budesonide 800 μg b.i.d.) there is a marked reduction in the number of low-density eosinophils, presumably reflecting inhibition of cytokine production in the airways [71].

## T Lymphocytes

An important target cell in asthma may be the T lymphocyte, since corticosteroids are very effective in inhibition of activation of these cells and in blocking the release of cytokines which are likely to play an important role in the recruitment and survival of inflammatory cells involved in asthmatic inflammation. Thus glucocorticoids potently inhibit the secretion of IL-5 from T lymphocytes [72].

## Mast cells

While corticosteroids do not appear to have a direct inhibitory effect on mediator release from lung mast cells [73], chronic corticosteroid treatment is associated with a marked reduction in mucosal mast cell number [74, 75]. This may be linked to a reduction in IL-5 and stem cell factor (SCF) production, which are necessary for mast cell expression at mucosal surfaces. Mast cells also secrete various cytokines (TNFα, IL-4, IL-5, IL-6, IL-8), but whether this is inhibited by corticosteroids has not yet been reported.

## Dendritic cells

Dendritic cells in the epithelium of the respiratory tract appear to play a critical role in antigen presentation in the lung as they have the capacity to take up allergen process it into peptides and present it via MHC molecules on the cell surface for presentation to uncommitted T lymphocytes [76]. In experimental animals the number of dendritic cells is markedly reduced by systemic and inhaled corticosteroids, thus dampening the immune response in the airways [77]. Topical corticosteroids markedly reduce the numbers of dendritic cell in the nasal mucosa [78], and it is likely that a similar effect would be seen in airways.

## Neutrophils

Neutrophils, which are not prominent in the bronchial biopsies of asthmatic patients, are not very sensitive to the effects of corticosteroids. Indeed, systemic corticosteroids increase peripheral neutrophil counts which may reflect an increased survival time due to an inhibitory action of neutrophil apoptosis (in complete contrast to the increased apoptosis seen in eosinophils) [79].

## Endothelial cells

GR gene expression in the airways is most prominent in endothelial cells of the bronchial circulation and airway epithelial cells. Corticosteroids do not appear to directly inhibit the expression of adhesion molecules, although they may inhibit cell adhesion indirectly by suppression of cytokines involved in the regulation of adhesion molecule expression. Corticosteroids may have an inhibitory action on airway microvascular leak induced by inflammatory mediators [80, 81]. This appears to be a direct effect on postcapillary venular epithelial cells. The mechanism for this antipermeability effect has not been fully elucidated, but there is evidence that synthesis of a 100 kDa protein distinct from lipocortin-1 termed vasocortin may be involved [82]. Although there have been no direct measurements of the effects of corticosteroids on airway microvascular leakage in asthmatic airways, regular treatment with inhaled corticosteroids decreases the elevated plasma proteins found in bronchoalveolar lavage fluid of patients with stable asthma [83].

## Epithelial cells

Epithelial cells may be an important source of inflammatory mediators in asthmatic airways and may drive and amplify the inflammatory response in the airways [84, 85]. Airway epithelium may be one of the most important targets for inhaled glucocorticoids in asthma [3, 86]. Corticosteroids inhibit the increased transcription of the IL-8 gene induced by TNFα in cultured human airway epithelial cells in vitro [87, 88] and the transcription of the RANTES gene in an epithelial cell line [89]. Inhaled corticosteroids inhibit the increased expression of GM-CSF and RANTES in the epithelium of asthmatic patients [84, 90, 91]. There is increased expression of iNOS in the airway epithelium of patients with asthma [92] and this may account for the increase in NO in the exhaled air of patients with asthma compared with normal subjects [93]. Asthmatic patients who are taking regular inhaled corticosteroid therapy, however do not show such an increase in exhaled NO [93], suggesting that glucocorticoids have suppressed epithelial iNOS expression. Furthermore double-blind randomised studies show that oral and inhaled glucocorticoids reduce the elevated exhaled NO in asthmatic patients to normal values [94, 95]. Glucocorticoids also decrease the transcription of other inflammatory proteins in airway epithelial cells, including COX-2, $cPLA_2$ and endothelin-1 [53, 56, 57]. Airway epithelial cells may be the key cellular target of inhaled corticosteroids; by inhibiting the transcription of several inflammatory genes inhaled corticosteroids may reduce inflammation in the airway wall (Fig. 6).

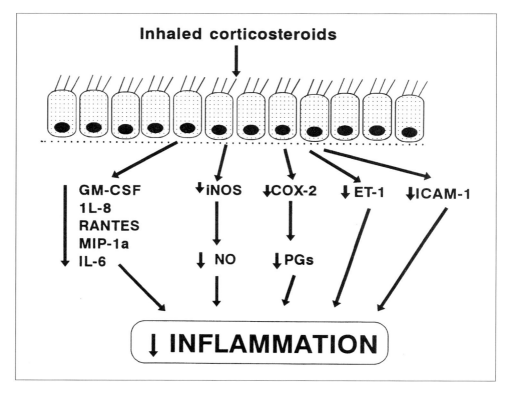

*Figure 6*
*Inhaled corticosteroids may inhibit the transcription of several "inflammatory" genes in airway epithelial cells and thus reduce inflammation in the airway wall.*

## Mucus secretion

Corticosteroids inhibit mucus secretion in airways and this may be a direct action of corticosteroids on submucosal gland cells [96]. Recent studies suggest that corticosteroids may also inhibit the expression of mucin genes, such as MUC2 and MUC5AC [97]. In addition, there are indirect inhibitory effects due to the reduction in inflammatory mediators that stimulate increased mucus secretion.

## Effects on astmatic inflammation

Glucocorticoids are remarkably effective in controlling the inflammation in asthmatic airways and it is likely that they have multiple cellular effects. Biopsy studies in patients with asthma have now confirmed that inhaled corticosteroids reduce the number and activation of inflammatory cells in the airway [74, 75, 91, 98, 99]. Similar results have been reported in bronchoalveolar lavage of asthmatic patients, with a reduction in both eosinophil number and eosinophil cationic protein concentrations, a marker of eosinophil degranulation, after inhaled budesonide [100]. These effects may be due to inhibition of cytokine synthesis in inflammatory and structural cells. There is also a reduction in activated CD4+ T-cells (CD4+/CD25+) in bronchoalveolar lavage fluid after inhaled glucocorticoids [101]. The disrupted epithelium is restored and the ciliated to goblet cell ratio is normalised after three months of therapy with inhaled corticosteroids [74]. There is also some evidence for a reduction in the thickness of the basement membrane [91], although in asthmatic patients taking inhaled corticosteroids for over 10 years the characteristic thickening of the basement membrane was still present [102].

## Effects on airway hyperresponsiveness

By reducing airway inflammation inhaled corticosteroids consistently reduce airway hyperresponsiveness (AHR) in asthmatic adults and children [103]. Chronic treatment with inhaled corticosteroids reduces responsiveness to histamine, cholinergic agonists, allergen (early and late responses), exercise, fog, cold air, bradykinin, adenosine and irritants (such as sulphur dioxide and metabisulphite). The reduction in AHR takes place over several weeks and may not be maximal until after several months of therapy. The magnitude of reduction is variable between patients and is in the order of one to two doubling dilutions for most challenges and often fails to return to the normal range. This may reflect suppression of the inflammation but persistence of structural changes which cannot be reversed by corticosteroids. Inhaled corticosteroids not only make the airways less sensitive to spasmogens, but they also limit the maximal airway narrowing in response to spasmogens [104].

## Clinical efficacy of inhaled corticosteroids

Inhaled corticosteroids are very effective in controlling asthma symptoms in asthmatic patients of all ages and severity [1, 105].

## Studies in adults

Inhaled corticosteroids were first introduced to reduce the requirement for oral corticosteroids in patients with severe asthma and many studies have confirmed that the majority of patients can be weaned off oral corticosteroids [106]. As experience has been gained with inhaled corticosteroids they have been introduced in patients with milder asthma, with the recognition that inflammation is present even in patients with mild asthma [107]. Inhaled anti-inflammatory drugs have now become first-line therapy in any patient who needs to use a $\beta_2$-agonist inhaler more than once a day, and this is reflected in national and international guidelines for the management of chronic asthma [108–110]. In patients with newly-diagnosed asthma inhaled corticosteroids (budesonide 600 µg twice daily) reduced symptoms and $\beta_2$-agonist inhaler usage and improved peak expiratory flows. These effects persisted over the two years of the study, whereas in a parallel group treated with inhaled $\beta_2$-agonists alone there was no significant change in symptoms or lung function [111]. In another study patients with mild asthma treated with a low dose of inhaled corticosteroid (budesonide 200 µg b.d.) showed fewer symptoms and a progressive improvement in lung function over several months and many patients became completely asymptomatic [112]. Similarly inhaled beclomethasone dipropionate (BDP, 400 µg b.d.) improved asthma symptoms and lung function and this was maintained over the 2.5 years of the study [113]. There was also a significant reduction in the number of exacerbations. Although the effects of inhaled corticosteroids on AHR may take several months to reach a plateau, the reduction in asthma symptoms occurs more rapidly [114].

High dose inhaled corticosteroids have now been introduced in many countries for the control of more severe asthma. This markedly reduces the need for maintenance oral corticosteroids and has revolutionised the management of more severe and unstable asthma [115–117]. Inhaled corticosteroids are the treatment of choice in nocturnal asthma, which is a manifestation of inflamed airways, reducing night time awakening and reducing the diurnal variation in airway function [118, 119]

Inhaled corticosteroids effectively control asthmatic inflammation but must be taken regularly. When inhaled corticosteroids are discontinued there is usually a gradual increase in symptoms and airway responsiveness back to pretreatment values [114], although in patients with mild asthma who have been treated with inhaled corticosteroids for a long time symptoms may not recur in some patients [120].

## Studies in children

Inhaled corticosteroids are equally effective in children. In an extensive study of children aged 7–17 years there was a significant improvement in symptoms, peak flow variability and lung function compared to a regular inhaled $\beta_2$-agonist which was maintained over the 22 months of the study [121], but asthma deteriorated when the inhaled corticosteroids were withdrawn [122]. There was a high proportion of drop-outs (45%) in the group treated with inhaled $\beta_2$-agonist alone. Inhaled corticosteroids are also effective in younger children. Nebulised budesonide reduced the need for oral corticosteroids and also improved lung function in children under the age of three [123]. Inhaled corticosteroids given via a large volume spacer improved asthma symptoms and reduced the number of exacerbations in preschool children and in infants [124, 125].

## Prevention of irreversible changes

Some patients with asthma develop an element of irreversible airflow obstruction, but the pathophysiological basis of this is not yet understood. It is likely that it is the result of chronic airway inflammation and that it may be prevented by treatment with inhaled corticosteroids. There is some evidence that the annual decline in lung function may be slowed by the introduction of inhaled corticosteroids [126]. Delay in starting inhaled corticosteroids may result in less overall improvement in lung function in both adults and children [127–129].

## Pharmacokinetics

The pharmacokinetics of inhaled corticosteroids are important in determining the concentration of drug reaching target cells in the airways and in the fraction of drug reaching the systemic circulation and therefore causing side-effects [1, 130, 131]. Beneficial properties in an inhaled corticosteroid are a high topical potency, a low systemic bioavailability of the swallowed portion of the dose and rapid metabolic clearance of any corticosteroid reaching the systemic circulation. After inhalation a large proportion of the inhaled dose (80–90%) is deposited on the oropharynx and is then swallowed and therefore available for absorption via the liver into the systemic circulation (Fig. 7). This fraction is markedly reduced by using a large volume spacer device with a metered dose inhaler (MDI) or by mouth washing and discarding the washing with dry powder inhalers. Between 10 and 20% of inhaled drug enters the respiratory tract, where it is deposited in the airways and this fraction is available for absorption into the systemic circulation. Most of the early studies on the distribution of inhaled corticosteroids were conducted in healthy volunteers, and it is not certain what effect inflammatory disease, airway obstruction, age of the patient or concomitant medication may have on the disposition of the inhaled dose. There may be important differences in the metabolism of different inhaled corticosteroids. BDP is metabolised to its more active metabolite beclomethasone monopropionate in many tissues including lung, but there is no information about the absorption or metabolism of this metabolite in humans. Flunisolide and budesonide are subject to extensive first-pass metabolism in the liver so that less reaches the systemic circulation [132, 133]. Little is known about the distribution of triamcinolone [134]. FP is almost completely metabolised by first-pass metabolism, which reduces systemic effects [135].

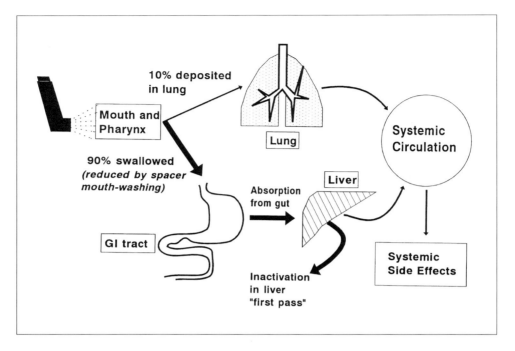

*Figure 7*
*Pharmacokinetics of inhaled corticosteroids.*

When inhaled corticosteroids were first introduced it was recommended that they should be given four times daily, but several studies have now demonstrated that twice daily administration gives comparable control [136, 137], although four times daily administration may be preferable in patients with more severe asthma [138]. However, patients may find it difficult to comply with such frequent administration unless they have troublesome symptoms. For patients with mild asthma who require ≤ 400 µg daily, once daily therapy may be sufficient [139].

## Side-effects of inhaled corticosteroids

The efficacy of inhaled corticosteroids is now established in short- and long-term studies in adults and children, but there are still concerns about side-effects, particularly in children and when high inhaled doses are needed. Several side-effects have been recognised.

## Local side-effects

Side effects due to the local deposition of the inhaled corticosteroid in the oropharynx may occur with inhaled corticosteroids, but the frequency of complaints depends on the dose and frequency of administration and on the delivery system used.

### *Dysphonia*

The commonest complaint is of hoarseness of the voice (dysphonia) and may occur in over 50% of patients using MDI [140, 141]. Dysphonia is not appreciably reduced by using spacers, but may be less with dry powder devices [142]. Dysphonia may be due to myopathy of laryngeal muscles and is reversible when treatment is withdrawn [141]. For most patients it is not troublesome but may be disabling in singers and lecturers.

### *Oropharyngeal candidiasis*

Oropharyngeal candidiasis (thrush) may be a problem in some patients, particularly in the elderly, with concomitant oral corticosteroids and more than twice daily administration [140]. Large volume spacer devices protect against this local side-effect by reducing the dose of inhaled corticosteroid that deposits in the oropharynx.

### *Other local complications*

There is no evidence that inhaled corticosteroids, even in high doses, increase the frequency of infections, including tuberculosis, in the lower respiratory tract [143, 144]. There is no evidence for atrophy of the airway epithelium and even after 10 years of treatment with inhaled corticosteroids there is no evidence for any structural changes in the epithelium [102]. Cough and throat irritation, sometimes accompanied by reflex bronchoconstriction, may occur when inhaled corticosteroids are given via a metered dose inhaler. These symptoms are likely to be due to surfactants in pressurised aerosols as they disappear after switching to a dry powder corticosteroid inhaler device [145].

## Systemic side-effects

The efficacy of inhaled corticosteroids in the control of asthma is undisputed, but there are concerns about systemic effects of inhaled corticosteroids, particularly as they are likely to be used over long periods and in children of all ages [105]. The safety of inhaled corticosteroids has been extensively investigated since their introduction 30 years ago [146]. One of the major problems is to decide whether a measurable systemic effect has any significant clinical consequence, and this necessitates careful long-term follow-up studies. As biochemical markers of systemic corticosteroid effects become more sensitive, then systemic effects may be seen more often, but this does not mean that these effects are clinically relevant. There are several case reports of adverse systemic effects of inhaled corticosteroids, and these are often idiosyncratic reactions, which may be due to abnormal pharmacokinetic handling of the inhaled corticosteroid. The systemic effect of an inhaled corticosteroid will depend on several factors, including the dose delivered to the patient, the site of delivery (gastrointestinal tract and lung), the delivery system used and individual differences in the patient's response to the corticosteroid.

## Effect of delivery systems

The systemic effect of an inhaled corticosteroid is dependent on the amount of drug absorbed into the systemic circulation. As noted above, approximately 90% of the inhaled dose from an MDI deposits in the oropharynx and is swallowed and subsequently absorbed from the gastrointestinal tract. Use of a large volume spacer device markedly reduces the oropharyngeal deposition, and therefore the systemic effects of inhaled corticosteroids [147]. For dry powder inhalers similar reductions in systemic effects may be achieved with mouth-washing and discarding the fluid. All patients using a daily dose of $\geq 800$ µg of an inhaled corticosteroid should therefore use either a spacer or mouth washing to reduce systemic absorption. Approximately 10% of an MDI enters the lung and this fraction (which presumably exerts the therapeutic effect) may be absorbed into the systemic circulation. As the fraction of inhaled corticosteroid deposited in the oropharynx is reduced, the proportion of the inhaled dose entering the lungs is increased. More efficient delivery to the lungs is therefore accompanied by increased systemic absorption, but this is offset by a reduction in the dose needed for optimal control of airway inflammation. For example, a multiple dry powder delivery system, the Turbohaler, delivers approximately twice as much corticosteroid to the lungs as other devices, and therefore has increased systemic effects. However this is compensated for by the fact that only half the dose is required [148].

## Hypothalamic-pituitary-adrenal axis

Glucocorticoids may cause hypothalamic-pituitary-adrenal (HPA) axis suppression by reducing corticotrophin (ACTH) production, which reduces cortisol secretion by the adrenal gland. The degree of HPA suppression is dependent on dose, duration, frequency and timing of corticosteroid administration. The clinical significance of HPA axis suppression is two-fold. Firstly, prolonged adrenal suppression may lead to reduced adrenal response to stress. There is no evidence that cortisol responses to the stress of an asthma exacerbation or insulin-induced hypoglycaemia are impaired, even with high doses of inhaled corticosteroids [149]. Secondly, measurement of HPA axis function provides evidence for systemic effects of an inhaled corticosteroid. Basal adrenal cortisol secretion may be measured by a morning plasma cortisol, 24 h urinary cortisol or by plasma cortisol profile over 24 h [150]. Other tests measure the HPA response following stimulation with tetracosactrin (which measures adrenal reserve) or stimulation with metyrapone and insulin (which measure the response to stress).

There are many studies of HPA axis function in asthmatic patients with inhaled corticosteroids, but the results are inconsistent as they have often been uncontrolled and patients have also been taking courses of oral corticosteroids (which may affect the HPA axis for weeks) [151]. BDP, budesonide and FP at high doses by conventional MDI (> 1600 µg daily) give a dose-related decrease in morning serum cortisol levels and 24 h urinary cortisol, although values still lie well within the normal range [152–154]. However, when a large volume spacer is used doses of 2000 µg daily of BDP or budesonide have little effect on 24 h urinary cortisol excretion [155]. Studies with inhaled flunisolide and triamcinolone in children show no effect on 24 h cortisol excretion at doses of up to 1000 µg daily [156, 157]. Stimulation tests of HPA axis function similarly show no consistent effects of doses of 1500 µg or less of inhaled corticosteroid. At high doses (> 1500 µg daily) budesonide and FP have less effect than BDP on HPA axis function [153, 158]. In children no suppression of urinary cortisol is seen with doses of BDP of 800 µg or less [159–161]. In studies where plasma cortisol has been measured at frequent intervals there was a significant reduction in cortisol peaks with doses of inhaled BDP as low as 400 µg daily [162], although this does not appear to be dose-related in the range 400–1000 µg [163, 164]. The clinical significance of these effects is not certain, however.

Overall, the studies which are not confounded by concomitant treatment with oral corticosteroids, have consistently shown that there are no significant suppressive effects on HPA axis function at doses of ≤ 1500 µg in adults and ≤ 400 µg in children.

## Effects on bone metabolism

Corticosteroids lead to a reduction in bone mass by direct effects on bone formation and resorption and indirectly by suppression of the pituitary-gonadal and HPA axes, effects on intestinal calcium absorption, renal tubular calcium reabsorption and secondary hyperparathyroidism [165]. The effects of oral corticosteroids on osteoporosis and increased risk of vertebral and rib fractures are well known, but there are no reports suggesting that long-term treatment with inhaled corticosteroids is associated with an increased risk of fractures. Bone densitometry has been used to assess the effect of inhaled corticosteroids on bone mass. Although there is evidence that bone density is less in patients taking high-dose inhaled corticosteroids, interpretation is confounded by the fact that these patients are also taking intermittent courses of oral corticosteroids [166].

Changes in bone mass occur very slowly and several biochemical indices have been used to assess the short-term effects of inhaled corticosteroids on bone metabolism. Bone formation has been measured by plasma concentrations of bone-specific alkaline phosphatase, serum osteocalcin, a non-collagenous 49-amino acid peptide secreted by osteoblasts, or by procollagen peptides. Bone resorption may be assessed by urinary hydroxyproline after a 12-h fast, urinary calcium excretion and pyridinium cross-link excretion. It is important to consider the age, diet, time of day and physical activity of the patient in interpreting any abnormalities. It is also necessary to choose appropriate control groups as asthma itself may have an effect on some of the measurements, such as osteocalcin [167]. Inhaled corticosteroids, even at doses up to 2000 µg daily, have no significant effect on calcium excretion, but acute and reversible dose-related suppression of serum osteocalcin has been reported with BDP and budesonide when given by conventional MDI in several studies [151]. Budesonide consistently has less effect than BDP at equivalent doses and only BDP increases urinary hydroxyproline at high doses [168]. With a large volume spacer even doses of 2000 µg daily of either BDP or budesonide are without effect on plasma osteocalcin concentrations, however [155]. Urinary pyridinium and deoxypyridinoline cross-links, which are a more accurate and stable measurement of bone and collagen degradation, are not increased with inhaled corticosteroids (BDP > 1000 µg daily), even with intermittent courses of oral corticosteroids [166]. It is important to monitor changes in markers of bone formation as well as bone degradation, as the net effect on bone turnover is important.

There has been particular concern about the effect of inhaled corticosteroids on bone metabolism in growing children. A very low dose of oral corticosteroids (prednisolone 2.5 mg) causes significant changes in serum osteocalcin and urinary hydroxyproline excretion, whereas daily BDP and budesonide at doses up to 800 µg daily have no effect [167, 169]. It is important to recognise that the changes in biochemical indices of bone metabolism are less than those seen with even low doses of oral corticosteroids. This suggests that even high doses of inhaled corticosteroids, particularly when used with a spacer device, are unlikely to have any long-term effect on bone structure. Careful long-term follow-up studies in patients with asthma are needed.

There is no evidence that inhaled corticosteroids increase the frequency of fractures. Long-term treatment with high dose inhaled corticosteroids has not been associated with any consistent change in bone density [170, 171]. Indeed, in elderly patients there may be an increase in bone density due to increased mobility [171].

## Effects on connective tissue

Oral and topical corticosteroids cause thinning of the skin, telangiectasiae and easy bruising, probably as a result of loss of extracellular ground substance within the dermis, due to an inhibitory effect on dermal fibroblasts. There are reports of increased skin bruising and purpura in patients using high doses of inhaled BDP, but the amount of intermittent oral corticosteroids in these patients is not known [172, 173]. Easy bruising in association with inhaled corticosteroids is more frequent in elderly patients [174] and there are no reports of this problem in children. Long-term prospective studies with objective measurements of skin thickness are needed with different inhaled corticosteroids.

## Ocular effects

Long-term treatment with oral corticosteroids increases the risk of posterior sub-capsular cataracts and there are several case reports describing cataracts in individual patients taking inhaled corticosteroids [146]. In a study of 48 patients who were exposed to oral and/or high dose inhaled corticosteroids the prevalence of posterior subcapsular cataracts (27%) correlated with the daily dose and duration of oral corticosteroids, but not with the dose and duration of inhaled corticosteroids [175]. In a recent cross-sectional study in patients aged 5–25 years taking either inhaled BDP or budesonide, no cataracts were found on slit-lamp examination, even in patients taking 2000 µg daily for over 10 years [176]. Recently there has been a report of a slight increase in the risk of glaucoma in patients taking very high doses of inhaled corticosteroids [177].

## Growth

There has been particular concern that inhaled corticosteroids may cause stunting of growth and several studies have addressed this issue. Asthma itself (as with other chronic diseases) may have an effect on the growth pattern and has been associated with delayed onset of puberty and decceleration of growth velocity that is more pronounced with more severe disease [178]. However, asthmatic children appear to grow for longer, so that their final height is normal. The effect of asthma on growth makes it difficult to assess the effects of inhaled corticosteroids on growth in cross-sectional studies, particularly as courses of oral corticosteroids are a confounding factor. Longitudinal studies have demonstrated that there is no significant effect of inhaled corticosteroids on statural growth in doses of up to 800 µg daily and for up to 5 years of treatment [121, 151, 179, 180]. A prospective study of inhaled BDP (400 µg daily) versus theophylline in children with mild to moderate asthma showed no effect on height, although there was some reduction in growth velocity compared to children treated with theophylline [181]. However it is not possible to relate changes in growth velocity to final height as other studies have demonstrated that there is a "catch up" period. In a longitudinal study in children aged 2–7 years with severe asthma, budesonide 200 μg daily had no effect on growth over 3–5 years [161]. In children with virally-induced wheezing BDP 400 μg daily has been reported to reduce growth compared with a placebo [182]. A meta-analysis of 21 studies, including over 800 children, showed no effect of inhaled BDP on statural height, even with higher doses and long duration of therapy [183].

Short-term growth measurements (knemometry) have demonstrated that even a low dose of an oral corticosteroid (prednisolone 2.5 mg) is sufficient to give complete suppression of lower leg growth. However inhaled budesonide up to 400 μg is without effect, although some suppression is seen with 800 μg and with 400 μg BDP [184, 185]. The relationship between knemometry measurements and final height are uncertain since low doses of oral corticosteroid that have no effect on final height cause profound suppression.

## Metabolic effects

Several metabolic effects have been reported after inhaled corticosteroids, but there is no evidence that these are clinically relevant at therapeutic doses. In adults fasting glucose and insulin are unchanged after doses of BDP up to 2000 μg daily [186] and in children with inhaled budesonide up to 800 μg daily [187]. In normal individuals high dose inhaled BDP may slightly increase resistance to insulin [188]. However, in patients with poorly controlled asthma high doses of BDP and budesonide paradoxically decrease insulin resistance and improve glucose tolerance, suggesting that the disease itself may lead to abnormalities in carbohydrate metabolism [189]. Neither BDP 2000 μg daily in adults nor budesonide 800 μg daily in children have any effect on plasma cholesterol or triglycerides [186, 187].

## Haematological effects

Inhaled corticosteroids may reduce the numbers of circulating eosinophils in asthmatic patients [71], possibly due to an effect on local cytokine generation in the airways. Inhaled corticosteroids may cause a small increase in circulating neutrophil counts [155, 190].

## Central nervous system effects

There are various reports of psychiatric disturbance, including emotional lability, euphoria, depression, aggressiveness and insomnia, after inhaled corticosteroids. Only eight such patients have so far been reported, suggesting that this is very infrequent and a causal link with inhaled corticosteroids has usually not been established [151].

*Table 2 - Side-effects of inhaled corticosteroids*

| Local side-effects | Systemic side-effects |
| --- | --- |
| Dysphonia | Adrenal suppression |
| Oropharyngeal candidiasis | Growth suppression |
| Cough | Bruising |
| | Osteoporosis |
| | Cataracts |
| | Glaucoma |
| | Metabolic abnormalities (glucose, insulin, triglycerides) |
| | Psychiatric disturbances |

## Safety in pregnancy

Based on extensive clinical experience, inhaled corticosteroids appear to be safe in pregnancy, although no controlled studies have been performed. There is no evidence for any adverse effects of inhaled corticosteroids on the pregnancy, the delivery or on the foetus [146]. It is important to recognise that poorly controlled asthma may increase the incidence of perinatal mortality and retard intra-uterine growth, so that more effective control of asthma with inhaled corticosteroids may reduce these problems.

## Clinical use of inhaled corticosteroids

Inhaled corticosteroids are now recommended as first-line therapy for all but the mildest of asthmatic patients [1]. Inhaled corticosteroids should be started in any patient who needs to use a β-agonist inhaler for symptom control more than once daily (or possibly three times weekly). It is conventional to start with a low dose of inhaled corticosteroid and to increase the dose until asthma control is achieved. However, this may take time and a preferable approach is to start with a dose of corticosteroids in the middle of the dose range (400 µg twice daily) to establish control of asthma more rapidly [191]. Once control is achieved (defined as normal or best possible lung function and infrequent need to use an inhaled $\mu_2$-agonist) the dose of inhaled corticosteroid should be reduced in a step-wise manner to the lowest dose needed for optimal control. It may take as long as three months to reach a plateau in response and any changes in dose should be made at intervals of three months or more. This strategy ("start high – go low") is emphasised in the revised BTS Guidelines for Asthma Management [110]. When doses of ≥ 800 µg daily are needed a large volume spacer device should be used with an MDI and mouth washing with a dry powder inhaler in order to reduce local and systemic side-effects. Inhaled corticosteroids are usually given as a twice daily dose in order to increase compliance. When asthma is more unstable four times daily dosage is preferable [138]. For patients who require ≤ 400 µg daily, once daily dosing appears to be as effective as twice daily dosing, at least for budesonide [139].

The dose of inhaled corticosteroid should be increased to 2000 µg daily if necessary, but higher doses may result in systemic effects and it may be preferable to add a low dose of oral corticosteroid, since higher doses of inhaled corticosteroids are expensive and have a high incidence of local side-effects. Nebulised budesonide has been advocated in order to give an increased dose of inhaled corticosteroid and to reduce the requirement for oral corticosteroids [192], but this treatment is expensive and may achieve its effects largely via systemic absorption.

Most of the guidelines for asthma treatment suggest that additional bronchodilators (slow-release theophylline preparations, inhaled and oral long-acting $\beta_2$-agonists and inhaled anticholinergics) should be introduced after increasing the dose of inhaled corticosteroid to 1600–2000 µg daily. However an alternative approach is to introduce these treatments when patients are taking 400–800 µg inhaled corticosteroid daily. Addition of the long-acting inhaled $\beta_2$-agonist salmeterol provides better control of asthma symptoms than doubling the dose of inhaled corticosteroids [193, 194]. Similarly, addition of low dose oral theophylline gives better control than doubling the dose of inhaled corticosteroid in patients not controlled on budesonide 800 µg daily [195].

Inhaled corticosteroids may be the most cost-effective way of controlling asthma, since reducing the frequency of asthma attacks will save on total costs [196, 197]. Inhaled corticosteroids improve the quality of life of patients with asthma and allow many patients a normal lifestyle [198].

## Systemic corticosteroids

Oral or intravenous corticosteroids may be indicated in several situations. Prednisolone, rather than prednisone, is the preferred oral corticosteroid as prednisone has to be converted in the liver to the active prednisolone. In pregnant patients prednisone may be preferable as it is not converted to prednisolone in the foetal liver, thus diminishing the exposure of the foetus to glucocorticoids. Enteric-coated preparations of prednisolone are used to reduce side-effects (particularly gastric side-effects) and give delayed and reduced peak plasma concentrations, although the bioavailability and therapeutic efficacy of these preparations are similar to uncoated tablets. Prednisolone and prednisone are preferable to dexamethasone, betamethasone or triamcinolone, which have longer plasma half-lives and therefore an increased frequency of adverse effects.

Short courses of oral corticosteroids (30–40 mg prednisolone daily for 1–2 weeks or until the peak flow values return to best attainable) are indicated for exacerbations of asthma, and the dose may be tailed off over 1 week once the exacerbation is resolved. The tail-off period is not strictly necessary [199], but some patients find it reassuring.

Maintenance oral corticosteroids are only needed in a small proportion of asthmatic patients with the most severe asthma that cannot be controlled with maximal doses of inhaled corticosteroids (2000 μg daily) and additional bronchodilators. The minimal dose of oral corticosteroid needed for control should be used and reductions in the dose should be made slowly in patients who have been on oral corticosteroids for long periods (e.g. by 2.5 mg per month for doses down to 10 mg daily and thereafter by 1 mg per month). Oral corticosteroids are usually given as a single morning dose as this reduces the risk of adverse effects since it coincides with the peak diurnal concentrations. There is some evidence that administration in the afternoon may be optimal for some patients who have severe nocturnal asthma [200]. Alternate day administration may also reduce adverse effects, but control of asthma may not be as good on the day when the oral dose is omitted in some patients.

Intramuscular triamcinolone acetonide (80 mg monthly) has been advocated in patients with severe asthma as an alternative to oral corticosteroids [201, 202]. This may be considered in patients in whom compliance is a particular problem, but the major concern is the high frequency of proximal myopathy associated with this fluorinated corticosteroid. Some patients who do not respond well to prednisolone are reported to respond to oral betamethasone, presumably because of pharmacokinetic handling problems with prednisolone [203].

## Corticosteroid-sparing therapy

In patients who have serious side-effects with maintenance corticosteroid therapy there are several treatments which have been shown to reduce the requirement for oral corticosteroids [204]. These treatments are commonly termed corticosteroid-sparing, although this is a misleading description that could be applied to any additional asthma therapy (including bronchodilators). The amount of corticosteroid sparing with these therapies is not impressive.

Several immunosuppressive agents have been shown to have corticosteroid effects, including methotrexate [205, 206], oral gold [207] and cyclosporin A [208, 209]. These therapies all have side-effects that may be more troublesome than those of oral corticosteroids and are therefore only indicated as an additional therapy to reduce the requirement of oral corticosteroids. None of these treatments is very effective, but there are occasional patients who appear to show a particularly good response. Because of side-effects these treatments cannot be considered as a way to reduce the requirement for inhaled corticosteroids. Side-effects are a problem with these immunosuppressive drugs and include nausea, vomiting, hepatic dysfunction, hepatic fibrosis, pulmonary fibrosis and increased infections for methotrexate and renal dysfunction for cyclosporin and oral gold. Several other therapies, including azathioprine, dapsone and hydroxychloroquine have not been found to be beneficial. The macrolide antibiotic troleandomycin is also reported to have corticosteroid-sparing effects, but this is only seen with methylprednisolone and is due to reduced metabolism of this corticosteroid, so that there is little therapeutic gain [210].

## Acute severe asthma

Intravenous hydrocortisone is given in acute severe asthma. The recommended dose is 200 mg i.v. [211]. While the value of corticosteroids in acute severe asthma has been questioned, others have found that they speed the resolution of attacks [212]. There is no apparent advantage in giving very high doses of intravenous corticosteroids (such as methylprednisolone 1 g). Indeed, intravenous corticosteroids have occasionally been associated with an acute severe myopathy [213]. In a recent study no difference in recovery from acute severe asthma was seen whether i.v. hydrocortisone in doses of 50, 200 or 500 mg every 6 h were used [214] and another placebo controlled study showed no beneficial effect of i.v. corticosteroids [215]. Intravenous corticosteroids are indicated in acute asthma if lung function is < 30% predicted and in it there is no significant improvement with nebulised $\beta_2$-agonist. Intravenous therapy is usually given until a satisfactory response is obtained and then oral prednisolone may be substituted. Oral prednisolone (40–60 mg) has a similar effect to intravenous hydrocortisone and is easier to administer [212, 216]. Oral prednisolone is the preferred treatment for acute severe asthma, providing there are no contraindications to oral therapy [110].

## Corticosteroid-resistant asthma

Although corticosteroids are highly effective in the control of asthma and other chronic inflammatory or immune diseases, a small proportion of patients with asthma fail to respond even to high doses of oral corticosteroids [217–219]. Resistance to the therapeutic effects of glucocorticoids is also recognised in other inflammatory and immune diseases, including rheumatoid arthritis and inflammatory bowel disease. Corticosteroid-resistant patients, although uncommon, present considerable management problems. Recently, new insights into the mechanisms whereby glucocorticoids suppress chronic inflammation have shed new light on the molecular basis of glucocorticoid resistance in asthma [217].

# Clinical features

Corticosteroid resistance (CR) in asthma was first described by Schwartz et al. in 1968, in six asthmatic patients who did not respond clinically to high doses of systemic corticosteroids and in whom there was also a reduced eosinopaenic response [220]. Carmichael and colleagues reported a larger group of patients with chronic asthma who were corticosteroid-resistant [221]. These patients failed to improve their mean peak expiratory flow (PEF) by > 15% after taking prednisolone 20 mg daily for at least 7 days. They differed clinically from corticosteroid-sensitive patients only in having a longer duration of symptoms, lower morning PEF values and a more frequent family history of asthma. These patients are not Addisonian and they do not suffer from the abnormalities in sex hormones described in familial glucocorticoid resistance. Plasma cortisol and adrenal suppression in response to exogenous cortisol are normal in these patients [222].

Absolute corticosteroid resistance in asthma is rare, but there are no population studies giving an estimate of the proportion of patients who are resistant. It is likely that most specialists would only have a few such patients in their clinic and the prevalence is probably < 1:1000 asthmatic patients. Much more common is a reduced responsiveness to corticosteroids, so that large inhaled or oral doses are needed to control asthma adequately. It is important to establish that the patient has asthma, rather than chronic obstructive pulmonary disease (COPD), "pseudoasthma" (a hysterical conversion syndrome involving vocal cord dysfunction), left ventricular failure or cystic fibrosis that do not respond to corticosteroids [223]. Asthmatic patients are characterised by a variability in PEF and, in particular, a diurnal variability of > 15% and episodic symptoms. It is also important to identify provoking factors (allergens, drugs, psychological problems) that may increase the severity of asthma and its resistance to therapy.

Distinction between corticosteroid-sensitive (CS) and CR asthmatics depends on the response to a high dose of oral corticosteroids given for a reasonable period. In research studies prednisolone is usually given in a dose of 40 mg daily for 2 weeks with twice daily monitoring of PEF. In SR asthma patients fail to improve the morning PEF or $FEV_1$ by > 15%. Patients with CR asthma show the typical diurnal variability in PEF and bronchodilate in response to inhaled $\beta_2$-agonists. Bronchial biopsy shows the typical inflammatory infiltrate of eosinophils in CR patients [224]. It is clearly important to establish that the patient is taking the oral corticosteroid by measurement of plasma cortisol, which is suppressed after high dose oral corticosteroids in both CS and CR patients [222] or by measurement of plasma prednisolone concentrations. Patients with COPD fail to improve lung function after a course of oral corticosteroids, but are distinguished from CR asthmatic patients by their lack of acute bronchodilator response and absence of diurnal variability in PEF.

Another group of patients with asthma is responsive to corticosteroids, but only in relatively high oral doses. These patients are best described as steroid-dependent (i.e. dependent on oral corticosteroids as opposed to inhaled corticosteroids). These patients deteriorate when the dose of oral corticosteroids is reduced. Rarely a maintenance dose of > 40 mg prednisolone daily may be required and such patients may mistakenly be classified as CR. Steroid-dependent asthmatic patients usually have severe disease and are presumed to have a high level of inflammation in their airways.

## Mechanisms of corticosteroid resistance

There may be several mechanisms for resistance to the effects of glucocorticoids [217–219]. Although a family history of asthma is more common in patients with SR than CS asthma, little is known of the inheritance of CR asthma. Resistance to the inflammatory and immune effects of glucocorticoids should be distinguished from the very rare familial glucocorticoid resistance, where there is an abnormality of glucocorticoid binding to GR.

### Familial glucocorticoid resistance

The rare inherited syndrome familial glucocorticoid resistance (FGR) is characterised by high circulating levels of cortisol without signs of symptoms of Cushing's syndrome [225]. Clinical manifestations, which may be absent, are due to an excess of non-glucocorticoid adrenal corticosteroids, stimulated by high ACTH levels, resulting in hypertension with hypokalaemia and/or signs of androgen excess (usually hirsutism and menstrual abnormalities in females). Only about 12 cases have so far been reported. Several abnormalities in GR function have been described in peripheral blood leukocytes or fibroblasts from these patients. These include a decreased affinity of GR for cortisol, a reduced number of GRs, GR thermolability and an abnormality in the binding of the GR complex to DNA. The molecular basis of the disease in four patients with a reduction in GR appears to be a point mutation in the corticosteroid-binding domain of GR.

### Resistance to anti-inflammatory actions of corticosteroids

Resistance to the anti-inflammatory and immunomodulatory effects of glucocorticoids differs from the familial glucocorticoid resistance described above, as it is not associated with high circulating concentrations of cortisol or ACTH, and is not accompanied by hypertension, hypokalaemia or androgen excess. Furthermore, these patients are not Addisonian and show normal adrenal suppression. This suggests that any abnormality is unlikely to be due to the same abnormalities in the corticosteroid-binding domain of GR, as described in FGR. Analysis of GR has failed to demonstrate any major abnormality in predicted structure in CR compared with

CS asthma [226]. Corticosteroid resistance may be primary (inherited or acquired of unknown cause) or secondary to some factor known to reduce glucocorticoid responsiveness (glucocorticoids themselves, cytokines, β-adrenergic agonists). There are several possible sites where abnormalities in the anti-inflammatory response to glucocorticoids in asthma may arise.

## Pharmacokinetic abnormalities

The initial suggestion of Schwartz et al. was that defective responses to corticosteroids were due to increased clearance of the glucocorticoid, resulting in reduced clinical and eosinopenic response [220]. There is no evidence for altered bioavailability or plasma clearance of prednisolone or methylprednisolone in patients with corticosteroid-resistant asthma [227, 228]. Metabolism of glucocorticoids may be increased by induction of P-450 enzymes in response to certain drugs (e.g. rifampicin, carbamazepine), which may thus lead to a secondary corticosteroid resistance [130].

## Antibodies to lipocortin-1

Some anti-inflammatory effects of glucocorticoids may be due to induction of lipocortin-1 [29]. In some patients with corticosteroid-resistant rheumatoid arthritis autoantibodies to lipocortin-1 have been described [229]. However, two independent studies have failed to demonstrate the presence of IgG or IgM lipocortin-1 antibodies in either SR or corticosteroid-dependent asthma [230, 231].

## Cellular abnormalities

Glucocorticoid resistance has been documented *in vitro* in monocytes and T-lymphocytes from CR asthmatic patients, with a reduction in the inhibitory effect of corticosteroids on cytokine production. These studies in circulating leukocytes suggest that the defect in glucocorticoid responsiveness extends outside the respiratory tract and is therefore unlikely to be secondary to inflammatory changes in the airways. In patients with SR asthma the reduced blanching response to topical glucocorticoids applied to the skin further indicates that there is a generalised abnormality that is unlikely to be secondary to local cytokine production [232].

## Abnormalities in GR function

In FGR there is an abnormality in GR structure that results in reduced glucocorticoid binding affinity. GR binding in monocytes and T lymphocytes of SR asthma shows either no difference in GR affinity and receptor density or a relative reduction in GR affinity [227, 233–235]. Corrigan et al. found some reduction of GR affinity in T cells from SR asthmatic patients but this could not account for the resistance to PHA-induced proliferative responses in cells from the same patients [227]. Sher et al. described two types of glucocorticoid resistance: a reduced affinity of GR binding confined to T lymphocytes which reverted to normal after 48 h in culture, and a much less common reduction in GR density (in only 2/17 SR patients) which did not normalise with prolonged incubation [235]. This suggests that there may be different types of corticosteroid resistance in asthma. The small reduction in GR affinity is unlikely to be of functional significance and is not associated with elevated plasma cortisol concentrations, as observed in patients with FGR. The small reduction in GR affinity may be secondary to cytokine exposure, since the normalisation of GR affinity *in vitro* is prevented by a combination of IL-2 and IL-4 [235] and this combination of cytokines reduces the binding affinity in nuclear GR in T lymphocytes, although either cytokine alone has no effect [236]. This suggests that corticosteroid resistance may occur in the airways of patients with asthma as a secondary phenomenon due to the local production of cytokines. In SR asthmatic patients there is a significant increase in the numbers of BAL cells expressing IL-2 and IL-4 mRNA compared to SS asthmatics, but no difference in IFNγ mRNA positive cells. After oral prednisone for 1 week there is a reduction in IL-4 expressing cells and a rise in IFNγ positive cells in SS asthma, whereas in SR asthma there was no fall in IL-4 positive cells and a fall in IFNγ positive cells [224]. This may indicate that there are different patterns of cytokine release that may contribute to corticosteroid resistance. Although this may account for the increased requirement for glucocorticoids in more severe asthma, it is unlikely to account for the reduced corticosteroid response seen in circulating mononuclear cells and in the skin of patients with no response to oral glucocorticoids.

There is, however, a marked reduction in GR-GRE binding in mononuclear cells of patients with CR asthma and Scatchard analysis has demonstrated a marked reduction in GR available for DNA binding compared with cells from patients with CS asthma [237].

*Interaction between GR and transcription factors*

In mononuclear cells of CS patients and normal control subjects the phorbol ester PMA, which activates AP-1, results in reduced GRE binding. This inhibitory effect is significantly abrogated in the PBMC of patients with SR asthma, indicating a likely abnormality in the interaction between GR and AP-1 [238]. This defect does not appear to apply to the other transcription factors, NF-κB and CREB, that also interact with GR [238]. The abnormality in the interaction between GR and AP-1 is unlikely to be due to a defect in GR, since the protein sequence of GR in patients with SR asthma is normal [226]. It is more likely to be due to a defect in AP-1 or its activation. Indeed, activation of c-Fos by phorbol esters is potentiated in the cells of patients with SR compared to SS asthma [239] and one of the key enzymes

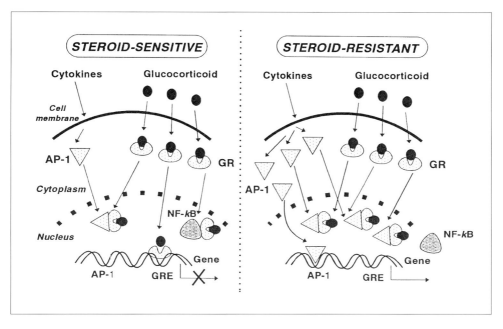

*Figure 8*
*Proposed mechanism of primary corticosteroid-resistance in asthma. Increased activation of activator protein-1 (AP-1) results in the consumption of glucocorticoid receptors (GR), thus preventing the anti-inflammatory action of corticosteroids, either through binding to GREs or through inhibition of NF-kB.*

involved in activation of AP-1, namely Jun N-terminal (JNK) kinase, is abnormally activated in these patients [240]. The increased basal and cytokine-induced AP-1 activity may lead to consumption of GR, so that corticosteroids are not able to suppress the inflammatory response, either through interacting with GRE or with other transcription factors, such as NF-κB (Fig. 8).

An abnormality in AP-1 may also account for the selective resistance to the effects of corticosteroid in SR asthma, since AP-1 is more likely to be important in the regulation of some genes than in others. It would also explain why resistance is seen to the antiinflammatory effects of corticosteroids, since such resistance can only arise when AP-1 is activated at the inflammatory site, whereas the hormonal effects of corticosteroids at uninflamed sites will not be impaired. Furthermore, there may also be differences in the corticosteroid resistance of different target cells, depending upon the relative balance of transcription factors.

## Secondary corticosteroid resistance

Although complete corticosteroid resistance is uncommon, there may be a spectrum of corticosteroid responsiveness in asthma. This may reflect several mechanisms that are secondary either to disease activity itself or to the effects of therapy.

### Down-regulation of GR

Down-regulation of GR in circulating lymphocytes after oral prednisolone has been demonstrated in normal individuals [241]. Whether high local concentrations of inhaled glucocorticoids reduce GR expression in surface cells of the airway, such as epithelial cells, is not yet certain. It is possible that certain individuals may be more susceptible to the effects of down-regulation. If effective GR density is reduced by direct interaction with other transcription factors, such as AP-1 and NF-κB, then the down-regulating effect of glucocorticoids on GR would be expected to have a greater functional consequence.

### Effects of cytokines

Several proinflammatory cytokines, including IL-1β, IL-6 and TNFα, activate AP-1 and NF-κB in human lung [13, 242]. As all these cytokines are known to be secreted in asthmatic inflammation, this suggests that these transcription factors will be activated in the cells of asthmatic airways. These activated transcription factors may then form protein-protein complexes with activated GR, both in the cytoplasm and within the nucleus, thus reducing the number of effective GR and thereby decreasing corticosteroid responsiveness [4] (Fig. 9). In a model in vitro system increased expression of c-Fos or c-Jun oncoproteins prevents the activation of mouse mammary tumour virus promoter by GR, thus creating a model of corticosteroid resistance [12]. Addition of recombinant c-Jun or c-Fos proteins to partially purified GR results in inhibition of DNA binding [12]. Phorbol esters, which activate AP-1, result in attenuation of glucocorticoid-mediated gene activation [243]. Any reduction in glucocorticoid responsiveness would be greater as the intensity of asthmatic inflammation increased and may contribute, for example, to the failure of oral or intravenous glucocorticoids to control acute exacerbations of asthma. Once the inflammation is brought under control with large doses of oral glucocorticoids, corticosteroid responsiveness increases again so that lower doses of inhaled or oral glucocorticoids are needed to control asthmatic inflammation. Increased resistance may also be due to the effects of cytokines on GR receptor function, since high concentrations of IL-2 and IL-4 have been shown to reduce GR affinity in T lymphocytes in vitro [236]. This effect would only be seen in mucosal T cells of patients with severe asthma and it is therefore difficulty to obtain evidence to support this possibility.

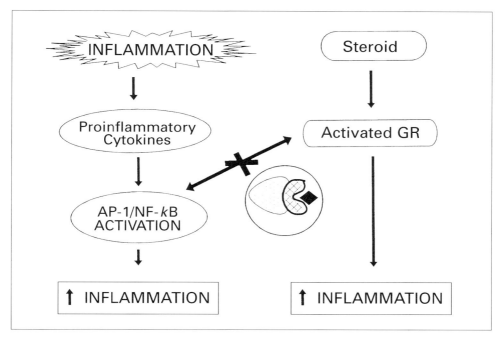

Figure 9
*Secondary corticosteroid resistance may arise in the presence of cytokine-mediated inflammation through an interaction between the cytokine-activated transcription factors, such as activator protein-1 (AP-1) and nuclear factor-κB (NF-κB), and the glucocorticoid receptor (GR), resulting in a reduced availability of GR for control of the inflammatory response. This can only be overcome by increasing the dose of glucocorticoid administered.*

## Effect of $\beta_2$-agonists

High concentrations of $\beta_2$-agonists activate CREB in rat and human lung and in inflammatory cells via an increase in cyclic AMP concentration [244, 245]. This results in reduced GRE binding due to the formation of GR-CREB complexes [246]. This predicts that high concentrations of $\beta_2$-agonists would induce corticosteroid resistance. In asthmatic patients, while 3 weeks of treatment with an inhaled corticosteroid blocked the airway response to inhaled allergen, concomitant treatment with inhaled corticosteroid and a relatively large dose of inhaled $\beta$-agonist appeared to provide no significant protection against allergen challenge [247]. This suggests that high doses of an inhaled $\beta_2$-agonists might interfere with the anti-asthma effect of inhaled glucocorticoids. It is possible that some patients who use very high doses of inhaled $\beta_2$-agonists (over two canisters per month of metered dose inhalers or regular nebulised doses), may develop a degree of corticosteroid resistance that is overcome by increasing the dose of inhaled or oral glucocorticoid. Corticosteroid responsiveness might be restored by reducing the dose of inhaled $\beta_2$-agonists. In an uncontrolled study in corticosteroid-dependent patients with severe asthma, gradual withdrawal of nebulised $\beta_2$-agonists resulted in a reduced requirement for oral prednisolone [248].

## References

1    Barnes PJ (1995) Inhaled glucocorticoids for asthma. *New Engl J Med* 332: 868–875
2    Barnes PJ (1996) Molecular mechanisms of steroid action in asthma. *J Allergy Clin Immunol* 97: 159–168
3    Barnes PJ (1996) Mechanism of action of glucocorticoids in asthma. *Am J Respir Crit Care Med* 154: S21–S27
4    Barnes PJ Adcock IM (1993) Anti-inflammatory actions of steroids: molecular mechanisms. *Trends Pharmacol Sci* 14: 436–441
5    Barnes PJ (1998) Antiinflammatory actions of glucocorticosteroids: molecular mechanisms. *Clin Sci* 94: 557–572
6    Bamberger CM, Bamberger AM, de Castro M, Chrousos GP (1995) Glucocorticoid receptor β, a potential endogenous inhibitor of glucocorticoid action in humans. *J Clin Invest* 95: 2435–2441
7    Muller M, Renkawitz R (1991) The glucocorticoid receptor. *Biochim Biophys Acta* 1088: 171–182
8    Encio PJ, Detgra-Wadleigh SD (1991) The genomic structure of the human glucocorticoid receptor. *J Biol Chem* 266: 7182–7188
9    Heck S, Kullmann M, Grast A, Ponta H, Rahmsdorf HJ, Herrlich P Cato ACB (1994) A distinct modulating domain in glucocorticoid receptor monomers in the repression of activity of the transcription factor AP-1. *EMBO J* 1994 13: 4087–4095
10   Gronemeyer H (1992) Control of transcription activation by steroid hormone receptors. *FASEB J* 6 (8): 2524–2529
11   Beato M, Herrlich P, Schutz G (1995) Steroid hormone receptors: many actors in search of a plot. *Cell* 83: 851–857
12   Yang-Yen H, Chambard J, Sun Y, Smeal T, Schmidt TJ, Drovin J, Karin M (1990) Transcriptional interference between c-Jun and the glucocorticoid receptor: mutual inhibition of DNA binding due to direct protein-protein interaction. *Cell* 62: 1205–1215
13   Adcock IM, Shirasaki H, Gelder CM, Peters MJ, Brown CR, Barnes PJ (1994) The effects of glucocorticoids on phorbol ester and cytokine stimulated transcription factor activation in human lung. *Life Sci* 55: 1147–1153
14   Adcock IM, Brown CR, Gelder CM, Shirasaki H, Peters MJ, Barnes PJ (1995) The effects of glucocorticoids on transcription factor activation in human peripheral blood mononuclear cells. *Am J Physiol* 37: C331–C338

15 Ray A Prefontaine KE (1994) Physical association and functional antagonism between the p65 subunit of transcription factor NF-kB and the glucocorticoid receptor. *Proc Natl Acad Sci USA* 91: 752–756

16 Scheinman RI, Gualberto A, Jewell CM, Cidlowski JA, Baldwin AS (1996) Characterization of the mechanisms involved in transrepression of NF-κB by activated glucocorticoid receptors. *Mol Cell Biol* 15: 943–953

17 Caldenhoven E, Liden J, Wissink S, Van De Stolpe A, Raaijmakers J, Koenderman L, Okret S, Gustafsson J, van der Saag P (1995) Negative cross-talk between RelA and the glucocorticoid receptor: a possible mechanism for the antiinflammatory action of glucocorticoids. *Mol Endocrinol* 9: 401–412

18 Imai E, Minger JN, Mitchell JA, Yamamoto KR, Granner DK (1993) Glucocorticoid receptor-cAMP response element-binding protein interaction and the response of the phosphoenolpyruvate carboxykinase gene to glucocorticoids. *J Biol Chem* 268: 5353–5356

19 Adcock IM, Barnes PJ (1996) Tumour necrosis factor-a causes retention of activated glucocorticoid receptor within the cytoplasm of A549 cells. *Biochem Biophys Res Commun* 225: 1127–1132

20 Janknecht R, Hunter T (1996) A growing coactivator network. *Nature* 383: 22–23

21 Kamei Y, Xu L, Heinzel T et al (1996) A CBP integrator complex mediates transcriptional activation and AP-1 inhibition by nuclear receptors. *Cell* 85: 403–414

22 Smith CL, Onate SA, Tsai MJ, O'Malley BW (1996) CREB binding protein acts synergistically with steroid receptor coactivator-1 to enhance steroid receptor-dependent transcription. *Proc Natl Acad Sci USA* 93: 8884–8888

23 Yao TP, Ku G, Zhou N, Scully R, Livingston DM (1996) The nuclear hormone receptor coactivator SRC-1 is a specific target of p300. *Proc Natl Acad Sci USA* 93: 10626–10631

24 Hong H, Kohli K, Garabedian MJ, Stallcup MR (1997) GRIP1, a transcriptional coactivator for the AF-2 transactivation domain of steroid, thyroid, retinoid, and vitamin D receptors. *Mol Cell Biol* 17: 2735–2744

25 Ogryzko VV, Schiltz RL, Russanova V, Howard BH, Nakatani Y (1996) The transcriptional coactivators p300 and CBP are histone acetyltransferases. *Cell* 87: 953–959

26 Wolffe AP (1997) Sinful repression. *Nature* 387: 16–17

27 Nagy L, Kao HY, Chakravarti D, Lin RJ, Hassig CA, Ayer DE, Schreiber SL, Evans RM (1997) Nuclear receptor repression mediated by a complex containing SMRT, mSin3A, and histone deacetylase. *Cell* 89: 373–380

28 Heinzel T, Lavinsky RM, Mullen TM et al (1997) A complex containing N-CoR, mSin3 and histone deacetylase mediates transcriptional repression. *Nature* 387: 43–48

29 Flower RJ Rothwell NJ (1994) Lipocortin-1: cellular mechanisms and clinical relevance. *Trends Pharmacol Sci* 15: 71–76

30 Abbinante-Nissen JM, Simpson LG, Leikauf GD (1995) Corticosteroids increase secretory leukocyte protease inhibitor transcript levels in airway epithelial cells. *Am J Physiol* 12: L601–L606

31 Levine SJ, Benfield T, Shelhamer JH (1996) Corticosteroids induce intracellular inter-leukin-1 receptor antagonist type I expression by a human airway epithelial cell line. *Am J Respir Cell Mol Biol* 15: 245–251

32 Sousa AR, Lane SJ, Nakhosteen JA, Lee TH, Poston RN (1996) Expression of inter-leukin-1 beta (IL-1b) and interleukin-1 receptor antagonist (IL-1ra) on asthmatic bronchial epithelium. *Am J Respir Crit Care Med* 154: 1061–1066

33 Colotta F, Re F, Muzio M, Bertini R, Polentarutti N, Sironi M, Giri JG, Dower SK, Sims JE, Mantovani A (1993) Interleukin-1 type II receptor: a decoy target for IL-1 that is regulated by IL-4. *Science* 261 (5120): 472–475

34 Wang P, Wu P, Siegel MI, Egan RW, Billah MM (1995) Interleukin (IL)-10 inhibits nuclear factor kappa B activation in human monocytes. IL-10 and IL-4 suppress cytokine synthesis by different mechanisms. *J Biol Chem* 270: 9558–9563

35 Borish L, Aarons A, Rumbyrt J, Cvietusa P, Negri J, Wenzel S (1996) Interleukin-10 reg-ulation in normal subjects and patients with asthma. *J Allergy Clin Immunol* 97: 1288–1296

36 John M, Lim S, Seybold J, Robichaud A, O'Connor B, Barnes PJ, Chung KF (1998) Inhaled corticosteroids increase IL-10 but reduce MIP-1α, GM-CSF and IFNγ release from alveolar macrophages in asthma. *Am J Respir Crit Care Med* 157: 256–262

37 Barnes PJ, Karin M (1997) Nuclear factor-κB: a pivotal transcription factor in chronic inflammatory diseases. *New Engl J Med* 336: 1066–1071

38 Auphan N, DiDonato JA, Rosette C, Helmberg A, Karin M (1995) Immunosuppression by glucocorticoids: inhibition of NF-κB activity through induction of IκB synthesis. *Science* 270: 286–290

39 Scheinman RI, Cogswell PC, Lofquist AK, Baldwin AS (1995) Role of transcriptional activation of IκBa in mediating immunosuppression by glucocorticoids. *Science* 270: 283–286

40 Brostjan C, Anrather J, Csizmadia V, Stoka D, Soares M, Bach FH, Winkler H (1996) Glucocorticoid-mediated repression of NFκB activity in endothelial cells does not involve induction of IkBa synthesis. *J Biol Chem* 271: 19612–19616

41 Newton R, Hart LA, Stevens DA, Bergmann M, Donnelly LE, Adcock IM, Barnes PJ (1998) Effect of dexamethasone on interleukin-1β-(IL-1β)-induced nuclear factor-κB (NF-κB) and κB-dependent transcription in epithelial cells. *Eur J Biochem* 254: 81–89

42 Heck S, Bender K, Kullmann M, Gottlicher M, Herrlich P Cato AC (1997) IκBα-inde-pendent downregulation of NF-κB activity by glucocorticoid receptor. *EMBO J* 16: 4698–4707

43 Borson DB, Jew S, Gruenert DC (1991) Glucocorticoids induce neutral endopeptidase in transformed human trachea epithelial cells. *Am J Physiol* 260: L83–89

44 Sont JK, van Krieken JH, van Klink HC, Roldaan AC, Apap CR, Willems LN, Sterk PJ (1997) Enhanced expression of neutral endopeptidase (NEP) in airway epithelium in biopsies from steroid- versus nonsteroid-treated patients with atopic asthma. *Am J Respir Cell Mol Biol* 16: 549–556

45 Collins S, Caron MG, Lefkowitz RJ (1988) β-Adrenergic receptors in hamster smooth

muscle cells are transcriptionally regulated by glucocorticoids. *J Biol Chem* 263: 9067–9070

46    Mak JCW, Nishikawa M, Barnes PJ (1995) Glucocorticosteroids increase $\beta_2$-adrenergic receptor transcription in human lung. *Am J Physiol* 12: L41–L46

47    Mak JCW, Nishikawa M, Shirasaki H, Miyayasu K, Barnes PJ (1995) Protective effects of a glucocorticoid on down-regulation of pulmonary $\beta_2$-adrenergic receptors *in vivo*. *J Clin Invest* 96: 99–106

48    Northrop JP, Ullman KS, Crabtree GR (1993) Characterization of the nuclear and cytoplasmic components of the lymphoid-specific nuclear factor of activated T cells (NF-AT). *J Biol Chem* 268: 2917–2923

49    Paliogianni F, Raptis A, Ahuja SS, Najjar SM, Boumpas DT (1993) Negative transcriptional regulation of human interleukin 2 (IL-2) gene by glucocorticoids through interference with nuclear transcription factors AP-1 and NF-AT. *J Clin Invest* 91: 1481–1489

50    Linden M, Brattsand R (1994) Effects of a corticosteroid, budesonide, on alveolar macrophages and blood monocyte secretion of cytokines: differential sensitivity of GM-CSF, IL-1b and IL-6. *Pulm Pharmacol* 7: 43–47

51    Robbins RA, Barnes PJ, Springall DR, Warren JB, Kwon OJ, Buttery LDK, Wilson AJ, Geller DA, Polak JM. Expression of inducible nitric oxide synthase in human bronchial epithelial cells. *Biochem Biophys Res Commun* 1994 203: 209–218

52    Xie Q, Kashiwarbara Y, Nathan C (1994) Role of transcription factor NF-κB/Rel in induction of nitric oxide synthase. *J Biol Chem* 269: 4705–4708

53    Mitchell JA, Belvisi MG, Akarasereemom P, Robbins RA, Kowon OJ, Croxtell J, Barnes PJ, Vane JR (1994) Induction of cyclo-oxygenase-2 by cytokines in human pulmonary epithelial cells: regulation by dexamethasone. *Br J Pharmacol* 113: 1008–1014

54    Yamamoto K, Arakawa T, Ueda N, Yamamoto S (1995) Transcriptional roles of nuclear factor kB and nuclear factor-interleukin 6 in the tumor necrosis-a-dependent induction of cyclooxygenase-2 in MC3T3-E1 cells. *J Biol Chem* 270: 31315–31320

55    Newton R, Kuitert LM, Bergmann M, Adcock IM, Barnes PJ (1997) Evidence for involvement of NF-κB in the transcriptional control of COX-2 gene expression by IL-1β. *Biochem Biophys Res Commun* 237: 28–32

56    Newton R, Kuitert LM, Slater DM, Adcock IM, Barnes PJ (1997) Induction of cPLA$_2$ and COX-2 mRNA by proinflammatory cytokines is suppressed by dexamethasone in human airway epitheial cells. *Life Sci* 60: 67–78

57    Vittori E, Marini M, Fasoli A, de Franchis R, Mattoli S (1992) Increased expression of endothelin in bronchial epithelial cells of asthmatic patients and effect of corticosteroids. *Am Rev Respir Dis* 1461: 1320–1325

58    Adcock IM, Peters M, Gelder C, Shirasaki H, Brown CR, Barnes PJ (1993) Increased tachykinin receptor gene expression in asthmatic lung and its modulation by steroids. *J Mol Endocrinol* 11: 1–7

59    Ihara H, Nakanishi S (1990) Selective inhibition of expression of the substance P receptor mRNA in pancreatic acinar AR42J cells by glucocorticoids. *J Biol Chem* 36: 22441–22445

60    Katsunuma T, Mak JCW, Barnes PJ (1998) Glucocorticoids reduce tachykinin NK$_2$-receptor expression in bovine tracheal smooth muscle. *Eur J Pharmacol; in press*

61    Owens GP, Hahn WE, Cohen JJ (1991) Identification of mRNAs associated with programmed cell death in immature thymocytes. *Mol Cell Biol* 11: 4177–4188

62    Cronstein BN, Kimmel SC, Levin RI, Martiniuk F, Weissmann G (1992) A mechanism for the antiinflammatory effects of corticosteroids: The glucocorticoid receptor regulates leukocyte adhesion to endothelial cells and expression of endothelial-leukocyte adhesion molecule 1 and intercellular adhesion molecule 1. *Proc Natl Acad Sci USA* 89: 9991–9995

63    Van De Stolpe A, Caldenhoven E, Raaijmakers JAM, Van Der Saag PT, Koendorman L (1993) Glucocorticoid-mediated repression of intercellular adhesion molecule-1 expression in human monocytic and bronchial epithelial cell lines. *Am J Respir Cell Mol Biol* 8: 340–347

64    Bergstrand H, Björnson A, Blaschuke E, Brattsand R, Eklund A, Larsson K, Linden M (1990) Effects of an inhaled corticosteroid, budesonide, on alveolar macrophage function in smokers. *Thorax* 45: 362–368

65    Standiford TJ, Kunkel SL, Rolfe MW, Evanoff HL, Allen RM, Srieter RW (1992) Regulation of human alveolar macrophage and blood monocyte-derived interleukin-8 by prostaglandin E$_2$ and dexamethasone. *Am J Respir Cell Mol Biol* 6: 75–81

66    Borish L, Mascali JJ, Dishuck J, Beam WR, Martin RJ, Rosenwasser LJ (1992) Detection of alveolar macrophage-derived IL-1β in asthma. Inhibition with corticosteroids. *J Immunol* 149: 3078–3082

67    Kita H, Abu-Ghazaleh R, Sanderson CJ, Gleich GJ (1991) Effect of steroids on immunoglobulin-induced eosinophil degranulation. *J Allergy Clin Immunol* 87: 70–77

68    Lamas AM, Leon OG, Schleimer RP (1991) Glucocorticoids inhibit eosinophil responses to granulocyte-macrophage colony-stimulating factor. *J Immunol* 147: 254–259

69    Wallen N, Kita H, Weiller D, Gleich GJ (1991) Glucocorticoids inhibit cytokine-mediated eosinophil survival. *J Immunol* 147: 3490–3495

70    Wempe JB, Tammeling EP, Köeter GH, Haransson L, Venge P, Postma DS (1992) Blood eosinophil numbers and activity during 24 hours effects of treatment with budesonide and bambuterol. *J Allergy Clin Immunol* 90: 757–765

71    Evans PM, O'Connor BJ, Fuller RW, Barnes PJ, Chung KF (1993) Effect of inhaled corticosteroids on peripheral eosinophil counts and density profiles in asthma. *J Allergy Clin Immunol* 91: 643–649

72    Rolfe FG, Hughes JM, Armour CL, Sewell WA (1992) Inhibition of interleukin-5 gene expression by dexamethasone. *Immunology* 77: 494–499

73    Cohan VL, Undem BJ, Fox CC, Adkinson NF, Lichtenstein LM, Schleimer RP (1989) Dexamethasone does not inhibit the release of mediators from human lung mast cells residing in airway, intestine or skin. *Am Rev Respir Dis* 140: 951–954

74    Laitinen LA, Laitinen A, Haahtela T (1992) A comparative study of the effects of an inhaled corticosteroid, budesonide, and of a β$_2$ agonist, terbutaline, on airway inflammation in newly diagnosed asthma. *J Allery Clin Immunol* 90: 32–42

75  Djukanovic R, Wilson JW, Britten YM, Wilson SJ, Walls AF, Poche WF, Howarth PH, Holgate ST (1992) Effect of an inhaled corticosteroid on airway inflammation and symptoms of asthma. *Am Rev Respir Dis* 145: 669–674

76  Holt PG. Regulation of antigen-presenting cell function(s) in lung and airway tissues. Eur Resp J 1993 6: 120–129

77  Nelson DJ, McWilliam AS, Haining S, Holt PG (1995) Modulation of airway intraepithelial dendritic cells following exposure to steroids. *Am J Respir Crit Care Med* 151: 475–481

78  Holm AF, Fokkens WJ, Godthelp T, Mulder PG, Vroom TM, Rinjntjes E (1995) Effect of 3 months' nasal steroid therapy on nasal T cells and Langerhans cells in patients suffering from allergic rhinitis. *Allergy* 50: 204–209

79  Cox G (1995) Glucocorticoid treatment inhibits apoptosis in human neutrophils. *J Immunol* 193: 4719–4725

80  Boschetto P, Rogers DF, Fabbri LM, Barnes PJ (1991) Corticosteroid inhibition of airway microvascular leakage. *Am Rev Respir Dis* 143: 605–609

81  Erjefalt I, Persson CGA (1991) Pharmacologic control of plasma exudation into tracheobronchial airways. *Am Rev Respir Dis* 143: 1008–1014

82  Carnuccio R, Di Rosa M, Guerrasio B, Iuvone T, Satebin L (1987) Vasocortin: a novel glucocorticoid-induced anti-inflammatory protein. *Br J Pharmacol* 90: 443–445

83  Van de Graaf EA, Out TA, Loos CM, Jansen HM (1991) Respiratory membrane permeability and bronchial hyperreactivity in patients with stable asthma. *Am Rev Respir Dis* 143: 362–368

84  Devalia JL, Wang JH, Sapsford RJ, Davies RJ (1994) Expression of RANTES in human bronchial epithelial cells and the effect of beclomethasone diproprionate (BDP). *Eur Resp J* 7 (Suppl 18): 98S

85  Levine SJ (1995) Bronchial epithelial cell -cytokine interactions in airway epithelium. *J Invest Med* 43: 241–249

86  Schweibert LM, Stellato C, Schleimer RP (1996) The epithelium as a target for glucocorticoid action in the treatment of asthma. *Am J Respir Crit Care Med* 154: S16–S20

87  Kwon OJ, Au BT, Collins PD, Baraniuk JN, Adcock IM, Chung KF, Barnes PJ (1994) Inhibition of interleukin-8 expression in human cultured airway epithelial cells. Immunology 81: 389–394

88  Kwon OJ, Au BT, Collins PD, Adcock IM, Mak JC, Robbins RA, Baraniuk JM, Chung KF, Barnes PJ (1994) Tumor necrosis factor-induced interleukin 8 expression in cultured human epithelial cells. *Am J Physiol* 11: L398–L405

89  Kwon OJ, Jose PJ, Robbins RA, Schall TJ, Williams TJ, Barnes PJ (1995) Glucocorticoid inhibition of RANTES expression in human lung epithelial cells. *Am J Respir Cell Mol Biol* 12: 488–496

90  Sousa AR, Poston RN, Lane SJ, Narhosteen JA, Lee TH (1993) Detection of GM-CSF in asthmatic bronchial epithelium and decrease by inhaled corticosteroids. *Am Rev Respir Dis* 147: 1557–1561

91  Trigg CJ, Manolistas ND, Wang J et al (1994) Placebo-controlled immunopathological

study of four months inhaled corticosteroids in asthma. *Am J Respir Crit Care Med* 150: 17–22

92    Hamid Q, Springall DR, Riveros-Moreno V, Chanez P, Howarth P, Redington A, Bousquet J, Godard P, Holgate S, Polak J (1993) Induction of nitric oxide synthase in asthma. *Lancet* 342: 1510–1513

93    Kharitonov SA, Yates D, Robbins RA, Logan-Sinclair R, Shinebourne E, Barnes PJ (1994) Increased nitric oxide in exhaled air of asthmatic patients. *Lancet* 343: 133–135

94    Yates DH, Kharitonov SA, Robbins RA, Thomas PS, Barnes PJ (1995) Effect of a nitric oxide synthase inhibitor and a glucocorticosteroid on exhaled nitric oxide. *Am J Resp Crit Care Med* 152: 892–896

95    Kharitonov SA, Yates DH, Barnes PJ (1996) Regular inhaled budesonide decreases nitric oxide concentration in the exhaled air of asthmatic patients. *Am J Resp Crit Care Med* 153: 454–457

96    Shimura S, Sasaki T, Ikeda K, Yamauchi K, Sasaki H, Takishima T (1990) Direct inhibitory action of glucocorticoid on glycoconjugate secretion from airway submucosal glands. *Am Rev Respir Dis* 141: 1044–1099

97    Kai H, Yoshitake K, Hisatsune A, Kido T, Isohama Y, Takahama K, Miyata T (1995) Dexamethasone suppresses mucus production and MUC-2 and MUC-5AC gene expression by NCI-H292 cells. *Am J Physiol* 271: L484–L488

98    Jeffery PK, Godfrey RW, Ädelroth E, Nelson F, Rogers A, Johansson S (1992) Effects of treatment on airway inflammation and thickening of basement membrane reticular collagen in asthma. *Am Rev Respir Dis* 145: 890–899

99    Burke C, Power CK, Norris A, Condez A, Schmekel B, Poulter LW (1992) Lung function and immunopathological changes after inhaled corticosteroid therapy in asthma. *Eur Respir J* 5: 73–79

100   Ädelroth E, Rosenhall L, Johansson S, Linden M, Venge P (1990) Inflammatory cells and eosinophilic activity in asthmatics investigated by bronchoalveolar lavage. *Am Rev Respir Dis* 142: 91–99

101   Wilson JW, Djukanovic R, Howarth PH, Holgate ST (1994) Inhaled beclomethasone diproprionate downregulates airway lymphocyte activation in atopic asthma. *Am J Respir Crit Care Med* 149: 86–90

102   Lungren R, Soderberg M, Horstedt P, Stenling R (1988) Morphological studies on bronchial mucosal biopsies from asthmatics before and after ten years treatment with inhaled steroids. *Eur Resp J* 1: 883–889

103   Barnes PJ (1990) Effect of corticosteroids on airway hyperresponsiveness. *Am Rev Respir Dis* 141: S70–S76

104   Bel EH, Timers MC, Zwinderman AH, Dijkman JH, Sterk PJ (1991) The effect of inhaled corticosteroids on the maximal degree of airway narrowing to methacholine. *Am Rev Respir Dis* 143: 109–113

105   Kamada AK, Szefler SJ, Martin RJ, Boushey HA, Chinchilli VM, Drazen JM, Fish JE, Israel E, Lazarus SC, Lemanske RF (1996) Issues in the use of inhaled steroids. *Am J Respir Crit Care Med* 153: 1739–1748

106 Reed CE (1990) Aerosol glucocorticoid treatment of asthma: adults. *Am Rev Respir Dis* 140: S82–S88

107 Barnes PJ (1989) A new approach to asthma therapy. *N Engl J Med* 321: 1517–1527

108 Sheffer AL (1992) International consensus report on diagnosis and management of asthma. *Clin Exp Allergy* 22 (Suppl 1): 1–72

109 Global Initiative for Asthma (1995) Global strategy for asthma management and prevention. NHLBI/WHO Workshop Report. Publication 95–3659

110 British Thoracic Society (1997) The British guidelines on asthma management. *Thorax* 52 (Suppl 1): S1–S21

111 Haahtela T, Jarvinen M, Kava T et al (1991) Comparison of a $\beta_2$-agonist terbutaline with an inhaled steroid in newly detected asthma. *New Engl J Med* 325: 388–392

112 Juniper EF, Kline PA, Vanzieleghem MA, Ramsdale EH, O'Byrne PM, Hargreave FE (1990) Effect of long-term treatment with an inhaled corticosteroid (budesonide) on airway hyperresponsiveness and clinical asthma in nonsteroid-dependent asthmatics. *Am Rev Respir Dis* 142: 832–836

113 Kerrebijn KF, Von Essen-Zandvliet EEM, Neijens HJ (1987) Effect of long-term treatment with inhaled corticosteroids and beta-agonists on bronchial responsiveness in asthmatic children. *J Allergy Clin Immunol* 79: 653–659

114 Vathenen AS, Knox AJ, Wisniewski A, Tattersfield AE (1991) Time course of change in bronchial reactivity with an inhaled corticosteroid in asthma. *Am Rev Respir Dis* 143: 1317–1321

115 Toogood JH (1989) High dose inhaled steroid therapy for asthma. *J Allergy Clin Immunol* 83: 528–536

116 Salmeron S, Guerin J, Godard P, Renon D, Michel H, Duroux P, Taytard A (1989) High doses of inhaled corticosteroids in unstable chronic asthma. *Am Rev Respir Dis* 140: 167–171

117 Lacronique J, Renon D, Georges D, Henry-Amar M, Marsac J (1991) High-dose beclomehtasone: oral steroid-sparing effect in severe asthmatic patients. *Eur Respir J* 4: 807–812

118 Dahl R, Pedersen B, Hägglöf B (1989) Nocturnal asthma: effect of treatment with oral sustained-release terbutaline, inhaled budesonide and the two in combination. *J Allergy Clin Immunol* 83: 811–815

119 Wempe JB, Tammeling EP, Postma DS, Auffarth B, Teengs JP, Koëter GH (1992) Effects of budesonide and bambuterol on circadian variation of airway responsiveness and nocturnal asthma symptoms of asthma. *J Allergy Clin Immunol* 90: 349–357

120 Juniper EF, Kline PA, Vanzielegmem MA, Hargreave FE (1991) Reduction of budesonide after a year of increased use: a randomized controlled trial to evaluate whether improvements in airway responsiveness and clinical asthma are maintained. *J Allergy Clin Immunol* 87: 483–489

121 van Essen-Zandvliet EE, Hughes MD, Waalkens HJ, Duiverman EJ, Pocock SJ, Kerrebijn KF (1992) Effects of 22 months of treatment with inhaled corticosteroids and/or

beta2-agonists on lung function, airway responsiveness and symptoms in children with asthma. *Am Rev Respir Dis* 146: 547–554

122 Waalkens HJ, van Essen-Zandvliet EE, Hughes MD, Gerritsen J, Duiverman EJ, Knol K, Kerrebijn KF. Cessation of long-term treatment with inhaled corticosteroids (budesonide) in children with asthma results in deterioration. *Am Rev Respir Dis* 1993 148: 1252–1257

123 Ilangovan P, Pedersen S, Godfrey S, Nikander K, Novisky N, Warner JO (1993) Nebulised budesonide suspension in severe steroid-dependent preschool asthma. *Arch Dis Child* 68: 356–359

124 Gleeson JGA, Price JF (1988) Controlled trial of budesonide given by Nebuhaler in preschool children with asthma. *Br Med J* 297: 163–166

125 Bisgard H, Munck SL, Nielsen JP, Peterson W, Ohlsson SV (1990) Inhaled budesonide for treatment of recurrent wheezing in early childhood. *Lancet* 336: 649–651

126 Dompeling E, Van Schayck CP, Molema J, Folgering H, van Grusven PM, van Weel C (1992) Inhaled beclomethasone improves the course of asthma and COPD. *Eur Resp J* 5: 945–952

127 Haahtela T, Järvinsen M, Kava T et al (1994) Effects of reducing or discontinuing inhaled budesonide in patients with mild asthma. *New Engl J Med* 331: 700–705

128 Agertoft L Pedersen S (1994) Effects of long-term treatment with an inhaled corticosteroid on growth and pulmonary function in asthmatic children. *Resp Med* 5: 369–372

129 Selroos O, Backman R, Forsen K, Löfroos A, Nieistö M, Pietinalcho A, Riska A (1994) When to start treatment of asthma with inhaled steroids? *Eur Resp J* 7 (Suppl 18): 151S

130 Szefler S (1991) Glucocorticoid therapy for asthma: clinical pharmacology. *J Allergy Clin Immunol* 88: 147–165

131 Johnson M (1996) Pharmacodynamics and pharmacokinetics of inhaled glucocorticoids. *J Allergy Clin Immunol* 97: 169–176

132 Chaplin MD, Rooks W, Svenson EW, Couper WC, Nerenberg C, Chu NI (1980) Flunisotide metabolism and dynamics of a metabolite. *Clin Pharmacol Ther* 27: 402–413

133 Ryrfeldt A, Andersson P, Edsbacker S, Tonnesson M, Davies D, Pauwels R (1982) Pharmacokinetics and metabolism of budesonide, a selective glucocorticoid. *Eur J Respir Dis* 63 (Supple 122): 86–95

134 Mollman H, Rohdewald P, Schmidt EW, Salomon V, Derendorf H (1985) Pharmacokinetics of triamcinolone acetonide and its phosphate ester. *Eur J Clin Pharmacol* 29: 85–89

135 Harding SM (1990) The human pharmacology of fluticasone diproprionate. *Resp Med* 84 (Suppl A): 25–29

136 Toogood JH, Baskerville JC, Jennings B, Lefcoe NM, Johansson SA (1982) Influence of dosing frequency and schedule on the response of chronic asthmatics to the aerosol steroid budesonide. *J Allergy Clin Immunol* 70: 288–298

137 Meltzer EO, Kemp JP, Welch MJ, Orgel HA (1985) Effect of dosing schedule on efficacy of beclomethasone diproprionate aerosol in chronic asthma. *Am Rev Respir Dis* 131: 732–736

138  Malo J, Cartier A, Merland N, Ghezzo H, Burke A, Morris J, Jennings BH (1989) Four-times-a-day dosing frequency is better than twice-a-day regimen in subjects requiring a high-dose inhaled steroid, budesonide, to control moderate to severe asthma. *Am Rev Respir Dis* 140: 624–628

139  Jones AH, Langdon CG, Lee PS, Lingham SA, Nankani JP, Follows RMA, Tollemar U, Richardson PDI (1994) Pulmicort Turbohaler once daily as initial prophylactic therapy for asthma. *Resp Med* 88: 293–299

140  Toogood JA, Jennings B, Greenway RW, Chung L (1980) Candidiasis and dysphonia complicating beclomethasone treatment of asthma. *J Allergy Clin Immunol* 65: 145–153

141  Williamson IJ, Matusiewicz SP, Brown PH, Greening AP, Crompton GK (1995) Frequency of voice problems and cough in patients using pressurised aerosol inhaled steroid preparations. *Eur Resp J* 8: 590–592

142  Selroos O, Backman R, Forsen KO, Lofroos AB, Niemsto M, Pietinalho A, Aikas C, Riska H (1994) Local side-effects during 4-year treatment with inhaled corticosteroids – a comparison between pressurized metered dose inhalers and Turbuhaler. *Allergy* 49: 888–890

143  Brogden RN, Heel RC, Speight TM, Avery GS (1984) Beclomethasone dipropionate. A reappraisal of its pharmacodynamic properties and therapeutic efficacy after a decade of use in asthma and rhinitis. *Drugs* 28: 99–126

144  Brogden RN, McTavish D. Budesonide (1992) An updated review of its pharmacological properties and therapeutic efficacy in asthma and rhinitis. *Drugs* 44: 375–407

145  Engel T, Heinig JH, Malling H-J, Scharing B, Nikander K, Masden F (1989) Clinical comparison of inhaled budesonide delivered either by pressurized metered dose inhaler or Turbuhaler. *Allergy* 44: 220–225

146  Barnes PJ, Pedersen S, Busse WW (1998) Efficacy and safety of inhaled corticosteroids: an update. *Am J Respir Crit Care Med* 157: S1–S53

147  Selroos O, Halme M (1991) Effect of a Volumatic spacer and mouth rinsing on systemic absorption of inhaled corticosteroids from a metered-dose inhaler and dry powder inhaler. *Thorax* 46: 891–894

148  Thorsson L, Edsbäcker S, Conradson T (1994) Lung deposition of budesonide from Turbohaler is twice that from a pressurized metered-dose inhaler P-MDI. *Eur Resp J* 7: 1839–1844

149  Brown PH, Blundell G, Greening AP, Crompton GK (1992) High dose inhaled corticosteroids and the cortisol induced response to acute severe asthma. *Respir Med* 86: 495–497

150  Holt PR, Lowndes DW, Smithies E, Dixon GT (1990) The effect of an inhaled steroid on the hypothalamic-pituitary-adrenal axis: which tests should be used? *Clin Exp Allergy* 20: 145–149

151  Barnes PJ, Pedersen S (1993) Efficacy and safety of inhaled steroids in asthma. *Am Rev Respir Dis* 148: S1–S26

152  Löfdahl CG, Mellstrand T, Svedmyr N (1989) Glucocorticosteroids and asthma – stud-

ies of resistance and systemic effects of glucocorticosteroids. *Eur J Resp Dis* 65 (Suppl 130): 69–79

153  Pedersen S, Fuglsang G (1988) Urine cortisol excretion in children treated with high doses of inhaled corticosteroids a comparison of budesonide and beclomethasone. *Eur Resp J* 1: 433–435

154  Clark DJ, Lipworth BJ (1997) Adrenal suppression with chronic dosing of fluticasone propionate compared with budesonide in adult asthmatic patients. *Thorax* 52: 55–58

155  Brown PH, Matusiewicz SP, Shearing C, Tibi L, Greening AP, Crompton GK (1993) Systemic effects of high dose inhaled steroids: comparison of beclomethasone diproprionate and budesonide in healthy subjects. *Thorax* 48: 967–973

156  Sly RM, Imseis M, Frazer M et al (1978) Treatment of asthma in children with triamcinolone acetonide aerosol. *J Allergy Clin Immunol* 62: 76–82

157  Placcentini G, Sette L, Peroni DG, Bonizatto C, Bonetti S, Boner AL (1990) Double blind evaluation of effectiveness and safety of flunisolide aerosol for treatment of bronchial asthma in children. *Allergy* 45: 612–616

158  Fabbri L, Burge PS, Croonenburgh L, Warlies F, Weeke B, Ciaccia A, Parker C (1993) Comparison of fluticasone proprionate with beclomethasone diproprionate in moderate to severe asthma treated for one year. *Thorax* 48: 817–823

159  Prahl P (1991) Adrenocortical suppression following treatment with beclomethasone and budesonide. *Clin Exp Allergy* 21: 145–146

160  Bisgaard H, Damkjaer Nielsen M, Andersen B et al (1988) Adrenal function in children with bronchial asthma treated with beclomethasone diproprionate or budesonide. *J Allergy Clin Immunol* 81: 1088–1095

161  Volovitz B, Amir J, Malik H, Kauschansky A, Varsano I (1993) Growth and pituitary-adrenal function in children with severe asthma treated with inhaled budesonide. *New Engl J Med* 329: 1703–1708

162  Law CM, Honour JW, Marchant JL, Preece MA, Warner JO (1986) Nocturnal adrenal suppression in asthmatic children taking inhaled beclomethasone dipropionate. *Lancet* 1: 942–944

163  Tabacknik E, Zadik Z (1991) Diurnal cortisol secretion during therapy with inhaled beclomethasone diproprionate in children with asthma. *J Pediatr* 118: 294–297

164  Philip M, Aviram M, Lieberman E, Zadik Z, Giat Y, Levy J, Tal A (1992) Integrated plasma cortisol concentration in children with asthma receiving long-term inhaled corticosteroids. *Pediatr Pulmonol* 12: 84–89

165  Hosking DJ (1993) Effect of corticosteroids on bone turnover. *Resp Med* 87 (Suppl A): 15–21

166  Packe GE, Douglas JG, MacDonald AF, Robins SP, Reid DM (1992) Bone density in asthmatic patients taking high dose inhaled beclomethasone dipropionate and intermittent systemic steroids. *Thorax* 47: 414–417

167  König P, Hillman L, Cervantes CI (1993) Bone metabolism in children with asthma treated with inhaled beclomethasone dipropionate. *J Pediatr* 122: 219–226

168 Ali NJ, Capewell S, Ward MJ (1991) Bone turnover during high dose inhaled corticosteroid treatment. *Thorax* 46: 160–164

169 Wolthers OD, Pedersen S (1993) Bone turnover in asthmatic children treated with oral prednisolone or inhaled budesonide. *Paediatr Pulmonol* 16: 341–346

170 Herrala J, Puolijoki H, Impivaara O, Liippo K, Tala E, Nieminen MM (1994) Bone mineral density in asthmatic women on high dose inhaled beclomethasone dipropionate. *Bone* 15: 621–623

171 Toogood JH, Baskerville JC, Markov AE, Hodsman AB, Fraher LJ, Jennings B, Haddad RG, Drost D (1995) Bone mineral density and the risk of fracture in patients receiving long-term inhaled steroid therapy for asthma. *J Allergy Clin Immunol* 96: 157–166

172 Capewell S, Reynolds S, Shuttleworth D, Edwards C, Finlay AY (1990) Purpura and dermal thinning associated with high dose inhaled corticosteroids. *Br Med J* 300: 1548–1551

173 Mak VHF, Melchor R, Spiro S (1992) Easy bruising as a side-effect of inhaled corticosteroids. *Eur Resp J* 5: 1068–1074

174 Roy A, Leblanc C, Paquette L, Ghezzo H, Cote J, Cartier A, Malo J (1996) Skin bruising in asthmatic subjects treated with high does of inhaled steroids: frequency and association with adrenal function. *Eur Respir J* 9: 226–231

175 Toogood JH, Markov AE, Baskerville J, Dyson C (1993) Association of ocular cataracts with inhaled and oral steroid therapy during long term treatment for asthma. *J Allergy Clin Immunol* 91: 571–579

176 Simons FER, Persaud MP, Gillespie CA, Cheang M, Shuckett EP (1993) Absence of posterior subcapsular cataracts in young patients treated with inhaled glucocorticoids. *Lancet* 342: 736–738

177 Garbe E, LeLorier J, Boivin J, Suissa S (1997) Inhaled and nasal glucocorticoids and the risks of ocular hypertension or open-angel glaucoma. JAMA 227: 722–727

178 Russell G (1993) Asthma and growth. *Arch Dis Child* 69: 695–698

179 Balfour-Lynn L (1986) Growth and childhood asthma. *Arch Dis Child* 61: 1049–1055

180 Ninan T, Russell G (1992) Asthma, inhaled corticosteroid treatment and growth. *Arch Dis Child* 67: 703–705

181 Tinkelman DG, Reed CE, Nelson HS, Offord KP (1993) Aerosol beclomethasone dipropionate compared with theophylline as primary treatment of chronic, mild to moderately severe asthma in children. *Pediatr* 92: 64–77

182 Doull IJ, Freezer NJ, Holgate ST (1995) Growth of prepubertal children with mild asthma treated with inhaled beclomethasone dipropionate. *Am J Respir Crit Care Med* 151: 1715–1719

183 Allen DB, Mullen M, Mullen B (1994) A meta-analysis of the effects of oral and inhaled corticosteroids on growth. *J Allergy Clin Immunol* 93: 967–976

184 Wolthers OD, Pedersen S (1993) Growth in asthmatic children treated with budesonide. *Pediatr* 90: 517–518

185 Wolthers O, Pedersen S (1993) Short term growth during treatment with inhaled fluticasone diproprionate and beclomethasone diproprionate. *Arch Dis Child* 68: 673–676

186  Ebden P, Jenkins A, Houston G, Davies BH (1986) Comparison of two high-dose corti-
     costeroid aerosol treatments, beclomethasone dipropionate (1500 mcg/day) and budes-
     onide (1600 mcg/day) for chronic asthma. *Thorax* 41: 869–874

187  Turpeinen M, Sorva R, Juntungen-Backman K (1991) Changes in carbohydrate and
     lipid metabolism in children with asthma inhaling budesonide. *J Allergy Clin Immunol*
     88: 384–389

188  Kruszynska YT, Greenstone M, Home PD (1987) Effect of high dose inhaled
     beclomethasone diproprionate on carbolydate and lipid metabolism in normal subjects.
     *Thorax* 42: 881–884

189  Kiviranta K, Turpeinen M (1993) Effect of eight months of inhaled beclomethascne
     diproprionate and budesonide on carbohydrate metabolism in adults with asthma. *Tho-
     rax* 48: 974–978

190  Toogood JH, Baskerville J, Jennings B (1984) Use of spacers to facilitate inhaled corti-
     costeroid treatment of asthma. *Am Rev Respir Dis* 129: 723–729

191  Barnes PJ (1996) Inhaled glucocorticoids: new developments relevant to updating the
     Asthma Management Guidelines. *Resp Med* 90: 379–384

192  Otulana BA, Varma N, Bullock A, Higenbottam T (1992) High dose nebulized steroid
     in the treatment of chronic steroid-dependent asthma. *Resp Med* 86: 105–108

193  Greening AP, Ind PW, Northfield M, Shaw G (1994) Added salmeterol versus higher-
     dose corticosteroid in asthma patients with symptoms on existing inhaled corticosteroid.
     *Lancet* 344: 219–224

194  Woolcock AJ, Barnes PJ (1996) Asthma: the important questions-part 3. *Am J Respir
     Crit Care Med* 153: S1–S31

195  Evans DJ, Taylor DA, Zetterstrom O, Chung KF, O'Connor BJ, Barnes PJ (1997) A
     comparison of low-dose inhaled budesonide plus theophylline and high-dose inhaled
     budesonide for moderate asthma. *New Engl J Med* 337: 1412–1418

196  Rutten-van Molken MPMH, van Doorslaer EKA, Jansen MCC, Kerstjens HAM, Rut-
     ten FFH (1995) Costs and effects of inhaled coricosteroids and bronchodilators in asth-
     ma and chronic obstructive pulmonary disease. *Am J Respir Crit Care Med* 151:
     975–982

197  Barnes PJ, Jonsson B, Klim J (1996) The costs of asthma. *Eur Respir J* 9: 636–642

198  van Schayk CP, Dompeling E, Rutten MP, Folgering H, van den Boom G, van Weel C
     (1995) The influence of an inhaled steroid on quality of life in patients with asthma or
     COPD. *Chest* 107: 1199–1205

199  O'Driscoll BR, Kalra S, Wilson M, Pickering CAC, Caroll KB, Woodcock AA (1993)
     Double blind trial of steroid tapering in acute asthma. *Lancet* 341: 324–327

200  Beam WR, Ballard RD, Martin RJ (1992) Spectrum of corticosteroid sensitivity in noc-
     turnal asthma. *Am Rev Respir Dis* 145: 1082–1086

201  McLeod DT, Capewell SJ, Law J, MacLaren W, Seaton A (1985) Intramuscular triam-
     cinolone acetamide in chronic severe asthma. *Thorax* 40: 840–845

202  Ogirala RG, Aldrich TK, Prezant DJ, Sinnett MJ, Enden JB, Williams MH (1991) High

dose intramuscular triamcinolone in severe life-threatening asthma. *New Engl J Med* 329: 585–589

203 Grandordy B, Beilmatoug N, Morelle A, De Lauture D, Marac J (1987) Effect of betamethasone on airway obstruction and bronchial response to salbutamol in prednisolone resistant asthma. *Thorax* 42: 65–71

204 Hill SJ, Tattersfield AE (1995) Corticosteroid sparing agents in asthma. *Thorax* 50: 577–582

205 Mullarkey MF, Lammert JK, Blumenstein BA (1990) Long-term methotrexate treatment in corticosteroid-dependent asthma. *Ann Intern Med* 112: 5777–581

206 Shiner RJ, Nunn AJ, Chung KF, Geddes DM (1990) Randomized, double-blind, placebo-controlled trial of methotrexate in steroid-dependent asthma. *Lancet* 336: 137–140

207 Nierop G, Gijzel WP, Bel EH, Zwinderman AH, Dijkman JH (1992) Auranofin in the treatment of steroid dependent asthma : a double blind study. *Thorax* 47: 349–354

208 Alexander AG, Barnes NC, Kay AB (1992) Trial of cyclosporin in corticosteroid-dependent chronic severe asthma. *Lancet* 339: 324–328

209 Szczeklik A, Nizankowska E, Dworski R, Domagala B, Pinis G (1991) Cyclosporin for steroid-dependent asthma. *Allergy* 46: 312–315

210 Nelson HS, Hamilos DL, Corsello PR, Levesque NV, Buchameier AD, Bucher BL (1993) A double-blind study of troleandamycin and methylprednisolone in asthmatic patients who require daily corticosteroids. *Am Rev Respir Dis* 147: 398–404

211 British Thorac Society (1993) Guidelines on the management of asthma. *Thorax* 48S (Suppl): S1–S24

212 Engel T, Heinig JH (1991) Glucocorticoid therapy in acute severe asthma – a critical review. *Eur Respir J* 4: 881–889

213 Decramer M, Lacquet LM, Fagard R, Rogiers P (1995) Corticosteroids contribute to muscle weakness in chronic airflow obstruction. *Am J Respir Crit Care Med* 150: 11–16

214 Bowler SD, Mitchell CA, Armstrong JG (1992) Corticosteroids in acute severe asthma: effectiveness of low doses. *Thorax* 47: 584–587

215 Morell F, Orkiols R, de Gracia J, Curul V, Pujol A (1992) Controlled trial of intravenous corticosteroids in severe acute asthma. *Thorax* 47: 588–591

216 Harrison BDN, Stokes TC, Hart GJ, Vaughan DA, Ali NJ, Robinson AA (1986) Need for intravenous hydrocortisone in addition to oral prednisolone in patients admitted to hospital with severe asthma without ventilatory failure. *Lancet* i: 181–184

217 Barnes PJ, Adcock IM (1995) Steroid-resistant asthma. *Q J Med* 88: 455–468

218 Barnes PJ, Greening AP, Crompton GK (1995) Glucocorticoid resistance in asthma. *Am J Respir Crit Care Med* 152: 125S–140S

219 Szefler SJ, Leung DY (1997) Glucocorticoid-resistant asthma: pathogenesis and clinical implications for management. *Eur Respir J* 10: 1640–1647

220 Schwartz HJ, Lowell FC, Melby JC (1968) Steroid resistance in bronchial asthma. *Am J Int Med* 69: 493–499

221 Carmichael J, Paterson IC, Diaz P, Crompton GK, Kay AB, Grant IWB (1981) Corticosteroid resistance in chronic asthma. *Br Med J* 282: 1419–1422

222 Lane SJ, Atkinson BA, Swimanathan R, Lee TH. Hypothalamic-pituitary axis in corti-costeroid-resistant asthma. *Am J Respir Crit Care Med* 1996 153: 1510–1514

223 Woolcock AJ (1993) Steroid resistant asthma: what is the clinical definition? *Eur Respir J* 6: 743–747

224 Leung DYM, Martin RJ, Szefler SJ, Sher ER, Ying S, Kay AB, Hamid Q (1995) Dys-regulation of interleukin 4, interleukin 5, and interferon γ gene expression in steroid-resistant asthma. *J Exp Med* 181: 33–40

225 Lamberts SWJ, Kioper JW, de Jong FH (1992) Familial and iatrogenic cortisol receptor resistance. *J Steroid Biochem Molec Biol* 43: 385–388

226 Lane SJ, Arm JP, Staynov DZ, Lee TH (1994) Chemical mutational analysis of the human glucocortiocoid receptor cDNA in glucocorticoid-resistant bronchial asthma. *Am J Resp Cell Mol Biol* 11: 42–48

227 Corrigan C, Brown PH, Barnes NC, Szefler SJ, Tsai J, Frew AJ, Kay AB (1991) Gluco-corticoid resistance in chronic asthma. *Am Rev Respir Dis* 144: 1016–1025

228 Lane SJ, Palmer JBD, Skidmore IF, Lee TH (1990) Corticosteroid pharmacokinetics in asthma. *Lancet* 336: 126S

229 Goulding NJ, Podgorski MR, Hall ND, Flower RJ, Browning JL, Pepinsky RB, Maddi-son PJ (1989) Autoantibodies to recombinant liportin-1 in rheumatoid arthritis and sys-temic lupus erythematosus. *Ann Rheum Dis* 48: 843–850

230 Wilkinson JR, Podgorski MR, Godolphin JL, Goulding NJ, Lee TH (1990) Bronchial asthma is not associated with auto-antibodies to lipocortin-1. *Clin Exp Allergy* 20: 189–192

231 Chung KF, Podgorski MR, Goulding NJ, Godolphin JL, Sharland PR, O'Connor B, Flower RJ, Barnes PJ (1991) Circulating autoantibodies to recombinant lipocortin-1 in asthma. *Resp Med* 95: 121–124

232 Brown PH, Teelucksingh S, Matusiewicz SP, Greening AP, Crompton GK, Edwards CRW (1991) Cutaneous vasoconstrictor responses to glucocorticoids in asthma. *Lancet* 337: 576–580

233 Corrigan CJ, Brown PH, Barnes NC, Tsai J, Frew AJ, Kay AB (1991) Peripheral blood T lymphocyte activation and comparison of the T lymphocyte inhibitory effects of glu-cocorticoids and cyclosporin A. *Am Rev Respir Dis* 144: 1026–1032

234 Lane SJ, Lee TH (1991) Glucocorticoid receptor characteristics in monocytes of patients with corticosteroid-resistant bronchial asthma. *Am Rev Respir Dis* 143: 1020–1024

235 Sher ER, Leung YM, Surs W, Kam JC, Zieg G, Kamada AK, Szefler SJ (1994) Steroid-resistant asthma. Cellular mechanisms contributing to inadequate response to glucocor-ticoid therapy. *J Clin Invest* 93: 33–39

236 Kam JC, Szefler SJ, Surs W, Sher FR, Leung DYM (1993) Combination IL-2 and IL-4 reduces glucocorticoid-receptor binding affinity and T cell response to glucocorticoics. *J Immunol* 151: 3460–3466

237 Adcock IM, Lane SJ, Brown CA, Peters MJ, Lee TH, Barnes PJ (1995) Differences in binding of glucocorticoid receptor to DNA in steroid-resistant asthma. *J Immunol* 154: 3000–3005

238  Adcock IM, Lane SJ, Brown CA, Lee TH, Barnes PJ (1995) Abnormal glucocorticoid receptor/AP-1 interaction in steroid resistant asthma. *J Exp Med* 182: 1951–1958

239  Adcock IM, Lane SJ, Barnes PJ, Lee TH (1996) Enhanced phorbol ester-induced c-Fos transcription and translation in steroid-resistant asthma. *Am J Respir Crit Care Med* 153: A682

240  Adcock IM, Brady H, Lim S, Karin M, Barnes PJ (1997) Increased JUN kinase activity in peripheral blood monocytes from steroid-resistant asthmatic subjects. *Am J Respir Crit Care Med* 155: A288

241  Rosewicz S, McDonald AR, Maddux BA, Godfine ID, Miesfeld RL, Logsden CD (1988) Mechanism of glucocorticoid receptor down-regulation by glucocorticoids. *J Biol Chem* 263: 2581–2584

242  Adcock IM, Brown CR, Shirasaki H, Barnes PJ (1994) Effects of dexamethasone on cytokine and phorbol ester stimulated c-Fos and c-Jun DNA binding and gene expression in human lung. *Eur Resp J* 7: 2117–2123

243  Vacca A, Screpanati I, Maroder M, Petrangeli E, Frati L, Guline A (1989) Tumor promoting phorbol ester and raw oncogene expression inhibit the glucocorticoid-dependent transcription from the mouse mammary tumor virus long terminal repeat. *Mol Endo* 3: 1659–1665

244  Peters MJ, Adcock IM, Brown CR, Barnes PJ (1995) β-Adrenoceptor agonists interfere with glucocorticoid receptor DNA binding in rat lung. *Eur J Pharmacol* (Molec Pharmacol Section) 289: 275–281

245  Stevens DA, Barnes PJ, Adcock IM (1995) β-Agonists inhibit DNA binding of glucocorticoid receptors in human pulmonary and bronchial epithelial cells. *Am J Resp Crit Care Med* 151: A195

246  Peters MJ, Adcock IM, Brown CR, Barnes PJ (1993) b-Agonist inhibition of steroid-receptor DNA binding activity in human lung. *Am Rev Respir Dis* 147: A772

247  Wong CS, Wamedna I, Pavord ID, Tattersfield AE (1994) Effect of regular terbutaline and budesonide on bronchial reactivity to allergen challenge. *Am J Resp Crit Care Med* 15047: 1268–1278

248  Peters MJ, Yates DH, Chung KF, Barnes PJ (1993) $\beta_2$-Agonist dose reduction: strategy and early results. *Thorax* 48: 1066

# Phosphodiesterases in asthma

*Hermann Tenor and Christian Schudt*

Byk Gulden Lomberg Chemische Fabrik GmbH, Byk Gulden Straße 2, D-78467 Konstanz, Germany

## Introduction

Airway obstruction and hyperreactivity in asthma are mainly caused by accumulation of inflammatory cells and their mediators promoting bronchoconstriction, airway oedema and airway remodeling. Cyclic AMP counteracts a huge variety of inflammatory cell functions involved in the development and maintenance of asthma. In addition, cyclic AMP has been shown to reverse bronchial constriction, airway oedema and smooth muscle proliferation and may therefore protect against airway remodeling in asthma. cAMP is generated from ATP by adenylate cyclases that are activated by G-protein coupled receptors such as the $\beta_2$-receptor. In fact, attenuating cAMP generation may aggravate clinical asthma as reported with $\beta_2$-antagonists. On the other hand, there is overwhelming evidence that $\beta_2$-agonists improve asthma. However, long-term administration of $\beta_2$-agonists may be hampered by the phenomenon of tachyphylaxis, e.g. receptor desensitization and post-receptor events. In particular, it was repeatedly demonstrated that continuous use of inhaled $\beta_2$-agonists is associated with an impairment of their acute protective effects against bronchoconstrictive stimuli [1–4]. Continuous inhalation of $\beta_2$-agonists impaired their bronchoprotective effect against AMP-induced hyperreactivity to a greater extent compared to hyperreactivity triggered by methacholine. These results may imply that $\beta_2$-agonists tend to desensitize mast cell responses more strongly than direct smooth muscle responses [4]. Apart from enhanced cAMP generation another option to increase cAMP is to inhibit its decay. Cyclic nucleotide hydrolysing phosphodiesterases (PDE) represent a superfamily of enzymes which break down cAMP and cGMP. Thus PDE inhibitors should increase cAMP in bronchial smooth muscle and inflammatory cells and have anti-asthmatic effects.

Seven PDE families have been characterized mainly based on substrate, activator or inhibitor sensitivities (Tab. 1) (families 8 and 9 have been identified recently). Several of these PDE families comprise subtypes encoded by different genes. As an example, four subtypes (PDE4A–D) have been identified for PDE4. mRNA-transcription of subtypes involves alternative splicing resulting in the expression of PDE

Anti-Inflammatory Drugs in Asthma, edited by A.P. Sampson and M.K. Church
© 1999 Birkhäuser Verlag Basel/Switzerland

*Table 1 - Classification of PDE isoenzyme families. Seven PDE families based on substrate preference and sensitivities to activators or inhibitors have been characterised.*

| PDE family | Preferred substrate | Activator | Inhibitor |
|---|---|---|---|
| PDE1 | cAMP, cGMP | $Ca^{2+}$-Calmodulin | |
| PDE2 | cAMP | cGMP | EHNA |
| PDE3 | cAMP | | cGMP, Milrinone |
| PDE4 | cAMP | | Rolipram |
| PDE5 | cGMP | | Sildenafil |
| PDE6 | cGMP | | |
| PDE7 | cAMP | | |

species with distinct N-terminal ends. This is exemplified by the five N-terminal splice variants so far described for PDE4D. As will be discussed below, N-terminal splicing may serve to direct intracellular localisation of the enzyme, post-translational modification or formation of distinct conformers. Phosphodiesterases share homologies in their amino acid sequence. A catalytic domain (~ 270 amino acids) is flanked by a hydrophilic C-terminus and an N-terminus that comprises regulatory sites. The catalytic core has a higher degree of homology within phosphodiesterases of one family (~ 80%) than with other families (~ 25%–40%). The catalytic core contains the PDE-specific sequence $HD(X)_2H(X_4)N$ and two $Zn^{2+}$-binding domains. The N-terminal domain contains the calmodulin-binding site (PDE1), the cGMP-binding site (PDE2 or 5), hydrophobic membrane association domains (PDE3) or membrane-targeting domains (PDE4) or other functionally relevant regions.

In humans, there is cell-specific expression of PDE families, subtypes or splice variants. Peripheral blood eosinophils, neutrophils, and monocytes contain almost exclusively PDE4. T lymphocytes, lung mast cells, and bronchial and vascular smooth muscle cells express PDE4 and 3. Human alveolar macrophages additionally exhibit PDE1 whereas human endothelial cells express PDE2, 3 and 4. Finally, PDE1 and 4 were detected in human bronchial epithelial cells. Regarding subtypes, PDE3A has been located in platelets, vascular smooth muscle and myocardium, whereas PDE3B was found in adipocytes, liver, pancreatic β-cells, the neuronal system and T lymphocytes. PDE4C was not found in peripheral blood cells, but it was abundant in the CNS. Studies examining whether expression of phosphodiesterase variants is up- or down-regulated in disease states such as asthma are at an early stage. Earlier studies implied that there may be an up-regulation of PDE in peripheral blood cells of patients with atopic dermatitis [5, 6], but others could not confirm these findings [7]. Results from studies investigating the pattern of PDE variants in eosinophils, T lymphocytes or neutrophils infiltrating the bronchial mucosa in asthmatics are eagerly awaited.

Recently, the interesting observation was made that distinct subtypes of PDE1 were increasingly expressed in maturing or proliferating cells. Firstly, it was shown that monocytes cultured with human AB serum for several days assume the phenotype of macrophages and this was associated with an enhanced expression of PDE1 that was absent in monocytes but detected in human alveolar macrophages [8, 9]. Secondly, PDE1B1 was expressed in proliferating T lymphocytes following incubation with PHA, but was absent in resting T cells. In fact, PDE1B1 antisense promotes apoptosis of lymphocytic cells, implying a functional role of PDE1B1 up-regulation in these cells [10]. Thirdly, proliferating human vascular smooth muscle cells express PDE1C but this was undetectable in quiescent cells [11]. From these latter findings the hypothesis may be raised that PDE1C up-regulation facilitates smooth muscle remodeling in vascular (pulmonary hypertension, atherosclerosis) disease and asthma and that PDE1C antisense or selective PDE1C inhibitors might reverse vascular or bronchial smooth muscle remodeling.

From the pattern of PDE isoenzymes decribed above it was concluded that particularly PDE4 inhibitors or dual-selective PDE3 and 4 inhibitors might provide benefit as efficient anti-asthma drugs since these families are found in almost all inflammatory cells. The development of new PDE4 or PDE3 and 4 inhibitors for asthma is greatly driven by the encouraging clinical experience with theophylline – a non-selective PDE inhibitor. In fact, although theophylline has been considered for decades as a pure bronchodilator, recent intensive research revealed and unequivocally confirmed that theophylline triggers a multitude of anti-inflammatory effects that certainly contribute to its effects in clinical asthma. *In vitro*, theophylline inhibits lipopolysaccharide (LPS)-induced TNFα formation in human monocytes and alveolar macrophages; human T lymphocyte proliferation, chemotaxis and cytokine generation; production of reactive oxygen species (ROS), degranulation, LTC$_4$ synthesis, and chemotaxis in human eosinophils; anti-IgE induced histamine release from human lung mast cells; degranulation and ROS formation in human neutrophils. Moreover, theophylline promotes human eosinophil apoptosis. Theophylline inhibited inflammatory cell accumulation in diverse allergen challenge models and attenuated airway oedema formation in experimental animals. Controlled clinical trials revealed that theophylline acts to reduce T lymphocyte infiltrates, to reduce IL-4 and IL-5 expression and to attenuate the number of activated eosinophils in bronchial biopsies obtained from asthmatics. There is certainty from a diversity of clinical trials that theophylline inhibits late and early responses to allergen challenge, again adding strong evidence to its anti-inflammatory profile [12–22]. Finally, two recent trials have shown that theophylline has steroid-sparing effects. Adding theophylline to budesonide 800 μg/day or beclomethasone 400 μg/day was at least equivalent and in some clinical parameters even significantly superior to a doubled steroid dose (i.e. budesonide 1600 μg/day or beclomethasone 800 μg/day) [23, 24]. In other trials it was shown that benefit from theophylline is still gained in those patients who do not further improve despite increasing steroid dose. It may be hypothesized that theophylline synergises with steroids also by inhibiting some of the inflammatory responses resistant to steroids.

New phosphodiesterase inhibitors for asthma are required in particular to improve the benefit-risk ratio. Originally, attention was paid to the hypothesis that family-selective PDE inhibitors i.e. PDE4 and PDE4 and 3 inhibitors might provide a solution. However, both disappointing clinical results with first generation selective inhibitors as well as considerable recent progress in PDE research fueled a slightly different concept, and the current paradigm has changed. Through post-translational regulation, association to other proteins or membranes PDEs are present in diverse functional states (conformations) and the second generation inhibitor should inhibit the state associated with inflammatory cells and processes but not the state assumed in non-inflammatory tissues (e.g. CNS, myocardium, vasculature).

This review will focus on PDE4 and PDE3 and recent progress with the development of selective (PDE4) or dual-selective (PDE3 and 4) inhibitors for asthma. Chemical structures of PDE4 inhibitors and dual-selective PDE3 and 4 inhibitors are illustrated in Figure 1 (see pages 110/111). Other PDE families which have so far not been in the focus of drug discovery for asthma have recently been extensively reviewed by others.

## Phosphodiesterase 4 family

PDE4 is a specific cyclic AMP hydrolysing phosphodiesterase activity that is potently inhibited by rolipram but not affected by cGMP. In early chromatographical investigations of heart and smooth muscle extracts, this phosphodiesterase activity eluted as the fourth activity from anion exchange columns [25]. Subsequent investigations revealed the ubiquitous presence of PDE4. In human peripheral blood eosinophils, monocytes, neutrophils, B cells but also neuronal cells, PDE4 represents the predominant isoenzyme. In other systems such as human alveolar macrophages, T cells, dendritic cells, endothelial cells, smooth muscle cells and bronchial epithelial cells, PDE4 was coexpressed with other PDE isoenzymes, in particular PDE3. This abundance of PDE4 in cells that orchestrate inflammation in bronchial asthma or rheumatoid arthritis was paralleled by evidence that PDE4 inhibitors such as rolipram potently suppressed a multitude of inflammatory cell functions e.g. ROS generation, cytokine synthesis, cysteinyl leukotriene-production, chemotaxis, and T lymphocyte proliferation. Hence, PDE4 or PDE3/4 inhibitors are thought to be capable of resolving inflammation in bronchial asthma or other inflammatory diseases.

However, the presence of PDE4 in neuronal cells implies that inhibitors of this isoenzyme family may induce CNS effects. In fact, the original intention with the classical PDE4 inhibitor rolipram was to develop an antidepressant drug. Moreover, clinical development of first generation PDE4 inhibitors failed due to CNS-induced adverse effects such as nausea or vomiting that occurred at therapeutic plasma concentrations. Therefore, it was necessary to elaborate strategies that allow to the dissociation of the anti-inflammatory actions of PDE4 inhibitors from their CNS-driven adverse effects based on the specific interaction of these second generation PDE4 inhibitors with PDE4 molecules. An intensive research campaign over the past decade revealed that PDE4 is encoded by four distinct genes (HSPDE4A–D). Transcription of mRNA from these genes is associated with alternate splicing of 5'-situated exons and finally PDE4 protein is expressed as a certain N-terminal splice variant of one of the four subtypes PDE4A–D. For human PDE4, thirteen splice variants have been characterised. Certainly, cellular systems may exhibit a different expression of these splice variants and it was reasoned that splice-variant selective PDE4 inhibitors may improve the ratio between anti-inflammatory potential and adverse effects.

The important breakthrough in PDE4 research is however, the discovery that PDE4 proteins may exist in two different conformational states. These conformations can be distiguished by their different affinity for the classical PDE4 inhibitor rolipram [26]. This discovery was the result of fundamental investigations to explain the early enigmatic finding that rolipram inhibits PDE4 catalytic activity with $K_i \approx 1$ $\mu$M, whereas rolipram binding affinity to PDE4 is in the range of $K_i \approx 1$ nM. Recent pharmacological studies suggest that the protein conformation with low affinity for rolipram (LAR-conformation) may predominate in inflammatory cells. On the other hand, in neuronal cells the PDE conformation with a high affinity for rolipram (HAR-conformation) may predominate. Indeed, there is an excellent correlation between interaction of PDE4 inhibitors with the LAR confirmation and inhibition of TNFα-generation from human monocytes [27, 28], IL-2 from murine splenocytes [29], superoxide from guinea pig eosinophils [30], degranulation of guinea pig mast cells [31], human T lymphocyte proliferation induced by antigen [32] and antigen-induced bronchoconstriction [33, 34]. In contrast, the correlation between association with HAR conformation and these functional responses is substantially weaker. On the other hand, interaction of PDE4 inhibitors with the HAR conformation strongly correlates with emesis [35, 36] and acid secretion from rabbit isolated gastric glands [37] (Tab. 2). In comparison, the correlation between association of PDE4 inhibitors with the LAR conformation and these functional responses is dramatically reduced. In conclusion, second generation PDE4 inhibitors designed to exhibit a more potent interaction with the LAR-conformer than with the HAR-conformer of the PDE4 molecule are suggested to dissociate therapeutic efficacy from adverse effects resulting in an improved ratio between anti-inflammatory potential and emesis threshold. Taking into account these encouraging conclusions it should not escape our attention that the PDE4-inhibitor induced suppression of certain inflammatory functions such as neutrophil degranulation [28] but also PDE4-inhibitor induced relaxation of methacholine-precontracted guinea pig trachea [38] may more closely correlate with HAR-conformer association than with LAR-conformer interaction.

*Table 2 - Correlation of inhibition of HAR or LAR conformation with functional effects. $IC_{50}$ values obtained for either inhibition of PDE4 catalysis (reflecting inhibition of the LAR conformer) or [$^3$H]rolipram binding to PDE4 (reflecting inhibition of the HAR conformer) were correlated to corresponding data for the inhibition or activation of functional responses. Higher degree of correlation between HAR or LAR and the functional response is depicted. Notably for some functional effects their correlation to one of the conformers depends on the stimulus. For example, reduction of human T-lymphocyte proliferation induced by antigen correlates to LAR-inhibition whereas suppression of PHA-stimulated proliferation appears to be more closely associated with HAR-inhibition.*

| | Correlation with | | |
|---|---|---|---|
| Cell/Tissue | HAR | LAR | Reference |
| Human monocytes | | LPS-induced TNFα release | [27, 28] |
| Mice splenocytes | | *Staph. aur.*-induced IL2 release | [29] |
| Human T lymphocytes | | Antigen-induced proliferation | [32] |
| Guinea pig mast cells | | PGD$_2$-release | [31] |
| Guinea pig eosinophils | | ROS generation | [30] |
| Guinea pig antigen-induced bronchoconstriction | | Relaxation | [33, 34] |
| Behavior, CNS | Emesis | | [35, 36] |
| Human T lymphocytes | PHA-induced proliferation | | [98] |
| Rabbit gastric glands | Acid secretion | | [37] |
| Human neutrophil | Degranulation | | [28] |
| Guinea pig peritoneal macrophages | cAMP-accumulation | | [45] |
| Guinea pig histamine/metacholine-induced tracheal constriction | Relaxation | | [38] |

In view of the pivotal role of the LAR and HAR conformers for the design of PDE4 inhibitors an intriguing aspect is to investigate for each of the PDE4 splice variants the LAR/HAR ratio or the interconvertibility of these conformers. In fact, currently available data indicate that the percentage of LAR conformer for human recombinant PDE4A5, PDE4B2 and PDE4D3 is 58% [39], 66% [40] and 47% [41], respectively. However, the extent to which a PDE4 variant assumes LAR or HAR conformation depends on the experimental conditions and may be different in intact cells.

Protein kinase A-triggered phosphorylation of PDE4D3 [42, 43] or membrane association of PDE4A5 [44, 45] may assist to augment the proportion of the corresponding HAR conformer. In addition, the hypothesis was raised that *in vitro* treatment of cellular extracts containing PDE4 with orthovanadate in combination with glutathione may result in an augmented amount of the HAR conformer reflected by an increased affinity of PDE4 to rolipram [45–47]. Orthovanadate in combination with glutathione also enhanced PDE4 activity in eosinophil membranes [47, 48]. In view of the fact that orthovanadate serves as a phosphotyrosine-phosphatase inhibitor it may be reasoned that orthovanadate acts by maintaining a tyrosine kinase-induced activated conformer of PDE4. Recent investigations give rise to the view that tyrosine kinases may stimulate PDE4 activity. The tyrosine kinase inhibitor genistein suppressed Ro20-1724-sensitive PDE4 activity in a neuronal cell line by 85% [49]. Genistein was shown to amplify GHRH-stimulated cAMP increase in rat anterior pituitary cells or rat pinealocytes. These effects were reversed by orthovanadate, occurred independently of the cAMP stimulus used and were not observed in the presence of phosphodiesterase inhibitors [50, 51]. Interestingly, strong suppression of PAF-induced human eosinophil LTC$_4$ and superoxide generation by tyrosine kinase inhibitors was demonstrated [52] which may also be explained by the proposed tyrosine kinase-PDE4 crosstalk. These data are corroborated by evidence that src tyrosine kinase activates PDE4 in rat thecal interstitial and mouse Leydig cells [53]. The tight association of SH3-binding domains located in the N-terminal end of PDE4A with SH3-domains in src-tyrosyl kinases [54], suggesting an *in situ* co-localization of certain PDE4 splice variants with tyrosine kinases, further supports the significance of this putative crosstalk between two major signalling cascades. In summary, based on available data the hypothesis arises that tyrosine kinases may activate PDE4 variants and augment the proportion of HAR conformers. In this respect, tyrosine kinases and protein kinase A comparably activate PDE4 by enhancing their phosphorylated form and the HAR fraction. Orthovanadate, by suppressing phosphotyrosine phosphatase imitates tyrosine kinase-mediated PDE4 modification.

The concept of optimising PDE4 inhibitors by screening for structures showing a high ratio of affinity for the LAR conformer compared to the HAR conformer has now been incorporated in the drug discovery strategies of leading pharmaceutical companies [34, 41, 55, 56]. A very promising candidate is SB207499 (Fig. 1) which associates 33-fold more potently with the LAR conformer versus the HAR conformer of PDE4A5, when compared to rolipram [41]. This compound is currently undergoing clinical investigations as an oral antiasthmatic.

## Gene and protein structure of PDE4 variants

Four PDE4 genes (PDE4A, B, C and D) have been distinguished. PDE4A and PDE4C genes are located on chromosome 19, whereas PDE4B and PDE4D genes are on chromosome 1 and chromosome 5, respectively. These genes are composed of a multitude of exons and introns. Hence, transcription from each of the four genes may result in several mRNA-products emerging from alternative splicing of exons situated near the 5'-end of the DNA open reading frame (ORF). cDNAs encoding different splice variants from rat and human PDE4 genes have been generated based on screening of cDNA libraries with oligonucleotides conservative for a specific PDE4 gene. cDNA was then transfected in cellular systems and corresponding PDE4 proteins were expressed. The amino acid sequences of expressed PDE4 protein variants have been analyzed. In addition, subcellular localisation and catalytic activity of PDE4 splice variants was characterized.

In general, PDE4 protein structures comprise three domains of amino acid sequences which are highly conserved within this enzyme family. A catalytic domain is flanked at its N-terminal end by two upstream conserved regions (UCR1 and UCR2) formed of about 60–100 amino acids. In human and rat PDE4 genes, two splice junctions have been identified. Alternative splicing at the junction next to the 5' end of the ORF results in protein structures that express both the UCR1 and UCR2 encoding regions (long form splice variants). On the other hand, PDE4 variants expressing the UCR2 but not the UCR1 region (short form splice variants) are elaborated by alternate splicing at the splice junction next to the 5' end of the region encoding the catalytic domain. The amino acid sequence at the N-terminal end may (i) serve to confer association to membranes and cytoskeletal proteins and hence, subcellular compartmentation, (ii) represent a site for phosphorylation, (iii) function as an endogenous inhibitor of catalytic activity, (iv) support interaction with other enzymes, and (v) affect sensitivity to exogenous PDE4 inhibitors. Hence, the diversity of PDE4 variants and their unique expression pattern in different cellular systems assists in cell-specific regulation of intracellular signalling and modulates the crosstalk of major signalling pathways.

Table 3 details the classification of currently characterized human PDE4 variants and their rat homologues.

## Phosphodiesterase 4A variants

In humans, a single PDE4A variant (PDE4A5) has been detected so far [44, 57–60]. The PDE4A5 protein consists of 886 amino acids and covers both N-terminal UCR1 and UCR2 conserved regions and the catalytic domain (long-form). cDNA for PDE4A5 was isolated from a human monocyte cDNA library [57]. PCR amplification with PDE4A5-specific oligonucleotide primers and Western blotting using antibodies specific for PDE4A5 located PDE4A5 mRNA-transcripts and protein in diverse systems e.g. human monocytes, T cells, B-cells, eosinophils and human brain [7, 61]. Recently, $Zn^{++}$-binding domains have been identified in the PDE4A5 protein structure and a strong association of PDE4A5 with $Zn^{++}$ was described

*Table 3 - Characteristics of PDE4 subtypes and splice variants.*
*Four different PDE4 genes are distinguished. Alternative splicing from at least two splice junctions results in short forms and long forms of PDE4.*

| Human PDE4 | Rat homologue | Structure | Comments |
|---|---|---|---|
| | 4A1 (RD1) | short-form | membrane-bound |
| ⌐A5 (PDE46) | 4A5 (RNPDE6) | long-form | cAMP → mRNA ↑, protein ↑ |
| | 4A8 (RNPDE39) | short-form | exclusively in rat testis |
| ⌐B1 | RPDE4B1 | long-form | |
| ⌐B2 | RPDE4B2 | short-form | cAMP → mRNA ↑, protein ↑ |
| ⌐B3 | 4B3 (pRPDE74) | long-form | |
| ⌐C-791 | | long-form | fetal human lung |
| ⌐C-426 | | | fetal human lung |
| ⌐C-D54 | | | human testis |
| ⌐C-D109 | | | human testis, inactive |
| ⌐D1 | RPDE4D1 | short-form | cAMP → mRNA ↑, protein ↑ |
| ⌐D2 | RPDE4D2 | short-form | cAMP → mRNA ↑, protein ↑ |
| ⌐D3 | RPDE4D3 | long-form | cAMP → phosphorylation |
| ⌐D4 | | long-form | |
| ⌐D5 | | long-form | |

($Kd = 0.4\ \mu M$). In fact, $Zn^{++}$ enhanced PDE4A activity, reduced the ability of inhibitors to suppress PDE4A activity by a factor of 10 and attenuated the association of rolipram with the enzyme by a factor of 30 [62].

Human recombinant PDE4A5 was engineered in COS-7 cells and PDE4 activity was detected in both cytosolic (88%) and particulate (12%) fractions [44]. Moreover, immunofluorescence studies were suggestive of an association with membrane structures such as cytoskeletal or cytoskeletal-associated proteins. From these studies it was speculated that the amount of PDE 4A5 associated to membrane or cytoskeletal structures *in situ* was higher than estimated by simple activity measurements in cytosolic and particulate fractions of cell lysates. In fact, studies with the rat homologue RNPDE6 (rat PDE4A5) of human PDE4A5 revealed that certain regions of the N-terminal end constitute SH3-binding domains [54]. These SH3-binding domains confer tight association with SH3-domains. Proteins with SH3-domains are tyrosyl kinases of the Src family but also structural proteins such as fodrin [63, 64]. It has been shown that complete src-kinases and isolated SH3-domains excised from these src-kinases bind to RNPDE6. The src-kinases lyn and fyn exhibit the strongest association to RNPDE6 reflected by a seven-fold higher binding affinity compared to v-src. Binding of these tyrosyl kinases does not affect

PDE activity. In contrast, src-kinases csk and crk inhibited PDE4 activity although their binding affinity was reduced compared to v-src [54].

Whether association with RNPDE6 modulates functions of src tyrosyl kinases has not yet been comprehensively explored. However, it merits attention that PDE association to src kinases directs capacity for cAMP hydrolysis to the immediate vicinity of these tyrosyl kinases. As an example, the tyrosyl kinase csk is phosphorylated and subsequently inactivated by cAMP-activated protein kinase [65]. Csk phosphorylates and inhibits other tyrosine kinases e.g. v-src resulting in suppression of expression of inflammation proteins such as TNFα, IL-1 or iNOS [66]. In this case, PDE association to csk may prevent cAMP-induced inactivation of this protein kinase and ultimately support the function of csk to counteract inflammatory processes. Apart from this indirect crosstalk mediated by catalytic PDE activity, it is unknown at present whether RPDE6 through protein-protein interaction directly modifies src kinases. Certainly, an additional function of enzymes distinct from their well-characterized catalytic activity is not uncommon which is illustrated by the immunophilins. In particular, the FK506-binding protein exhibits catalytic activity as peptidyl-prolyl *cis-trans* isomerase and associates to calcineurin phosphatase resulting in inhibition of the phosphatase activity [67, 68]. Moreover, the interaction of the synaptic vesicle phosphoprotein synapsine I with src SH3-domains attenuates tyrosine phosphorylating capacity [69]. These findings show that direct interaction of proteins with SH3 domains of src may modify tyrosine kinase activity. In view of cAMP-dependent up-regulation of PDE4A mRNA transcripts and protein [70] and considering an orchestrating role of src-kinases in cellular functions as diverse as T lymphocyte proliferation [71], monocyte TNFα generation [72], apoptosis [73, 74], and eosinophil degranulation [75] it would be attractive to hypothesise that PDE4A protein may regulate src tyrosyl kinase activity independently from cAMP breakdown.

PDE4A5 engineered in COS-7 cells that is bound to the particulate fraction of cell lysates exhibits only about half the maximum enzyme activity determined for PDE4A5 found in the cytosolic fraction. Moreover, the potency of rolipram in inhibiting particulate PDE4A5 activity ($K_i = 37$ nM) was about 43-fold higher than its potency in suppressing cytosolic enzyme activity ($K_i = 1.6$ μM). Whereas inhibition by rolipram of cytosolic PDE4 activity was purely competitive, inhibition data obtained with the particulate enzyme were best fitted by a partial competitive model [44]. Although the authors did not measure rolipram binding, they formulated the hypothesis that the cytosolic and particulate enzyme fractions have a different proportion of PDE4A5 conformers. Expression of PDE4A5 deletion mutants in COS cells revealed that UCR1 and UCR2 was required for high affinity rolipram binding whereas inhibition of catalytic activity was still found in an enzyme truncated to the catalytic core. Rolipram inhibition of the full-length PDE4A5 followed a shallow log dose-inhibition curve ($N = 0.69$) and was about five-fold more potent compared to suppression of the truncated core enzyme that followed competitive kinetics with a Hill coefficient close to unity [60]. These results are consistent with the hypothesis that full-length recombinant PDE4A5 coexists in two distinct conformers e.g. HAR and LAR. In contrast the core enzyme may only adopt the LAR conformation. The amino acid sequence located N-terminal to the catalytic domain is required for constitution of the HAR conformer.

Analysis of rolipram and RP73401 binding to PDE4A5 deletion mutants further extended these results [59]. RP73401 represents a benzamide originally designed as an anti-asthmatic drug [76]. In contrast to rolipram, this compound associated to the PDE4-high affinity rolipram binding site at concentrations comparable to those required for inhibition of catalysis ($IC_{50} \approx 0.6$ nM) [59, 77]. In consequence the hypothesis was raised that RP73401 exhibits similar capacity to label LAR and HAR [46]. This hypothesis is supported by the finding that deletion of 331 amino acids at the N-terminal end of PDE4A5 retains high affinity binding of RP73401 whereas rolipram high affinity binding is lost [59]. In parallel, RP73401-induced inhibition of catalysis is not affected by N-terminal deletion of 331 amino acids whereas such a truncation impairs rolipram inhibition of cAMP-hydrolysis by a factor of ~6 [59]. In addition, these authors detected high ($K_d \approx 1$ nM) and low affinity ($K_d \approx 100$ nM) rolipram binding to the full length human recombinant PDE4A5 (Met1-886) [78] as well as to a fully active truncated form of PDE4A5 (Met265-836) using an equilibrium filter binding technique. Inhibition of cAMP hydrolysis by rolipram was found to be in a range comparable to low-affinity rolipram binding. This indicates that standard measurement of inhibition of PDE4-induced cAMP hydrolysis by rolipram may predominantly reflect catalytic inhibition of the LAR conformer. A strong argument for the concept of two PDE4A5 conformers with different affinities for rolipram but similar affinities for RP73401 is provided by the finding that the $B_{max}$ value for [$^3$H]RP73401 binding is two to three-fold higher than that for [$^3$H]rolipram binding [39]. These data based on standard filtration technique are consistent with the view that RP73401 labels HAR and LAR whereas with rolipram only binding to HAR is detectable under these experimental conditions. Taken together, there is considerable evidence that for human PDE4A5 two conformers can be distinguished. Rolipram discriminates between these conformers whereas RP73401 binds and inhibits catalytic activity of both conformers with identical affinity. Rolipram and RP73401 bind to the catalytic site of the conformers since cAMP is a competitive inhibitor of association of these compounds with PDE4A5 [59].

However, the structural requirements within the central conserved region for inhibitor association compared to cAMP binding to PDE4A5 are different. PDE4A5 point mutants where either His505 or His506 were replaced by Asn using site directed mutagenesis displayed an increase in cAMP-$K_M$. In parallel, the $IC_{50}$ for cAMP competition of [$^3$H]rolipram and [$^3$H]RP73401 binding reflected a decrease in cAMP affinity for the enzyme. On the other hand, binding and inhibition curves for rolipram and RP73401 were not affected [39].

From the PDE4 variants expressed in rat tissue the short form RNPDE4A1 (RD1) is of interest since a 24 amino acid residue confers complete membrane association in its native state in rat cerebellum [79] and when engineered in COS cells [80, 81] or a human carcinoma thyroid cell line [82]. Deletion of the 24 amino acid residue flanking the N-terminal end of the core region results in an enzyme which is completely located in the cytosol [80]. On the other hand, a chimeric construct of the N-terminal domain of RD1 with chloramphenicol-acetyltransferase, which is cytosolic in its native state, was exclusively expressed in a membrane associated form [83]. In addition, deletion of the N-terminal end results in a substantial increase in $V_{MAX}$ suggesting that this unique 24 amino acid chain acts as an endogenous inhibitor of PDE4 activity [79, 80]. Notably, neither $K_M$ nor rolipram inhibition was affected by deletion of the N-terminal 24 amino acids [80]. Immunofluorescent studies revealed that RD1 primarily associated to the Golgi apparatus [79, 82]. Interestingly, RD1 engineered in human thyroid carcinoma FTC cell lines was accompanied by a down-regulation of endogenous PDE1C mRNA transcript and enzyme activity [82]. It remains an open question whether transcription of PDE1C mRNA is regulated by cAMP.

## Phosphodiesterase 4B variants

Three PDE4B variants can be distinguished in humans. PDE4B1 and PDE4B3 are long forms, whereas PDE4B2 represents a short form [58, 84–86]. The rat homologue of PDE4B2 was completely associated to membranes, whereas rat PDE4B1 was cytosolic [87]. In contrast, each of the human PDE4B1-3 splice variants engineered in COS7 cells was expressed in both cytosolic and particulate fractions [86]. However, PDE4B1 and B2 but not PDE4B3 were released from the microsomal particulate fraction following exposure to Triton X-100 suggesting a different mechanism of enzyme association to membrane fractions for PDE4B1 and 4B2 in comparison to PDE4B3. This hypothesis is corroborated by the finding that $V_{MAX}$ values determined for particulate PDE4B1 and PDE4B2 were substantially reduced compared to the cytosolic forms, whereas particulate PDE4B3 showed similar maximum enzyme activity to the cytosolic enzyme [86]. Comprehensive kinetic analysis of cytosolic PDE4B1-3 expressed in COS-7 cells revealed a higher $V_{MAX}$ of the short form PDE4B2 compared to the long forms PDE4B1 and PDE4B3 [86]. These data support the view that the N-terminal end and also membrane association may depress enzyme activity. In contrast to the long forms where rolipram-induced inhibition of PDE4 activity was roughly identical for the cytosolic and particulate species, the selective PDE4 inhibitor attenuated PDE4B2 more potently when expressed in the cytosolic ($IC_{50} \approx 20$ nM) than in the particulate fraction ($IC_{50} \approx 200$ nM) [86]. Although the shallow log dose inhibition curves were suggestive of co-existence of the HAR and LAR conformers for both membrane-associated and cytosolic PDE4 forms, it may be hypothesized that the cytosolic PDE4B2 species is dominated by the HAR conformer whereas the LAR conformer represents the predominant folding of PDE4B2 in its membrane-bound state.

That PDE4B2 protein forms HAR and LAR conformations has recently been unequivocally demonstrated [40]. These authors separated high-affinity rolipram binding ($K_d \approx 7$ nM) paralleled by high-affinity enzyme inhibition ($K_i \approx 5$–10 nM) from low-affinity rolipram binding ($K_d \approx 210$ nM) paralleled by low-affinity enzyme inhibition ($K_i \approx 200$–400 nM). Rolipram bound with stoichiometries of 0.3 and 0.6 molecules rolipram per molecule of PDE4B2 to the HAR conformer and LAR conformer, respectively. In contrast, an N-terminal and C-terminal deletion mutant of PDE4B2 encompassing amino acids 152–528 of the 564 amino acid sequence exclusively assumed the LAR conformation. Rolipram association to this deletion mutant fit to a low-affinity, single site ($K_d \approx 1$ µM). In parallel, rolipram-induced inhibition of PDE4B2 (152–528) activity gave a single low-affinity inhibition constant ($K_i \approx 400$ nM). Stoichiometry of rolipram binding to the PDE4B2 (152–528) deletion mutant was 0.9 molecules rolipram per PDE4B2 molecule. Stoichiometry of rolipram binding strongly supports the concept that full-length PDE4B2 protein assumes two conformations that are discriminated by their different affinity for rolipram whereas the PDE4B2 (152–528) deletion mutant exclusively exists in the LAR conformer. Similar to these data are findings with PDE4A5 discussed in the previous section, where deletion of the N-terminal end was associated with a loss of high affinity rolipram binding [59, 78]. Hence, domains in the N-terminal end of PDE4 variants appear indispensable to form the HAR conformer.

The distinct characterisation of HAR and LAR conformers of highly purified human recombinant PDE4B2 in this study [40] is based on techniques for the measurement of enzyme activity and rolipram binding different from those used in previous investigations. To assess cAMP hydrolysing capacity PDE4B2 preparations were preincubated with rolipram for 1 h before the activity assay was performed. Notably, this protocol imitates conditions in the rolipram binding experiments. This technique gave two distinct inhibition constants whereas PDE activity measurement immediately after addition of rolipram i.e. according to the standard common protocol gave a single (low affinity) inhibition constant only. Isothermal titration calorimetry served to assess rolipram binding to PDE4B2. This technique described the binding of rolipram to PDE4B2 protein by evaluating measurements of the energy generated through association of rolipram to the enzyme. Following this technique two distinct binding constants were obtained whereas standard filter binding experiments exclusively detected high affinity rolipram binding.

In conclusion, these experiments add further evidence that rolipram binding is associated with inhibition of catalytic activity. The apparent discrepancy between high affinity rolipram binding and low affinity rolipram inhibition of enzyme catalysis observed previously derives from the limitations of standard protocols for assessment of rolipram inhibition of PDE4 catalysis and rolipram binding to PDE4.

Point mutations within the catalytic core region of rat PDE4B1 resulted in phosphodiesterase species that were resistant to rolipram inhibition. Moroever, these point mutations did not show high affinity rolipram binding. In contrast, the modified enzymes demonstrated $K_M$ and $V_{MAX}$ values comparable to native rat PDE4B1 [88]. These findings reiterate the view that structural elements required for rolipram interaction with the phosphodiesterase 4 protein may be at least in part different from those required for cyclic AMP association [39].

## Phosphodiesterase 4C variants

cDNA encoding human PDE4C was first isolated from a substantia nigra cDNA library and transfection of PDE4C cDNA resulted in expression of corresponding PDE4 activity [89]. Northern blotting with PDE4C specific riboprobes and RT PCR with PDE4C specific oligonucleotide primers revealed that PDE4C is located in diverse human systems e.g. brain, liver, lung, heart. However, PDE4C was completely absent in peripheral blood leukocytes e.g. neutrophils, eosinophils, T cells, B-lymphocytes [89, 90]. Recently, cDNA from two different human PDE4C splice variants encompassing 791 and 426 amino acids have been isolated from human fetal lung cDNA library. Screening of human testis cDNA library revealed the presence of another splice variant. Proteins encoded by these three splice variants displayed PDE activity sensitive to phosphodiesterase 4 inhibitors. A fourth splice variant was identified in human testis mRNA. This variant lacked 55 amino acids in the catalytic domain and was inactive [91]. The significance of PDE4C splice variants remains to be investigated.

## Phosphodiesterase 4D variants

There are at least five splice variants of PDE4D. The variants PDE4D1 and PDE4D2 are short forms whereas PDE4D3-5 are long forms. PDE4D species were first detected in rat [92–94] and have now also been found in human tissue [58, 95]. PDE4D1-3 transcripts and corresponding PDE4D1 and PDE4D2 proteins were identified in human mononuclear cells [96, 97]. Other sources of human PDE4D variants are monocytes [7, 27], CD4+- and CD8+-T cells [7, 98], TH2-T lymphocytes [99], Jurkat T cells (PDE4D1 and 2) [100], B lymphocytes and eosinophils [7]. cDNA encoding human PDE4D1–5 has recently been isolated from HeLa cell cDNA libraries using riboprobes specific for PDE4D [101]. Transfection of cDNA in COS-7 cells resulted in the expression of five enzymatically active PDE4D species. The PDE4D variants obtained differed based on their subcellular distribution and inhibition by rolipram. Whereas the short forms PDE4D1 and PDE4D2 were exclusively cytosolic, the additional N-terminal extension in the long forms PDE4D3-5 conferred partial association to the particulate fraction (30–60% of total PDE4 protein). Rolipram inhibited all cytosolic PDE4D activities except PDE4D3 with comparable high potency ($IC_{50} \approx 50$–80 nM) accompanied by a shallow concentration-inhibition curve (Hill coefficient $n \approx 0.5$). In contrast, the log concentration inhibition curve for rolipram-induced inhibition of PDE4D3 activity was substantially more steep reflected by a Hill coefficient close to unity. Moreover, rolipram less potently depressed PDE4D3 activity ($IC_{50} \approx 140$ nM) compared to the other PDE4D species. Notably, particulate PDE4D5 activity is less sensitive to rolipram by a factor of ~7 than its cytosolic homologue. This rightward shift of the log concentration inhibition curve is accompanied by an increased curve steepness. These results may indicate that in this study PDE4D3 and particulate PDE4D5 predominantly form the LAR conformations, whereas other species are present in both LAR and HAR conformers. Recent work raised the hypothesis that protein kinase A - induced phosphorylation of PDE4D3 directs transition of the LAR into the HAR conformer [43]. If phosphorylation is the pivotal event that converts LAR into HAR it is conceivable that PDE4D3 is completely dephosphorylated in the ATP-deprived state of cell-free extracts and therefore, the LAR conformer predominates. In consequence the conclusion may be drawn that for PDE4D3 the proportion of HAR / LAR conformers is different in cell-free extracts compared to *in situ* conditions.

Deletion of an N-terminal end encompassing 121 amino acids from PDE4D1 resulted in a six-fold increase in $V_{MAX}$. These findings complement data obtained with PDE4A species where an inhibitory N-terminal end has also been described [102].

In summary, four different genes encode PDE4. mRNA-transcription from these genes results in a diversity of N-terminal splice variants. N-terminal ends are versatile tools that direct PDE4-localisation or association with other proteins or regulate PDE4 activity. Ultimately the diversity of N-terminal ends serves to translocate and regulate PDE4 activity in defined intracellular compartments where the enzyme affords precise regulation of cAMP and consequently, protein kinase A activity.

There is now ample evidence that PDE4A, 4B and 4D species are present in at least two different conformers. Rolipram binds and inhibits the PDE conformers with different potency. In contrast, RP73401 does not discriminate between the conformers. Rolipram and RP73401 act at the (catalytic) cAMP-binding site. These claims are supported by experimental results.

(i)   In standard assays rolipram shows high affinity binding to PDE4 but low affinity catalytic PDE4 inhibition. In most systems, log-dose inhibition curves for rolipram are shallow.
(ii)  High affinity rolipram binding sites have been localized on highly purified, recombinant PDE4 [40, 84, 103]
(iii) cAMP competitively inhibits [³H]rolipram and [³H]RP73401 binding to PDE4A [59, 103]

(iv) Rolipram binding to PDE4A reveals high and low affinity binding sites, whereas RP73401 binding kinetics would fit to a homogenous population of binding sites.

(v) $B_{MAX}$ for high affinity rolipram binding to PDE4A is about half the $B_{MAX}$ for RP73401 binding.

(iv) Convincing data suggest that PDE4B2 forms two conformers. One conformer shows high affinity rolipram binding sites and hence, is inhibited by low concentrations of rolipram. The other conformer is characterized by low affinity rolipram binding sites and is inhibited by higher concentrations of rolipram.

(v) Compared to other PDE4D variants rolipram exhibits less potency to suppress PDE4D3. On the other hand, log concentration inhibition curves for rolipram-inhibition of PDE4D3 are substantially steeper (Hill coefficient close to unity) compared to the other PDE4D species. This implies that under cell free conditions LAR represents the predominant conformation of PDE4D3.

Regarding standard assays of rolipram binding and catalytic inhibition it appears that rolipram binding detects HAR whereas catalytic inhibition visualizes predominantly the LAR conformation. However, both assays are conducted in cell free systems and the ultimate relevance of rolipram binding and catalytic inhibition *in situ* remains largely unknown.

Interaction of PDE4 inhibitors with LAR or HAR conformers correlates with different cellular responses. Whereas HAR correlates with behavioral effects, LAR may be more strongly associated with the gating of inflammatory responses.

## PDE4 regulation

Expression and activity of the diverse PDE4 variants is selectively regulated by a sophisticated network of cellular messengers. cAMP has been found to enhance mRNA transcription of certain PDE4 splice variants. In addition, some PDE4 variants may be subject to posttranslational modification such as protein kinase A dependent phosphorylation resulting in increased PDE4 activity. Phosphatidic acid has also been described to up-regulate enzyme activity of PDE4 species. PDE4 variants interact with tyrosine kinases or other SH3-domain comprising proteins which may modulate their catalytic activity (see previous section for discussion). In this chapter, regulation by enhanced mRNA transcription, phosphorylation and phosphatidic acid will be reviewed.

### cAMP-dependent transcriptional regulation of PDE4 subtypes

Up-regulation of PDE4 activity by long-term incubation with cAMP-increasing agents was detected almost two decades ago (Tab. 4). Incubation of rat Sertoli cells

Table 4 - Cell-specific cAMP-induced transcriptional up-regulation of PDE4 variants. Enhanced mRNA transcription for PDE4 variants by cAMP appears to depend on the cell-type indicating a role of cell-specific cofactors. In the case of PDE4D, the short forms PDE4D1 and PDE4D2 are transcriptionally up-regulated by cAMP. In contrast, the long-form PDE4D3 is resistant to this type of up-regulation. Instead, PDE4D3 activity is increased as a consequence of protein kinase A-dependent phosphorylation.

| Tissue | PDE isoenzyme | Reference |
|---|---|---|
| Rat brain | 4A | [124] |
| Rat Sertoli cells | 4D, 4B | [104], [113] |
| Rat aortic smooth muscle cells | 3/4 | [107] |
| U937 cells, human monocytes | 4A, 4B | [105], [61] |
| Mono Mac 6 cells | 4A, 4B, 4D | [70] |
| Guinea pig macrophages | 4 | [108] |
| HaCaT cells | 4 | [109] |
| Myoblasts | 4 | 110] |
| Rat PC12 cells | 4 | [111] |
| Jurkat cells | 3, 4D1, 4D2 | [100] |
| Myocardium | 1C, 4B | [123] |

with FSH, dibutyryl cAMP or 3-isobutyl-1-methylxanthine for several hours result-ed in an approximate 10-fold increase in PDE4 activity [104]. More recently it was found that 1 µM salbutamol in combination with 30 µM rolipram added to human monocytic U937 cells over 4 h induced an up to four-fold up-regulation of PDE4 [105]. These data were extended by findings that dibutyryl cAMP over 18-24 h induced a two to three-fold increase in PDE4 activity from human peripheral blood monocytes and human monocytic MonoMac6 cells [70]. Long-term cAMP-depen-dent up-regulation of PDE4 was also shown in other systems (summarized in Tab. 4), e.g. rat aortic vascular smooth muscle cells [106, 107], guinea pig macrophages [108], human keratinocyte HACAT cells [109], myoblast cell lines [110] and rat phaeochromocytoma (PC12) cells [111]. Protein kinase A inhibitors reversed long-term PDE4 upregulation which suggests that this process is mediat-ed by protein kinase A [109]. This hypothesis is further corroborated by data show-ing that L6 myoblasts expressing an inhibitory mutant of the regulatory subunit of protein kinase A were not capable of causing cAMP-dependent PDE4 up-regulation 110]. Regarding the mechanism of long-term cAMP-induced PDE4 up-regulation, it was found that incubation with cycloheximide or actinomycin D inhibited this up-regulation [104, 105, 109]. These results indicated that mRNA transcription and *de novo* protein synthesis were involved. In fact, following incubation of rat sertoli cells with FSH there was a time and concentration dependent increase in PDE4 mRNA [112] followed by augmented PDE4 protein and activity [113]. Later it was shown under identical experimental conditions that the amount of PDE4D mRNA transcripts increased, whereas the amount of PDE4B mRNA transcripts was less affected [113]. Identification of the amazing number of splice variants of PDE4A-D subtypes was paralleled by findings that some but not all splice variants were transcriptionally regulated by cAMP. Among the PDE4D splice variants, cAMP increased mRNA transcripts of the short forms PDE4D1 and PDE4D2. In contrast, mRNA transcription of the long form PDE4D3 was not affected by cAMP [114]. In human monocytic MonoMac-6 cells exposed to dibutyryl cAMP mRNA transcripts for PDE4A5, PDE4B2 and PDE4D1 increased [70]. Notably, although PDE4A5 represents a long form splice variant its mRNA transcription appears to be regulated by cAMP. These findings are corroborated by data obtained in human monocytic U-937 cells [90, 115] and human monocytes [61] where increases in PDE4A and PDE4B mRNA transcripts and protein were observed following long-term combined exposure to rolipram and salbutamol although in these cells PDE4D was not affected. On the other hand, incubation of Jurkat-T cells with forskolin augmented the amount of mRNA transcripts for PDE4D1 and PDE4D2 but also PDE3, whereas PDE4D3, PDE4D4, PDE4B and PDE4C were not affected and mRNA transcription of a PDE4A variant decreased [100]. The mechanism of cAMP-dependent up-regulation of PDE4D1-mRNA transcripts has recently been investigated [116]. An intronic, cAMP-responsive promoter region has been identified in the PDE4D gene. Activation of this 5' upstream intronic promoter region directs transcription of truncated mRNA products from the PDE4D gene – the short forms PDE4D1 and PDE4D2. A TATA-box was not detected in this promoter sequence but instead GC-rich regions were found which may also serve to signal the transcription start site. RNAse protection assays revealed at least two cap sites for transcription initiation. DNA-sequence encompassing 1500 bp 5' upstream of the translation start site coupled to a luciferase reporter gene resulted in ~five-fold activation of baseline luciferase expression. cAMP further increased luciferase expression in this construct by a factor of ~4.5. These results demonstrated that the intron 5' upstream of the PDE4D1 open reading frame acts as promoter and confers cAMP responsiveness. A cAMP response element (CRE) was identified in the 5' untranslated region of the transcribed PDE4D1 mRNA. No further CRE were detected up to 1500 bp 5'upstream of the translation initiation site. However, deletion of a region comprising the CRE within the 1500 bp 5' upstream of the translation initiation site resulted in a fragmented promoter that still conferred cAMP-inducibility of a luciferase reporter gene. Hence, cAMP may act to increase PDE4D1 mRNA transcription by mechanisms independent from CREB-induced CRE activation. AP-consensus sites have been identified upstream of the proximal cap site and there is evidence that cAMP may be capable of amplifying AP-mediated transcription. In fact, c-fos expression, AP-binding to DNA and AP-directed transcription of reporter genes may be enhanced by cAMP [117–119]. In view of these findings the observation may be of interest that TPA – a potent stimulus of AP-induced transcription – synergistically potentiated cAMP-induced luciferase expression directed by the PDE4D1 promoter [116]. In parallel to PDE4D1, mRNA transcription of PDE4B2 is also regulated by a cAMP-responsive intronic promoter. However, this promoter includes a TATA-box that confers efficient baseline mRNA transcription [116]. A more rapid cAMP-responsive up-regulation of PDE4B2 mRNA compared to PDE4D1 mRNA was observed in human monocytic MonoMac 6 cells [70].

## Heterologous desensitization by PDE4 up-regulation

cAMP-dependent transcriptional regulation of PDE4 may cause heterologous desensitization of cellular responses induced by $\beta_2$-agonists or other cAMP-generating drugs. In human monocytic U-937 cells exposed to rolipram in combination with salbutamol over 4 h, $PGE_2$-induced cAMP accumulation was dramatically reduced compared to control cells. The additional presence of rolipram restored this impaired cAMP accumulation indicating that it was operated by PDE4 up-regulation. In parallel, the capacity of $PGE_2$ to suppress monocytic $LTD_4$-induced $Ca^{2+}$-mobilisation was substantially reduced in U937 cells exposed to salbutamol and rolipram for 4 h compared to control cells. Again, rolipram reversed this functional desensitization [115]. An impaired capacity for cellular cAMP accumulation as a consequence of protracted cAMP elevation has also been shown in Jurkat-T lymphocytes [120], rat aortic smooth muscle cells [107] and the human keratinocyte HaCaT cells [109]. In these systems, cAMP-dependent PDE4 up-regulation based on *de novo* protein synthesis has been shown and PDE inhibitors could reverse the concomitant desensitization of cAMP accumulation.

Heterologous desensitisation following prolonged administration of $\beta_2$-agonists may have therapeutic implications in asthma [121]. In asthmatics, regular treatment with $\beta_2$-agonists resulted in tachyphylaxis to their protective effects against methacholine- or AMP-induced bronchoconstriction [1–4]. Although part of these effects may originate in $\beta$-receptor desensitisation, the hypothesis was raised that PDE4 up-regulation may also be involved [121]. Future clinical trials may investigate whether PDE inhibitors e.g. theophylline restore the impaired bronchoprotective effects of $\beta_2$-agonists caused by their regular administration.

cAMP-dependent transcriptional regulation of PDE4 may drive the cardioprotective effects of prostacyclin in the ischaemic myocardium. In an experimental approach, hearts removed from rats pretreated intramuscularly with 7-oxo $PGI_2$ for 48 h exhibited a substantially impaired inotropic reponse to isoproterenol associated with reduced isoproterenol-induced cAMP accumulation compared to sham-treated animals. Whereas the capacity of the cAMP-generating system was found to be unaffected, exposure of intact rats to 7-oxo $PGI_2$ induced a marked alteration in the pattern of myocardial PDE subtypes. Strong increases in PDE1C and PDE4E3 transcripts were described accompanied by reduced expression of PDE4D1–3 species. These alterations in PDE transcripts were paralleled by changes in protein levels and by increased PDE4 and PDE1 activities [122, 123]. The increased PDE1C expression induced by 7-oxo prostacyclin may limit $Ca^{2+}$-induced myocardial damage by enhancing $Ca^{2+}$-dependent down-modulation of myocardial cAMP. Other experiments demonstrated that pharmacologically induced impaired or activated noradrenergic signalling in the intact rat is associated with reduced or enhanced PDE4A protein, respectively in cerebral cortex [124]. These latter studies with intact animals provide convincing evidence for the physiological relevance of cAMP-operated transcriptional PDE4 up-regulation.

## Protein kinase A-induced phosphorylation and up-regulation of PDE4

A substantial but transient increase in cAMP content of U937 cells is induced by salbutamol or $PGE_2$. In fact, cAMP levels returned to baseline after 15 min exposure to salbutamol or $PGE_2$. However, the combination of salbutamol with rolipram exerts a profound cAMP increase lasting over > 4 h [42, 105]. Desensitization of the cAMP-generating system may provide an explanation for these findings. Alternatively, a short-term up-regulation of PDE4 may be involved. This hypothesis is particularly supported by the marked protracted cAMP increase induced by the addition of rolipram. Indeed, Torphy and colleagues [105] observed a significant increase of PDE4 activity after only 15 min incubation of U937 cells with $PGE_2$ (10 µM) or salbutamol (10 µM). Corroborating these data, PDE4 in human keratinocyte HaCaT cells was significantly up-regulated after 30 min incubation with rolipram (10 µM) and salbutamol (1 µM) and PDE4 up-regulation was only partly inhibited by cycloheximide [109]. In addition, the PDE4 activity increase following incubation of rat thyroid FRTL-5 cells with TSH, dibutyryl cAMP or forskolin over 10–15 min was resistant to cycloheximide, supporting the concept that short-term PDE4 up-regulation was independent from *de novo* protein synthesis [125]. On the other hand, the phosphatase inhibitor okadaic acid enhanced PDE4 up-regulation in FRTL-5 cells and in consequence the concept arose that short-term cAMP-induced increase in PDE4 activity may be driven by PDE4 phosphorylation. Indeed, protein kinase A phosphorylates PDE4 which was paralleled by an increase in PDE4 activity in rat thyroid FRTL-5 cells [43, 125] and human monocytic U937 cells [42]. Protein kinase A-induced short-term up-regulation of PDE4 activity has also been described in rat parotid tissue [126], UMR-106 osteoblast like cells [127], LRM 55 astroglial cells [128] or bovine vascular smooth muscle cells [129] indicating that PDE4 activity regulation by cAMP-mediated phosphorylation represents an ubiquitous event. However, protein kinase A-triggered PDE4 phopshorylation is restricted to particular splice variants. As an example, within the PDE4D subfamily PKA phosphorylates the long form PDE4D3 but not the short forms PDE4D1 and PDE4D2 [42, 43, 125]. Meanwhile, based on elegant experiments using site directed mutagenesis, Sette and Conti [43] discovered that protein-kinase A mediated PDE4D3 activity increase is associated with phosphorylation of serine 54 at the N-terminal end of the enzyme. In fact, substitution of serine 54 by alanine completely abolished phosphorylation and PDE-activity increase. Furthermore, as a consequence of protein kinase A-triggered phosphorylation of PDE4D3, altered sensitivity of the enzyme to PDE4 inhibitors occurred. RS-25344, a highly specific PDE4 inhibitor blocked activity of the phosphorylated PDE4D3 form with ~100-fold higher potency than the non-phosphorylated enzyme [42]. From experiments with rolipram the hypothesis was raised that PDE4D3 phosphorylation tips the balance of HAR to LAR conformers in favour of the HAR conformer [43]. Careful analysis of log concentration inhibition curves revealed that rolipram displayed high ($IC_{50} \sim 1$ nM) and low ($IC_{50} \sim 1$ µM) affinity inhibition of basal PDE4D3 catalytic activity. These $IC_{50}$ values are close to those obtained for rolipram binding to HAR and LAR. Phosphorylation-induced PDE4D3 activity increment was almost entirely based on an increase in the PDE activity that was inhibited by low nanomolar rolipram concentrations. In contrast, activity of the PDE4D3 conformer inhibited by micromolar rolipram concentrations was not affected. These findings imply an increase in HAR conformation induced by PDE4D3 phosphorylation. Rolipram log concentration-inhibition curves suggest that 72% of basal PDE4D3 assumes the LAR conformer with the remaining 28% in the HAR state. In contrast, regarding the phosphorylated PDE4D3 62% of the enzyme forms the HAR state with only 38% in the LAR conformation [43]. In view of the concept that anti-inflammatory effects of PDE4 inhibitors are related to LAR whereas unwanted CNS effects are based on their interaction with HAR those PDE4 inhibitors which lock PDE4D3 in the non-phosphorylated state should provide anti-inflammatory drugs with reduced side-effects.

## Regulation of PDE4 activity by phosphatidic acid

Phosphatidic acid (PA) was found to up-regulate PDE4 activity of some but not all variants, most probably based on a direct interaction. In particular, incubation of the long forms PDE4A5, PDE4B2 and PDE4D3 with PA resulted in a 1.5–2-fold up-regulation of PDE4 activity. On the other hand, activities of the short forms PDE4B2, PDE4D1 and PDE4D2 were not affected. PA-induced PDE4 up-regulation may facilitate Con-A stimulated proliferation of rat thymocytes [130, 131].

## Candidate PDE4 inhibitors as antiasthmatics

Based on the fact that PDE4 was localized in almost all inflammatory cells and also in bronchial smooth muscle, and that PDE4 inhibitors have the capacity to suppress diverse inflammatory cell functions, it was anticipated that PDE4 inhibitors would be potent anti-asthmatic drugs. As discussed before, although an abundance of PDE4 inhibiting structures were synthesized and exhibited anti-inflammatory potency *in vitro* and in experimental animals none of them has been licensed or reached phase III clinical trials mainly due to intolerable CNS side-effects. In fact, definite proof of antiasthmatic potency of PDE4 inhibitors in large-scale controlled clinical studies is still awaited. However, based on the concept that a beneficial ratio of LAR/HAR inhibition should improve the benefit-risk ratio there are some promising PDE4 inhibitors which recently reached phase I or II clinical trials. These compounds designed in consideration of the LAR/HAR-concept have been denominated as "second generation PDE4 inhibitors". Chemical structures of the compounds are depicted in Figure 1. Affinity ratios to HAR and LAR of these compounds related to rolipram are given in Table 5.

### SB207499 (Ariflo®)

SB207499 (Ariflo®) represents a second generation PDE4 inhibitor. The potency ratios for inhibition of the HAR vs LAR conformers of PDE4A, PDE4B2 and PDE4D3 are at least four-fold higher than for rolipram implying that SB207499 in comparison to rolipram preferentially inhibits PDE4 in its LAR conformer (see also Tab. 5). Whereas rolipram inhibits the HAR conformer of all PDE4 variants tested with at least 20-fold higher potency than the LAR conformers, SB204799 inhibits the LAR conformer of PDE4A with two-fold higher potency than its HAR conformer and for PDE4B2 and PDE4D3 inhibition of HAR was only about two-fold and five-fold more potent than for LAR. In fact, binding experiments revealed that SB207499 adhered to a two-fold higher number of binding sites on PDE4 than rolipram. This finding reiterates that SB207499 has the capacity to bind to both HAR and LAR [41].

This distinct profile of SB207499 affinity to the PDE4 conformers is reflected by its *in vitro* effects. SB207499 inhibits T cell proliferation and monocyte TNFα generation with comparable potency as rolipram. This is in accordance with earlier findings that inhibition of these inflammatory functions is mediated by LAR. In contrast, SB207499 proves to be ~160-fold less potent than rolipram in attenuating gastric gland acid secretion [132]. On the other hand, anti-IgE induced basophil degranulation was clearly more potently inhibited by rolipram than by SB207499 and this implies that similar to neutrophil degranulation, inhibition of basophil degranulation requires blocking of the HAR conformer. The compound is currently being clinically tested as an oral anti-asthmatic drug.

Table 5 - Inhibition of HAR and LAR by PDE4 inhibitors.

PDE4 inhibitors may be distinguished by their affinities to the two PDE4 conformers. $IC_{50}$ [µM] values for inhibition of catalysis ($IC_{50}$) reflecting affinity to LAR as well as for inhibition of [$^3$H]rolipram binding (RB) reflecting affinity to HAR are given. Results from different authors (references in brackets) are documented. The relative ratios were calculated from the ratios $IC_{50}$/RB for each of the compounds related to 100% which was defined as the ratio $IC_{50}$/RB for rolipram. It becomes evident that particularly SB207499, CDP840, RP73401 and benafentrine exhibit preferential affinity to LAR compared to rolipram, Ro-201724, denbufylline or RS25344.

| | [27] | | [34] | | [133] | | [37] | | relative ratio | | | |
| | $IC_{50}$ | RB | $IC_{50}$ | RB | $IC_{50}$ | RB | $IC_{50}$ | RB | [27] | [34] | [133] | [37] |
|---|---|---|---|---|---|---|---|---|---|---|---|---|
| Rolipram | 0.31 | 0.0017 | 0.103 | 0.005 | 2.2 | 0.006 | 0.63 | 0.007 | 100 | 100 | 100 | 100 |
| Ro 20-1724 | 2.4 | 0.0170 | | | | | 9.34 | 0.1 | 77 | | | 104 |
| Denbufylline | 0.2 | 0.0041 | 0.123 | 0.019 | | | 0.54 | 0.021 | 27 | 31 | | 28.6 |
| CDP840 | | | 0.007 | 0.06 | 0.143 | 0.008 | | | | 0.6 | 4.8 | |
| SB207499 | | | 0.05 | 0.077 | 0.149 | 0.077 | | | | 3.2 | 0.5 | |
| RP 73401 | 0.0012 | 0.0004 | 0.0005 | 0.005 | 0.008 | 0.001 | | | 1.6 | 0.5 | 2.1 | |
| CP80366 | | | | | 0.5 | 0.008 | | | | | 16.7 | |
| RS25344 | | | 0.011 | 0.001 | | | | | | 53 | | |
| Zardaverine | | | | | | | 1.11 | 0.45 | | | | 2.7 |
| Benzafentrine | | | | | | | 2.19 | 7.5 | | | | 0.3 |

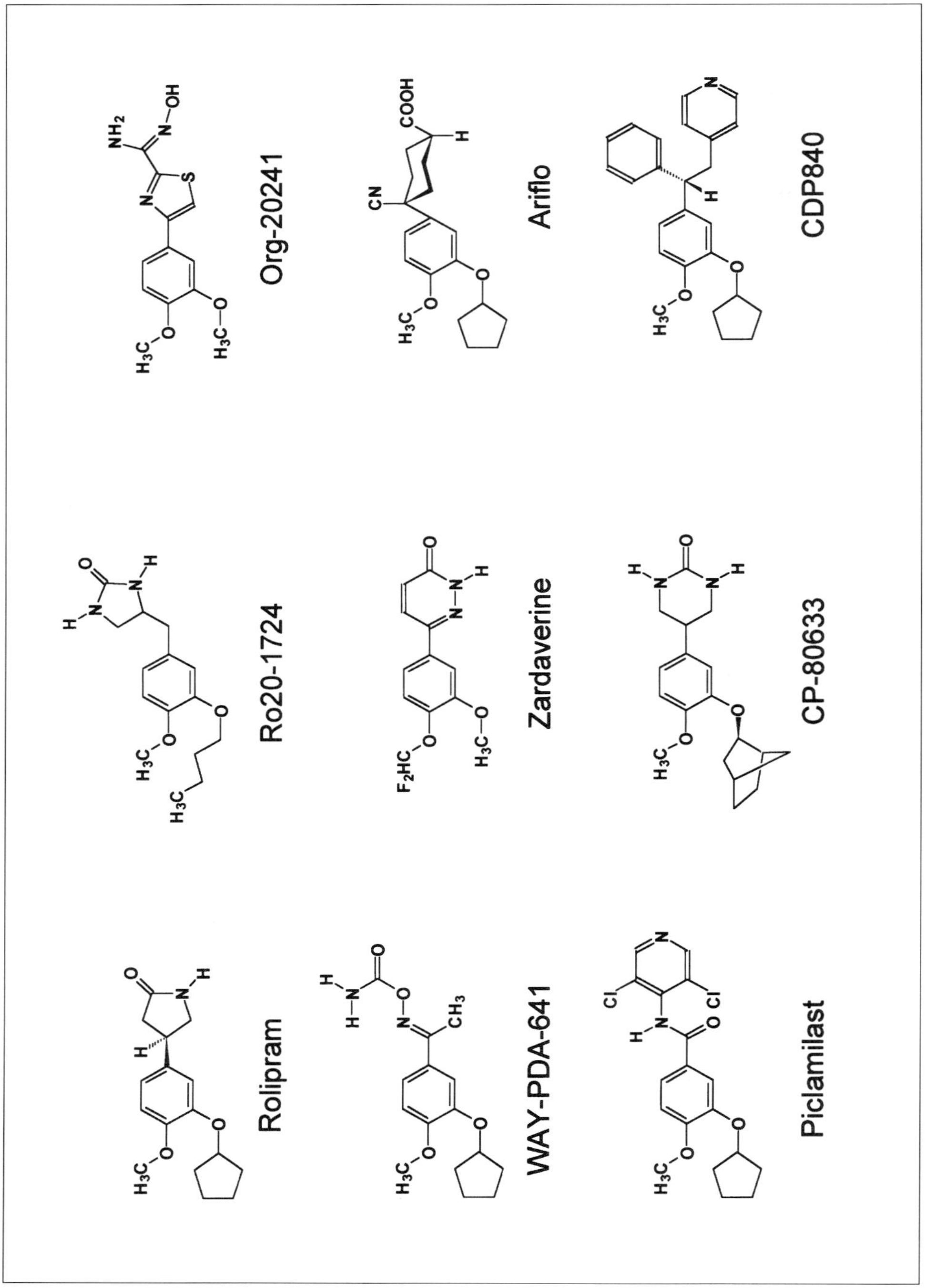

Org-20241

Ariflo

CDP840

Ro20-1724

Zardaverine

CP-80633

Rolipram

WAY-PDA-641

Piclamilast

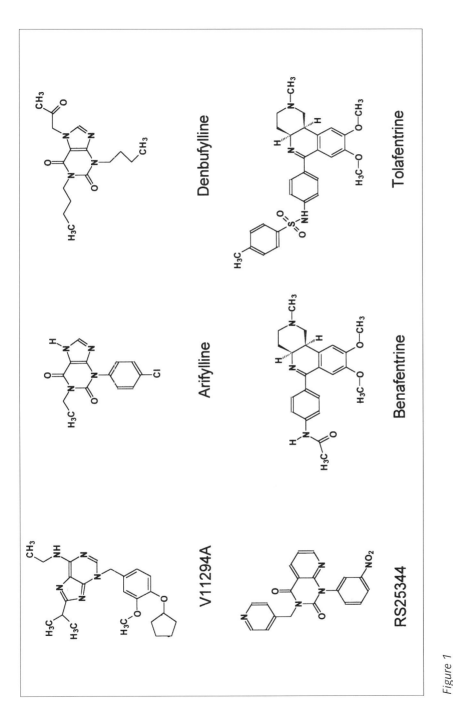

Figure 1

*Chemical structures of PDE4 inhibitors. Zardaverine, tolafentrine, benafentrine and Org-20241 are dual-selective PDE3&4 inhibitors. The other compounds are selective inhibitors of PDE4. Most structures are related to rolipram e.g. piclamilast (RP73401), ariflo (SB207499), CP-80633, WAY-PDA-641, CDP840 or V11284A. Tolafentrine and benafentrine are benzonaphthyridines.*

## CDP840

CDP840 was shown to suppress PDE4 hydrolysing capacity of subtypes A, B and D with comparable potency ($IC_{50}$ = 2.9–4.3 nM) whereas the compound inhibited PDE4C ~25-fold less potently. In addition, CDP840 was less efficient in competing for [$^3$H]rolipram binding to guinea pig brain membranes ($IC_{50}$ = 60 nM) than in inhibiting PDE4 activity (Tab. 5). CDP840 had a fairly high oral bioavailability. These findings should predict a favorable profile of CDP840 [34]. However, other recent investigations came to different conclusions based on their findings that CDP840 inhibited catalytic PDE4 activity (reflecting LAR) less potently than the compound competed with [$^3$H]rolipram binding to brain membranes [133]. In the above studies, competition of [$^3$H]rolipram binding has not been measured with the recombinant human PDE4 variants that served for determination of PDE4 catalysis but with guinea pig and mice brain membranes. The discrepancy between the two studies emphasizes that PDE4 catalysis and [$^3$H]rolipram-binding should be assessed with identical human recombinant PDE4 variants.

In animal models CDP840 mostly given by the intraperitoneal route has been shown to reduce antigen-induced pulmonary eosinophil accumulation and bronchoconstriction and to attenuate ozone-triggered airway hyperreactivity [34, 134–136]. Finally, in mild-moderate asthmatic humans CDP840 given orally at a daily dose of 30 mg over 10 days significantly suppressed late airway obstruction to allergen challenge. An oral dose of 30 mg/day was well tolerated as reflected by the absence of adverse events [137]. However, development of CDP840 was discontinued.

## CP80366

CP80633 inhibits PDE4A, B and D with comparable $IC_{50}$ values (0.3–0.5 µM), whereas [$^3$H]rolipram binding to brain membranes is competed at substantially lower concentrations (8 nM) (Tab. 5) [133]. Therefore, CP80633 does not represent a second generation PDE4 inhibitor. The compound stimulated $PGE_1$-facilitated cAMP increase in human monocytes, inhibited LPS-triggered human monocytic TNFα-generation and zymosan-stimulated human eosinophil ROS release with $IC_{50}$ values close to those required for suppression of catalysis [133]. The capacity of CP-80633 to counteract allergen-challenge induced bronchoconstriction and bronchoalveolar cellular infiltration in animal models further adds to the anti-inflammatory profile of the compound. In another system it was found that CP-80633 given by the oral route (10 mg/kg) to mice elevated plasma cAMP by a factor of 6 and inhibited LPS-induced systemic TNFα production by 95% [138]. The compound has been tested in phase II trials in patients with atopic dermatitis. It was found that topical application of CP-80633 over 28 days significantly reduced skin inflammation in these patients. Oral administration of CP80633 to humans resulted in emesis at plasma concentrations above 0.16 µg/ml [139].

## RP73401

The benzamide RP73401 (Piclamilast) was the first described second generation PDE4 inhibitor. In fact, in the catalytic assay (reflecting LAR) RP73401 suppressed human recombinant PDE4D3 with $IC_{50}$ of 0.1 nM and the benzamide exhibited a comparable affinity to PDE4D3 ($K_d = 0.08$ nM) as determined in the [$^3$H]RP73401 binding assay (reflecting HAR). RP73401 attenuated catalytic activity of PDE4A and PDE4B with comparable efficacy as PDE4D and competed for [$^3$H]rolipram binding to brain membranes with $IC_{50} = 1$ nM i.e. in the range of PDE4 catalysis inhibition [34, 41, 133]. In conclusion, RP73401 does not discriminate between the HAR and LAR conformers whereas in contrast rolipram exhibits clear preference for the HAR conformer (Table 5).

*In vitro*, RP73401 enhanced $\beta_2$-agonist facilitated eosinophil and monocyte cAMP increase and consequently inhibited eosinophil $LTC_4$ and ROS generation, eosinophil degranulation [20, 77, 140], LPS-induced TNFα expression in human monocytes [27], and IL-2 release from *Staph. aureus* enterotoxin stimulated CD3-differentiated splenocytes [29] in the lower nanomalor range. Rolipram was substantially less potent than RP73401 in attenuating monocyte TNFα generation and splenocyte differentiation, reiterating that these functional responses are inhibited by interaction with the LAR (where rolipram is less potent than RP73401) rather than the HAR conformer (where rolipram shows comparable potency to RP73401) of PDE4 (Tab. 5). On the other hand RP73401 counteracted methacholine-induced contraction of guinea pig trachea which is considered as an HAR-correlated response [38] (Tab. 2) in a dose range comparable to rolipram [46]. In animal models of airway inflammation RP73401 given by the intratracheal route dose-dependently inhibited antigen-induced bronchoconstriction and bronchoalveolar inflammatory cell influx. In addition, RP73401 counteracted histamine-induced microvascular leakage into the guinea pig lung [141]. The compound is currently being developed for rheumatoid arthritis [139].

## Phosphodiesterase 3

PDE3 is also described as the cGMP-inhibited PDE activity. In fact, although PDE3 exhibits similar affinity for cAMP and cGMP as substrates ($K_M = 0.1$–0.8 µM), the $V_{MAX}$ for cAMP is about 4–10 times higher compared to cGMP. Abundant PDE3 activity is found in the myocardium where it may be tightly associated with the sarcoplasmic reticulum. Therefore, there was considerable interest from the pharmaceutical industry in developing selective PDE3 inhibitors as inotropics in chronic heart failure (CHF) culminating in the clinical development of amrinone, milrinone and enoximone. Whilst these compounds have meanwhile been licensed in some regions for acute treatment of otherwise refractory CHF where they result in some improvement of systemic haemodynamics, its chronic administration has been discouraged based on clinical trials demonstrating a variety of haemodynamic adverse events and finally, increased mortality [142–144]. Indeed, in the severely damaged ischemic myocardium cAMP increase may facilitate the generation of arrhythmias.

So far two different PDE3 subtypes encoded by different genes have been identified. PDE3A is located on chromosome 12 and PDE3B on chromosome 11 [145]. PDE3A and PDE3B have a different cellular expression pattern. PDE3A is predominantly found in myocardium, vasculature, bronchial smooth muscle, platelets. In contrast, human lymphocytes [146] but also adipocytes, hepatocytes, pancreatic B cells and renal epithelial cells [145] contain PDE3B. Hence, the hypothesis arises that selective inhibition of PDE3B should support anti-inflammatory effects without cardiovascular adverse effects.

Subtypes are distinguished by a 44 amino acid insert in the N-terminal end of the catalytic core which is highly homologous for one subtype among different species but shows substantially less homology if the two subtypes are compared. This 44 amino acid insert is unique for PDE3 species. Binding of PDE3 selective inhibitors is exclusively mediated by the catalytic domain since it is not affected by either N-terminal mutants or site directed mutants in the 44 amino acid insert [147]. The N-terminal region contains a hydrophobic site that directs membrane association. Expression of full-length human recombinant PDE3A and PDE3B in SF9 cells results in membrane associated PDE3 activity. On the other hand, expression of PDE3 forms truncated at their N-terminal end results in predominant cytosolic expression [148]. It is not known so far whether the platelet PDE3A species which is cytosolic represents a splice variant that omits the hydrophobic membrane association region. The occurrence of multiple splice products from PDE3A has been proposed based on the use of different initiation sites in the PDE3A gene [149]. The N-terminal region also comprises the protein kinase A phosphorylation site. In rat adipocytes PDE3B serine 302 has been identified as a target for PKA-induced phosphorylation [150]. PKA-induced phosphorylation is associated with up-regulation of PDE3 activity. In addition to phosphorylation, transcriptional regulation of PDE3 has been observed. In Jurkat cells, chronic cAMP-exposure resulted in a biphasic PDE3 up-regulation [100]. The initial PDE3 increase based on phosphorylation whereas the later PDE3 up-regulation was reversed by prior incubation with actinomycin D indicating that enhanced mRNA transcription was involved. Exposure of vascular smooth muscle cells in culture to forskolin or 8-bromo cAMP also enhanced PDE3 activity based on *de novo* protein synthesis [107]. In an animal model of pulmonary hypertension induced by chronic hypoxia there was an up-regulation of PDE3A paralleled by an elevation of the corresponding mRNA detected by Northern blot technique [151].

PDE3 occurs in macrophages and T lymphocytes, endothelial cells, mast cells, bronchial and vascular smooth muscle cells. Selective PDE3 inhibitors may have some functional effects in animal models relevant to asthma. In particular, selective PDE3 inhibitors may cause bronchodilation as a consequence of the occurrence of PDE3 in human bronchi. In fact, it was found that the selective PDE3 inhibitor SKF94120 reduced the basal tone of human bronchial rings [152]. In a clinical setting, the PDE3 selective inhibitor cilostazol attenuated methacholine-induced bronchial hyperresponsiveness [153].

Whilst exclusive inhibition of PDE3 does not represent a promising strategy for drug development in asthma the fact that additional inhibition of PDE3 frequently amplifies the effects of PDE4 inhibitors implies that dual selective type PDE3 and 4 inhibitors could be an attractive concept in asthma-related drug discovery. This may be of particular interest since compounds such as benafentrine interact predominantly with LAR (Tab. 5). In the last section of this chapter, synergisms between PDE3 and PDE4 inhibition will be briefly discussed.

## Synergistic and additive effects of PDE3 and 4 inhibition

PDE3 and PDE4 inhibitors may act synergistically to enhance intracellular cAMP and consequently, to modulate functional responses in cells orchestrating the inflammatory response (Fig. 2). Quiescent human peripheral blood CD4+ and CD8+-T lymphocytes expressed PDE3B [145], PDE4A, PDE4B and PDE4D and PDE7. On the other hand, PDE1, PDE2 and PDE5 were absent in these cells [98, 154, 155]. Following PHA stimulation for several hours however, there was an induction of PDE1B [10]. PDE3 inhibitors, whilst almost inactive by themselves, synergistically enhanced reduction of T lymphocyte proliferation and IL-2 generation by inhibition of PDE4. 100 nM rolipram inhibited PHA-induced [3H]thymidine incorporation in human CD4+-T lymphocytes by about 20%. The selective PDE3 inhibitor SKF95654 (10 µM) did not affect [3H]thymidine incorporation. Adding 10 µM SKF95654 to 100 nM rolipram resulted in about 50% reduction of PHA-induced [3H]thymidine incorporation. Similarly, addition of 10 µM SKF95654 which by itself did not affect IL-2 generation to 10 nM rolipram that induced 25% inhibition of IL-2 synthesis resulted in 60% reduction of PHA-induced IL-2-generation in CD4+-T lymphocytes [98].

In human alveolar macrophages there is coexpression of PDE1, PDE3 and PDE4 [9]. Rolipram or the PDE3-selective inhibitor motapizone suppressed LPS-stimulated TNFα generation dose-dependently following biphasic log concentration inhibition curves. These biphasic curves reflect functional effects of selective PDE3 or PDE4 inhibition at lower inhibitor concentrations, whereas at higher con-

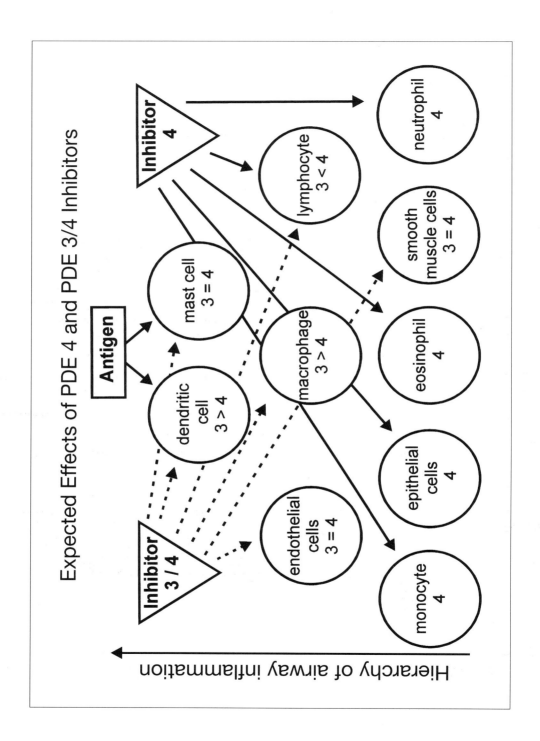

centrations rolipram or motapizone lost their selectivity and additionally inhibited other isoenzymes. At concentrations < 1 µM motapizone synergistically amplified the reduction of TNFα release induced by rolipram [156]. These data were corroborated by findings that in human monocyte-derived macrophages LPS-stimulated TNFα generation was synergistically reduced by exposure to a combination of PDE3 and 4 inhibitors (40–50% reduction) when compared to each of the selective inhibitors alone (< 15% reduction) [8]. Monocyte-derived macrophages showed a PDE isoenzyme profile comparable to human alveolar macrophages; PDE1, 3 and 4 were expressed [8]. In contrast, LPS-induced TNFα synthesis in human monocytes (i.e. the precursor cells of monocyte derived macrophages) was almost completely inhibited by rolipram reflecting the predominant expression of PDE4 in these cells [8].

Rolipram synergistically enhanced inhibition of serum-stimulated [³H]thymidin incorporation into vascular smooth muscle cells by the PDE3 inhibitor cilostamide [157]. With 1 µM cilostamide and 10 µM rolipram, [³H]thymidine incorporation was attenuated by about 25% and 20%, respectively. Combined administration resulted in 80% reduction. Rat aortic rings precontracted with phenylephrine showed less than 20% relaxation to either 3 µM milrinone (PDE3 selective) or 10 µM rolipram. However, the combined inhibition of PDE3 and PDE4 by these compounds resulted in > 90% relaxation. Human pulmonary artery precontracted with $PGF_{2\alpha}$ did not respond to 1 µM rolipram. Exposure to 1 µM motapizone (selective PDE3 inhibitor) induced about 30% relaxation. However, 1 µM rolipram was synergistic to 1 µM motapizone resulting in 75% relaxation [158]. Similarly, in human bronchi, combined exposure to rolipram and the PDE3-selective inhibitor SKF94120 showed a trend for overadditive reduction of inherent airway tone [152].

*Figure 2*

*Targets of PDE4 and PDE3/4 inhibitors. A multitude of cells are involved in airway inflammation. Dendritic cells function as antigen presenting cells whereas antigen directly activates mast cells. Lymphocytes orchestrate airway inflammation. Eosinophils or neutrophils predominantly constitute terminal effector cells i.e. cytotoxic proteins (ECP, EDN) are released as a consequence of eosinophil activation. Smooth muscle cells may not only exhibit a contractile phenotype but they may also assume proliferative, motile or synthetic (cytokine producing) phenotypes. Epithelial and endothelial cells generate a multitude of cytokines and other mediators apart form their barrier function. Terminal effector cells e.g. eosinophils exclusively express PDE4. On the other hand in cells orchestrating inflammation e.g. T-lymphocytes or in antigen-presenting cells e.g. dendritic cells PDE3 and PDE4 are detected. In these cells selective PDE4 inhibitors partially but not completely inhibit functional responses. However, complete inhibition is attained by dual-selective PDE3&4 inhibitors. Dual-selective PDE3&4 inhibitors are therefore an attractive approach in asthma management.*

cAMP-dependent transcriptional and post-translational up-regulation (PKA-dependent phosphorylation) of PDE3 and PDE4 may be one explanation for the synergistic functional effects of PDE3 and PDE4 inhibitors. One may postulate that exclusive selective inhibition of PDE3 may provide a cAMP-signal that phosphorylates PDE4 or stimulates transcription of PDE4 mRNA. Increased PDE4 activity masks functional effects of PDE3 inhibitors by down-regulating cAMP. Simultaneous PDE4 inhibition would then result in synergistic cAMP response and functional effect.

Synergisms between PDE3 and PDE4 inhibitors and the occurrence of both PDE3 and PDE4 in diverse cellular systems involved in asthma were decisive for the design of dual-delective PDE3 and 4 inhibitors. Preclinical and some clinical experience with the dual-selective inhibitors zardaverine, AH21-132 and tolafentrine will be briefly reviewed.

## Zardaverine

The pyridazinone derivative zardaverine inhibited PDE3 from human platelets and PDE4 from human neutrophils with $IC_{50}$ values of 0.6 and 0.2 µM, respectively [159]. Other isoenzymes were hardly affected up to 100 µM. Zardaverine inhibited human monocyte PDE4 with $IC_{50}$ 1.1 µM. For competition of zardaverine with [$^3$H]rolipram binding to rat brain membranes an $IC_{50}$ of 0.45 µM was calculated (Tab. 5) [37]. However, zardaverine more strongly inhibited [$^3$H]rolipram binding to PDE4 of human origin. Zardaverine counteracted the contraction of guinea pig trachea in response to a variety of spasmogens (e.g. histamine, ovalbumin, U46619, and $LTC_4$) [160]. In addition, zardaverine potently reduced endogenous tone of isolated human bronchi [152]. In the anaesthesized guinea pig zardaverine given intravenously (1–60 µmol/kg) inhibited histamine induced bronchoconstriction, and following oral application (1–100 µmol/kg) attenuated acetylcholine- or ovalbumin-induced dyspnoea [160]. In the rat, oral zardaverine (3–30 µmol/kg) shows bronchodilator activity [161].

Zardaverine protects against a multitude of inflammatory responses (for review refer to [162]). In particular, zardaverine inhibited LPS-stimulated $TNF\alpha$ release from human alveolar macrophages and human T lymphocyte proliferation with monophasic log concentration-inhibition curves, corresponding to $IC_{50}$ values of 1.85 and 1.7 µM, respectively [156]. Zardaverine inhibited the increase in endothelial permeability of HUVEC (human umbilical vein endothelial cell) monolayers induced by thrombin or E. coli haemolysin and this effect was further accentuated in combination with adenylate cyclase activators [163]. In cultured porcine pulmonary artery endothelial cells, zardaverine at concentrations up to 10 µM had no effect on $H_2O_2$-induced endothelial hyperpermeability. Endothelial cells from porcine pulmonary artery expressed PDE1, 2, 3 and 4, and PDE3 and 4 should have been strongly inhibited by 10 μM zardaverine. However, in the presence of 1 μM $PGE_1$ that was inactive on its own, 10 nM zardaverine completely inhibited $H_2O_2$-induced increase in endothelial permeability. Hence, $PGE_1$ synergistically potentiated the efficacy of zardaverine by a factor of > 10,000. In addition, in the presence of $PGE_1$, synergistic suppression of endothelial hyperpermeability by combined PDE3 and PDE4 inhibition may be deduced from the experimental findings. 10 nM rolipram or 10 nM motapizone did not reduce the $H_2O_2$-induced increase in endothelial permeability in the presence of 1 μM $PGE_1$. However, 10 nM zardaverine completely inhibited $H_2O_2$-induced increased endothelial permeability. 10 nM zardaverine afforded only ~10% inhibition of PDE3 and 4 which is less than the extent of PDE3 and 4 inhibition obtained by combining 10 nM rolipram and 10 nM motapizone (25% inhibition) [164].

Provided salbutamol (1 μM) was present, zardaverine inhibited C5a-stimulated human eosinophil degranulation and chemoluminescence with $IC_{50}$ values (0.4–0.9 μM) in the range of those obtained for PDE3 and PDE4 inhibition. In contrast, zardaverine up to 10 μM was inactive when salbutamol was absent [20]. On the other hand zardaverine attenuated fMLP-stimulated human eosinophil $LTC_4$ synthesis in the absence of salbutamol ($IC_{50} = 0.3$ μM) [140].

The finding that cAMP-triggered inhibition of some functional responses (e.g. eosinophil $LTC_4$ generation) is operated by PDE inhibition alone whereas reduction of other responses (e.g. eosinophil degranulation, endothelial hyperpermeability) requires the additional presence of an adenylate cyclase enhancing stimulus merits attention. The following explanations may be provided. Firstly, cAMP-triggered modulation of different functional responses may require different thresholds of protein kinase A activation. Secondly, cells and membrane compartments may differ regarding their expression of "high cycling" and "low cycling" adenylate cyclase subtypes. "High cycling" adenylate cyclase offers high baseline cAMP generation whereas "low cycling" adenylate cyclase elaborates less cAMP under baseline conditions. It appears evident that coincidence of "low cycling" conditions with a high threshold of PKA-activation requires both inhibition of PDE activity and stimulation of cAMP generation to modulate a functional response [165]. In fact, in an elegant experimental setting, Underwood and collegues recently demonstrated [166] that endogenous catecholamines were required for rolipram-induced inhibition of antigen-induced bronchial obstruction in the anaesthetized guinea pig to be apparent. Both $β_2$-antagonists and adrenalectomy dramatically reduced the anti-obstructive potency of intravenously given rolipram [166]. On the other hand, PDE inhibition alone may suppress functional responses in the case of "high cycling" conditions accompanied by a low "functional" PKA activation threshold [165]. Thirdly, cells may release endogenously formed stimulants of adenylate cyclase activity, in particular following stimulation. This is illustrated by data showing adenosine release from human neutrophils incubated with fMLP [167] and PAF-induced $PGE_2$ generation in human eosinophils [18]. In this context, it is of interest that fMLP stimulation of neutrophils resulted in a transient cAMP increase that was potentiated by the PDE4-selective inhibitor Ro 20-1724 and abolished by adenosine deaminase [167]. Extending these data, Schudt and colleagues [159] reported that 1 μM zardaverine, that only slightly and insignificantly increased the cAMP content of quiescent neutrophils, dramatically potentiated cAMP increase following fMLP stimulation by about three-fold. Taken together, these data suggest that adenosine released by stimulated human neutrophils supports modulation of functional responses by PDE inhibitors such as zardaverine in these cells.

In the isolated perfused rat lung, zardaverine inhibited LPS-induced bronchoconstriction ($IC_{50} = 1.8$ μM) and in parallel, reduced $TXA_2$ release in the perfusate [168]. 10 μM zardaverine protected against increased endothelial cell permeability and oedema formation in the isolated perfused rabbit lung challenged with $H_2O_2$ [169]. Furthermore, it was demonstrated that zardaverine inhibits antigen-induced accumulation of eosinophils in guinea pig airways [170–172]. Zardaverine given by the oral route attenuated LPS-induced liver injury in mice [173].

In clinical trials, single doses of zardaverine (1.5–6 mg) given by the inhaled route (MDI) afforded a modest increase in $FEV_1$ in mild-moderate asthmatics. About 55% of the asthmatics responded to zardaverine with an $FEV_1$ increase of at least 10% [162, 174–176]. Zardaverine protected against the early airway reaction to allergen challenge but only slightly reduced the extent of the late airway reaction [162]. Administration of zardaverine was associated with the occasional occurrence of nausea and vomiting typically associated with first generation PDE4 inhibitors. Clinical development of zardaverine was discontinued.

## AH21-132 (Benafentrine)

The benzonaphtyridine benafentrine (AH21-132) inhibited PDE3 (human platelets) and PDE4 (human neutrophils) with $IC_{50}$ values of 1.74 and 1.76 μM, respectively. Bronchodilatory, anti-inflammatory and clinical effects of this compound have been recently extensively reviewed [162]. Briefly, AH21-132 reversed human bronchus contractility induced by histamine, carbachol or endogenous spasmogens with $IC_{50}$ values of 4.0, 8.0, and 4.7 μM, respectively. In the anaesthesized, ventilated guinea pig the benzonaphthyridine protected against bombesin-induced airway obstruction. The anti-inflammatory potential of benafentrine is reflected by the finding that the compound inhibited PAF- or antigen-induced airway eosinophil accumulation [162]. AH21-132 showed some clinical efficacy in asthmatics where the benzonaphthyridine induced transient bronchodilation and protected against allergen-challenge induced late airway obstruction [162]. Interestingly, single daily doses of 800 mg or repeated daily doses of 200 mg over 14 days given orally were well tolerated. The high oral tolerability of benafentrine may originate in the LAR-specificity of this compound (Tab. 5).

*Table 6 - Summary of expected adverse effects with classical PDE3 or PDE4 inhibitors and strategies for design of PDE inhibitors avoiding these unwanted effects.*

*PDE3 and PDE4 are expressed in diverse cellular systems apart from those relevant in airway inflammation. PDE3 is abundant in the cardiovascular system and cAMP increase followed by inhibition of PDE3 results in enhanced myocardial contractility, vascular smooth muscle relaxation and inhibition of platelet aggregation. Nausea and vomiting may origin in cAMP increase in the area postrema as a consequence of PDE4 inhibition. On the other hand, gastric acid hypersecretion may represent a peripheral effect of PDE4 inhibition. Hence, non-selective PDE3 and 4 inhibition would result in a variety of unwanted effects. However, implementing recent findings regarding cell-specific prevalence of conformers or subtypes of PDE3 or PDE4 in drug discovery strategies would minimize the occurrence of these unwanted effects.*

|  | PDE3 | PDE4 |
|---|---|---|
| Adverse events | Tachycardia | Nausea |
|  | Arrhythmia | Vomiting |
|  | SVRI-reduction | Gastric acid secretion |
|  | CI-increase | Headache |
|  | Platelet inhibition |  |
| Avoidance strategy | PDE3B inhibition | PDE4-LAR inhibition |

*SVRI, systemic vascular resistance index; CI, cardiac index*

## Tolafentrine

Tolafentrine is another benzonaphtyridine. The compound inhibits PDE1–5 with $IC_{50}$ values of 18, 0.8, 0.09, 0.06 and 2 µM, respectively. Tolafentrine relaxes isolated human bronchial smooth muscle *in vitro* [177] and inhibits histamine-induced bronchoconstriction in the anaesthesized guinea pig *in vivo* [178]. Tolafentrine inhibits LPS-stimulated TNFα-generation in human alveolar macrophages, proliferation of human lymphocytes [156], degranulation and chemoluminescense of human eosinophils (when combined with salbutamol) [20], and fMLP-stimulated eosinophil $LTC_4$ synthesis [140]. These *in vitro* findings might predict an anti-inflammatory potential of tolafentrine *in vivo*.

Although dual-selective PDE3/4 inhibitors are considered as promising new drugs in asthma, there are some concerns regarding cardiovascular side-effects due to the PDE3 inhibiting component (Tab. 6). However, in clinical trials with dual selective inhibitors, haemodynamic effects were not observed. Regarding the potential of PDE3 inhibitors to induce cardiovascular effects such as those in milrinone trials [142, 143] it should be taken into account that patients included in those trials had severe cardiac failure i.e. these studies targeted a completely different population from asthma trials. However, since PDE3B is abundant in human lymphocytes but not in the cardiovascular system the safety profile may be increased by selectively inhibiting PDE3B. In fact, an ideal second generation dual selective PDE3/4 inhibitor for asthma should selectively inhibit PDE3B but not PDE3A and show selectivity for the LAR conformer of PDE4 subtypes. A dual selective PDE3B/4-LAR inhibitor with high oral bioavailability would represent a cutting edge strategy for future drug development in asthma.

## References

1    Cockcroft DW, O'Byrne PM, Swystun VA, Bhagat R (1995) Regular use of inhaled albuterol and the allergen-induced late asthmatic response. *J Allergy Clin Immunol* 96: 44–49

2    Yates DH, Sussman HS, Shaw MJ, Barnes PJ, Chung KF (1995) Regular formoterol treatment in mild asthma. Effect on bronchial responsiveness during and after treatment. *Am J Respir Crit Care Med* 152: 1170–1174

3    Cheung D, Timmers MC, Zwinderman AH, Bel EH, Dijkman JH, Sterk PJ (1992) Long-term effects of a long-acting beta 2-adrenoceptor agonist, salmeterol, on airway hyperresponsiveness in patients with mild asthma. *N Engl J Med* 327: 1198–1203

4    O'Connor BJ, Aikman SL, Barnes PJ (1992) Tolerance to the nonbronchodilator effects of inhaled beta 2-agonists in asthma. *N Engl J Med* 327: 1204–1208

5    Butler JM, Chan SC, Stevens S, Hanifin JM (1983) Increased leukocyte histamine release with elevated cyclic AMP-phosphodiesterase activity in atopic dermatitis. *J Allergy Clin Immunol* 71: 490–497

6    Chan SC, Reifsnyder D, Beavo JA, Hanifin JM (1993) Immunochemical characterization of the distinct monocyte cyclic AMP-phosphodiesterase from patients with atopic dermatitis. *J Allergy Clin Immunol* 91: 1179–1188

7    Gantner F, Tenor H, Gekeler V, Schudt C, Wendel A, Hatzelmann A (1997) Phosphodiesterase profiles of highly purified human peripheral blood leukoyte populations from normal and atopic individuals: a comparative study. *J Allergy Clin Immunol* 100: 527–535

8    Gantner F, Kupferschmidt R, Schudt C, Wendel A, Hatzelmann (1997) *In vitro* differentation of human monocytes to macrophages: change of PDE profile and its relationship to suppression of tumor necrosis factor-alpha release by PDE inhibitors. *Br J Pharmacol* 121: 221–231

9    Tenor H, Hatzelmann A, Kupferschmidt R, Stanciu L, Djukanovic R, Schudt C, Wendel A, Church MK, Shute JK (1995) Cyclic nucleotide phosphodiesterase isoenzyme activities in human alveolar macrophages. *Clin Exp Allergy* 25: 625–633

10   Jiang X, Li J, Paskind M, Epstein PM (1996) Inhibition of calmodulin-dependent phos-

phodiesterase induces apoptosis in human leukemic cells. *Proc Natl Acad Sci USA* 93: 1236–1241

11    Rybalkin SD, Bornfeldt KE, Sonnenburg WK, Rybalkina IG, Kwak KS, Hanson K, Krebs EG, Beavo JA (1997) Calmodulin-stimulated cyclic nucleotide phosphodiesterase (PDE1C) is induced in human arterial smooth muscle cells of the synthetic, proliferative phenotype. *J Clin Invest* 100: 2611–2621

12    Banner KH, Page CP (1996) Anti-inflammatory effects of theophylline and selective phosphodiesterase inhibitors. *Clin Exp Allergy* 26 (Suppl 2): 2–9

13    Jaffar ZH, Sullivan P, Page C, Costello J (1996) Low-dose theophylline modulates T-lymphocyte activation in allergen-challenged asthmatics. *Eur Respir J* 9: 456–462

14    Banner KH, Page CP (1995) Immunomodulatory actions of xanthines and isoenzyme selective phosphodiesterase inhibitors. *Monaldi Arch Chest Dis* 50: 286–292

15    Banner KH, Page CP (1995) Theophylline and selective phosphodiesterase inhibitors as anti-inflammatory drugs in the treatment of bronchial asthma. *Eur Respir J* 8: 996–1000

16    Finnerty JP, Lee C, Wilson S, Madden J, Djukanovic R, Holgate ST (1996) Effects of theophylline on inflammatory cells and cytokines in asthmatic subjects: a placebo-controlled parallel group study. *Eur Respir J* 9: 1672–1677

17    Djukanovic R, Finnerty JP, Lee C, Wilson S, Madden J, Holgate ST (1995) The effects of theophylline on mucosal inflammation in asthmatic airways: biopsy results. *Eur Respir J* 8: 831–833

18    Tenor H, Hatzelmann A, Church MK, Schudt C, Shute JK (1996) Effects of theophylline and rolipram on leukotriene C4 (LTC4) synthesis and chemotaxis of human eosinophils from normal and atopic subjects. *Br J Pharmacol* 118: 1727–1735

19    Schudt C, Tenor H, Hatzelmann A (1995) PDE Isoenzymes as targets for anti-asthma drugs. *Eur Respir J* 8: 1179–1183

20    Hatzelmann A, Tenor H, Schudt C (1995) Differential effects of non-selective and selective phosphodiesterase inhibitors on human eosinophil functions. *Br J Pharmacol* 114: 821–831

21    Dent G, Giembycz MA, Rabe KF, Wolf B, Barnes PJ, Magnussen H (1994) Theophylline suppresses human alveolar macrophage respiratory burst through phosphodiesterase inhibition. *Am J Respir Cell Mol Biol* 10: 565–572

22    Kidney J, Dominguez M, Taylor PM Rose M, Chung KF, Barnes PJ (1995) Immunomodulation by theophylline in asthma. Demonstration by withdrawal of therapy. *Am J Respir Crit Care Med* 151: 1907–1914

23    Evans DJ, Taylor DA, Zetterstrom O, Chung KF, O'Connor BJ, Barnes PJ (1997) A comparison of low-dose inhaled budesonide plus theophylline and high-dose inhaled budesonide for moderate asthma. *N Engl J Med* 337: 1412–1418

24    Ukena D, Harnest U, Sakalauskas R, Magyar P, Vetter N, Steffen H, Leichtl S, Rathgeb F, Keller A, Steinijans VW (1997) Comparison of addition of theophylline to inhaled steroid with doubling of the dose of inhaled steroid in asthma. *Eur Respir J* 10: 2754–2760

25 Reeves ML, Leigh BK, England PJ (1987) The identification of a new cyclic nucleotide phosphodiesterase activity in human and guinea pig cardiac ventricle. Implications for the mechanism of action of selective phosphodiesterase inhibitors. *Biochem J* 214: 535–541

26 Rocque WJ, Holmes WD, Patel IR, Dougherty RW, Ittoop O, Overton L, Hoffman CR, Wisely GB, Willard DH, Luther MA (1997) Detailed characterization of a purified type 4 phosphodiesterase, HSPDE4B2B: differentiation of high- and low- affinity (R)-rolipram binding. *Protein Expr Purif* 9: 191–202

27 Souness JE, Griffin M, Maslen C, Ebsworth K, Scott LC, Pollock K, Palfreyman MN, Karlsson JA (1996) Evidence that cyclic AMP phosphodiesterase inhibitors suppress TNF alpha generation from human monocytes by interacting with a "low-affinity" phosphodiesterase 4 conformer. *Br J Pharmacol* 118: 649–658

28 Barnette MS, Bartus JO, Burman M, Christensen SB, Cieslinski LB, Esser KM, Prabhakar US, Rush JA, Torphy TJ (1996) Association of the anti-inflammatory activity of phosphodiesterase 4 (PDE4) inhibitors with either inhibition of PDE4 catalytic activity or competition for [3H]rolipram binding. *Biochem Pharmacol* 51: 949–956

29 Souness JE, Houghton C, Sardar N, Withnall MT (1997) Evidence that cyclic AMP phosphodiesterase inhibitors suppress interleukin-2 release from murine splenocytes by interaction with a "low-affinity" phosphodiesterase 4 conformer. *Br J Pharmacol* 121: 743–750

30 Barnette MS, Manning CD, Cieslinski LB, Burman M, Christensen SB, Torphy TJ (1995) The ability of phosphodiesterase IV inhibitors to suppress superoxide production in guinea pig eosinophils is correlated with inhibition of phosphodiesterase IV catalytic activity. *J Pharmacol Exp Ther* 273: 674–679

31 Underwood DC, Osborn RR, Novak LB, Matthews JK, Newsholme SJ, Undem BJ, Hand J, Torphy TJ (1993) Inhibition of antigen-induced bronchoconstriction and eosinophil infiltration in the guinea pig by the cyclic AMP-specific phosphodiesterase inhibitor, rolipram. *J Pharmacol Exp Ther* 266: 306–313

32 Essayan DM, Huang SL, Undem BJ, Kagey-Sobotka A, Lichtenstein LM (1994) Modulation of antigen- and mitogen-induced proliferative responses of peripheral blood mononuclear cells by nonselective and isoenzyme selective cyclic nucleotide phosphodiesterase inhibitors. *J Immunol* 153: 3408–3416

33 Barnette MS, Christensen SB, Underwood DC, Torphy TJ (1996) Phosphodiesterase 4: Biological underpinnings for the design of improved inhibitors. *Pharmacol Rev Comm* 8: 65–73

34 Hughes B, Owens R, Perry M, Warrelow G, Allen R (1997) PDE4 inhibitors: the use of molecular cloning in the design and development of novel drugs. *Drug Dis Today* 2: 89–101

35 Schmiechen R, Schneider HH, Wachtel H (1990) Close correlation between behavioural response and binding *in vivo* for inhibitors of the rolipram-sensitive phosphodesterase. *Psychopharmacol* 102: 17–20

36 Duplantier AJ, Biggers MS, Chambers RJ, Cheng JB, Cooper K, Damon DB, Eggler JF,

Kraus KG, Marfat A, Masamune H et al (1996) Biarylcarboxylic acids and amides: inhibition of phosphodiesterase type IV versus [$^3$H]rolipram binding activity and their relationship to emetic behaviour in the ferret. *J Med Chem* 39: 120–125

37    Barnette MS, Grous M, Cieslinski LB, Burman M, Christensen SB, Torphy TJ (1995) Inhibitors of phosphodiesterase IV (PDE IV) increase acid secretion in rabbit isolated gastric glands: correlation between function and interaction with a high-affinity rolipram binding site. *J Pharmacol Exp Ther* 273: 1396–1402

38    Harris AL Connell MJ, Ferguson EW, Wallace AM, Gordon RJ Pagani ED, Silver PJ (1989) Role of low Km cyclic AMP phosphodiesterase inhibition in tracheal relexation and bronchodilation in the guinea pig. *J Pharmacol Exp Ther* 251: 199–206

39    Jacobitz, S, Ryan MD, Mc Laughlin MM, Livi GP, DeWolf WE, Torphy TJ (1997) Role of conserved histidines in catalytic activity and inhibitor binding of human recombinant phosphodiesterase 4A. *Mol Pharmacol* 51: 999–1006

40    Rocque WJ, Tian G, Wiseman JS, Holmes WD, Zajac-Thompson I, Willard DH, Indravaden R, Patel G, Wisely B, Clay WC et al (1997) Human recombinant phosphodiesterase 4B2B binds (R)-rolipram at a single site with two affinities. *Biochemistry* 36: 14250–14261

41    Torphy TJ, Christensen SB, Barnette MS, Burman M., Cieslinski LB, DeWolf WE (1997) Molecular basis for an improved therapeutic index of SB 207499, a second generation phosphodiesterase 4 inhibitor. *Eur Respir J* 10 (Suppl 25): 3135

42    Alvarez R, Sette C., Yang D, Eglen R, Wilhelm R, Shelton ER, Conti M (1995) Activation and selective inhibition of a cyclic AMP-specific phosphodiesterase, PDE-4D3. *Mol Pharmacol* 48: 616–622

43    Sette C, Conti M (1996) Phosphorylation and activation of a cAMP-specific phosphodiesterase by the cAMP-dependent protein kinase. *J Biol Chem* 271: 16526–16530

44    Huston E, Pooley L, Julien P, Scotland G, McPhee I, Sullivan M, Bolger G, Houslay MD (1996) The human cyclic AMP-specific phosphodiesterase PDE-46 (HSPDE4A4B) expressed in transfected COS7 cells occurs as both particulate and cytosolic species that exhibit distinct kinetics of inhibition by the antidepressant rolipram. *J Biol Chem* 271: 31334–31344

45    Kelly JJ, Barnes PJ, Giembycz MA (1996) Phosphodiesterase 4 in macrophages: relationship between cAMP accumulation, suppression of cAMP hydrolysis and inhibition of [3H]R-(–)rolipram binding by selective inhibitors. *Biochem J* 318: 425–436

46    Souness JE, Rao S (1997) Proposal for pharmacologically distinct conformers of PDE4 cyclic AMP phosphodiesterases. *Cell Signal* 9: 227–236

47    Souness JE, Scott LC (1993) Stereospecifity of rolipram actions on eosinophil cyclic AMP-specific phosphodiesterase. *Biochem J* 291: 389–395

48    Souness JE, Maslen C, Scott LC (1992) Effects of solubilization and vanadate/glutathione complex on inhibitor potencies against eosinophil cyclic AMP-specific phosphodiesterase. *FEBS Lett* 302: 181–4

49    Stringfield TM, Morimoto BH (1997) Modulation of cyclic AMP levels in a clonal neur-

al cell line by inhibitors of tyrosine phosphorylation. *Biochem Pharmacol* 53: 1271–1278

50    Ogiwara T, Chik CL, Ho AK (1997) Tyrosine kinase inhibitors enhance GHRH-stimulated cAMP accumulation and GH release in rat anterior pituitary cells. *J Endocrinol* 152: 193–199

51    Ho A, Wiest R, Ogiwara T, Murdoch G, Chik CL (1995) Potentiation of agonist-stimulated cyclic AMP accumulation by tyrosine kinase inhibitors in rat pinealocytes. *J Neurochem* 65: 1597–1603

52    Dent G, Munoz NM, Zhu X, Rühlmann E, Leff AR, Magnussen H, Rabe KF (1997) Tyrosine kinase inhibition by genistein blocks PAF-induced respiratory burst and leukotriene C4 production in human eosinophils. *Eur Resp J* 10 (Supp 25): 265s

53    Taylor CC, Limback D, Terranova PF (1997) Src tyrosine kinase activity in rat thecal-interstitial cells and mouse TM3 Leydig cells is positively associated with cAMP-specific phosphodiesterase activity. *Mol Cell Endocrinol* 126: 91–100

54    O'Connell JC, McCallum JF, McPhee I, Wakefield J, Houslay ES, Wishart W, Bolger G, Frame M, Houslay MD (1996) The SH3 domain of Src tyrosyl protein kinase interacts with the N-terminal splice region of the PDE4A cAMP-specific phosphodiesterase RPDE-6 (RNPDE4A5). *Biochem J* 318: 255–261

55    Masamune H, Cheng JB, Cooper K, Eggler JF, Marfat A, Marshall SC, Shirley JT, Tickner JE, Umland JP, Vazquez E (1995) Discovery of micromolar PDE4 inhibitors that exhibit much reduced affinity for the [$^3$H]rolipram binding site: 3-norbornyloxy-4-methoxyphenylmethylene oxindoles. *Bioorgan & Med Chem Lett* 5: 1965–1968

56    Cheng JB, Cooper K, Duplantier AF, Eggler JF, Kraus KG, Marshall SC, Marfat A, Masamune H, Shirley J et al (1995) Synthesis and *in vitro* profile of a novel series of catechol benzimidazoles. The discovery of potent, selective phosphodiesterase type IV inhibitors with greatly attenuated affinity for the [$^3$H]rolipram binding site. Bioorgan & Med Chem Lett 5: 1969–1972

57    Livi GP, Kmetz P, McHale MC, Cieslinski LB, Sathe GM, Taylor DP, Davis RL, Torphy TJ, Balcarek JM (1990) Cloning and expression of cDNA for a human low-Km, rolipram-sensitive cyclic AMP phosphodiesterase. *Mol Cell Biol* 6: 2678–2686

58    Bolger C, Michaelil T, Martin T, St. John T, Steiner B, Rodgers L, Riggs M, Wigler M, Ferguson K (1993) A family of human phosphodiesterases homologous to the dunce learning and memory gene product of drosophila melanogaster are potential targets for antidepressant drugs. *Mol Cell Biol* 13: 6558–6571

59    Jacobitz S, McLaughlin MM, Livi GP, Burman M, Torphy TJ (1996) Mapping the functional domains of human recombinant phosphodiesterase 4A: structural requirements for catalytic activity and rolipram binding. *Mol Pharmacol* 50: 891–899

60    Owens RJ, Catterall C, Batty D, Jappy J, Russell A, Smith B, O'Connell J, Perry MJ (1997) Human phosphodiesterase 4A: characterization of full-length and truncated enzymes expressed in COS cells. *Biochem J* 326: 53–60

61    Manning CD McLaughlin MM, Livi GP, Cieslinski B, Torphy TJ, Barnette MS (1996) Prolonged Beta-adrenoceptor stimulation up-regulates cAMP phosphodiesterase activi-

ty in human monocytes by increasing mRNA and protein for phosphodiesterases 4A and 4B. *J Pharmacol Exp Ther* 276: 810–818

52  Percival MD, Yeh B, Falgueyret JP (1997) Zinc dependent activation of cAMP-specific phosphodiesterase (PDE4A). *Biochem Biophys Res Comm* 241: 175–180

53  Houslay M, Scotland G, Erdogan S, Huston E, Mackenzie S, McCallum J, McPhee I, Pooley L, Rena G, Ross A et al. (1996) Intracellular targeting, interaction with Src homology 3 (SH3) domains and rolipram-detected conformational switches in cAMP-specific PDE4A phosphodiesterase. *Biochem Soc Trans* 25: 374–379

54  Houslay MD (1996) The N-terminal alternately spliced regions of PDE4A cAMP-specific phosphodiesterases determine intracellular targeting and regulation of catalytic activity. *Biochem Soc Trans* 24: 980–986

55  Sun G, Ke S, Budde RJ (1997) Csk phosphorylation and inactivation *in vitro* by the cAMP-dependent protein kinase. *Arch Biochem Biophys* 343: 194–200

56  Iwabuchi K, Hatakeyama S, Takahashi A, Ato M, Okada M, Kajino Y, Kajino K, Ogasawara K, Takami K, Nakagawa H et al. (1997) CsK overexpression reduces several monokines and nitric oxide productions but enhances prostaglandin E2 production in response to lipopolasaccharide in the macrophage cell line J774A.1. *Eur J Immunol* 27: 742–749

57  Thomson AW, Bonham C, Zeevi A (1995) Mode of action of tracrolimus (FK506): molecular and cellular mechanisms. *Ther Drug Monit* 6: 584–591

58  Itoh S, Navia MA (1995) Structure comparison of native and mutant human recombinant FKBP12 complexes with the immunosupresssant drug FK506 (tracolimus). *Protein Sci* 11: 2261–2268

59  Onofri F, Giovedi S, Vaccaro P, Czernik AP, Valtorta F, De Camilli P, Greengard P, Benfenati F (1997) Synapsin I interacts with c-Src and stimulates its tyrosine kinase activity. *Proc Natl Acad Sci* 94: 12168–12173

70  Verghese MW, McDonnell RT, Lenhard JM, Hamacher L, Jin SLC (1995) Regulation of distinct cyclic AMP-specific phosphodiesterase (phosphodiesterase Type 4) isozymes in human monocytic cells. *Mol Pharmacol* 47: 1164–1171

71  Miyazaki T, Taniguchi T (1996) Coupling of the IL2 receptor complex with non-receptor protein tyrosine kinases. *Cancer Surv* 27: 25–40

72  Beaty CD, Franklin TL, Uehara Y, Wilson CB (1994) Lipopolysaccharide-induced cytokine production in human monocytes: role of tyrosine phosphorylation in transmembrane signal transduction. *Eur J Immunol* 24: 1278–1284

73  Schlottmann KE, Gulbins E, Lau SM, Coggeshall KM (1996) Activation of Src-family tyrosine kinases during Fas-induced apoptosis. *J Leukoc Biol* 60: 546–554

74  Yousefi S, Hoessli DC, Blaser K, Mills GB, Simon HU (1996) Requirement of Lyn and Syk tyrosine kinases for the prevention of apoptosis by cytokines in human eosinophils. *J Exp Med* 183: 1407–1414

75  Kato M, Kita H, Morikawa A (1997) Role of tyrosine kinases in human eosinophil degranulation. *Int Arch Allergy Immunol* 114 (Suppl 1): 14–17

76  Ashton MJ, Cook DC, Fenton G, Karlsson JA, Palfreyman MN, Raeburn D, Ratcliffe

AJ, Souness JE, Thurairatnam S, Vicker N (1994) Selective type IV phosphodiesterase inhibitors as antiasthmatic agents. The syntheses and biological activities of 3-(cyclopentyloxy)-4-methoxybenzamides and analogues. *J Med Chem* 37: 1696–1703

77  Souness JE, Maslen C, Webber S, Foster M, Raeburn D, Palfreyman MN, Ashton MJ, Karlsson JA (1995) Suppression of eosinophil function by RP73401, a potent and selective inhibitor of cyclic AMP-specific phosphodiesterase: comparison with rolipram. *Br J Pharmacol* 115: 39–46

78  Jacobitz S, McLaughlin MM, Livi GP, Ryan MD, Torphy TJ (1994) The role of conserved histidine residues on cAMP hydrolyzing activity and rolipram binding of human phosphodiesterase IV. *FASEB J* 8: A371

79  Shakur Y, Wilson M, Pooley L, Lobban M, Griffiths S, Campbell A, Beattie J, Daly S, Houslay M (1995) Identification and characterization of the type-IVA cyclic AMP-specific phosphodiesterase RD1 as a membrane-bound protein expressed in cerebellum. *Biochem J* 306: 801–9

80  Shakur Y, Pryde JG, Houslay MD (1993) Engineered deletion of the unique N-terminal domain of the cyclic AMP-specific phosphodiesterase RD1 prevents plasma membrane association and the attainment of enhanced thermostability without altering its sensitivity to inhibition by rolipram. *Biochem J* 292: 677–686

81  McPhee I, Pooley L, Lobban M, Bolger G, Houslay MD (1995) Identification, characterization and regional distribution in brain of RPDE-6 (RNPDE4A5), a novel splice variant of the PDE4A cyclic AMP phosphodiesterase family. *Biochem J* 310: 965–974

82  Pooley L, Shakur Y, Rena G, Houslay MD (1997) Intracellular localization of the PDE4A cAMP-specific phosphodiesterase splice variant RD1 (RNPDE4A1A) in stably transfected human thyroid carcinoma FTC cell lines. *Biochem J* 321: 177–185

83  Scotland G, Houslay M (1995) Chimeric constructs show that the unique N-terminal domain of the cyclic AMP phosphodiesterase RD1 (RNPDE4A1A; rPDE-IVA1) can confer membrane association upon the normally cytosolic protein chloramphenicol acetyltransferase. *Biochem J* 308: 673–681

84  Mc Laughlin MM, Cieslinski LB, Burman M, Thorphy TJ, Livi GP (1993) A low-Km, rolipram sensitive, cAMP-specific phosphodiesterase from human brain. *J Biol Chem* 268: 6470–6476

85  Obernolte R, Bhakta S, Alvarez R, Bach C, Zuppan P, Mulkins M, Jarnagin K, Shelton ER (1993) The cDNA of a human lymphocyte cyclic-AMP phosphodiesterase (PDE IV) reveals a multigene family. *Gene* 129: 239–247

86  Huston E, Lumb S, Russell A, Catterall C, Ross AH, Steele MR, Bolger GB, Perry MJ, Owens RF, Houslay MD (1997) Molecular cloning and transient expression in COS7 cells of a novel human PDE4B cAMP-specific phosphodiesterase HSPDE4B3. *Biochem J* 328: 549–558

87  Lobban M, Shakur Y, Beattie J, Houslay MD (1994) Identification of two splice variant forms of type-IVB cyclic AMP phosphodiesterase, DPD (rPDE IVB1) and PDE-4 (rPDE-IVB2) in brain: selective localization in membrane and cytosolic compartments and differential expression in various brain regions. *Biochem J* 304: 399–406

88    Pillai R, Kytle K, Reyes A, Colicelli J (1993) Use of a yeast expression system for the isolation and analysis of drug-resistant mutants of a mammalian phosphodiesterase. *Proc Natl Acad Sci* 90: 11970–11974

89    Engels P, Sullivan M, Muller T, Lubbert H (1995) Molecular cloning and functional expression in yeast of human cAMP-specific phosphodiesterase subtype (PDE IV-C). *FEBS-Lett* 358: 305–310

90    Engels P, Fichtel K, Lubbert H (1994) Expression and regulation of human and rat phosphodiesterase type IV isogenes. *FEBS Lett* 350: 291–295

91    Obernolte R, Ratzliff J, Baecker PA, Daniels DV, Zuppan P, Jarnagin K, Shelton ER (1997) Multiple splice variants of phosphodiesterase PDE4C cloned from human lung and testis. *Biochem Biophys Acta* 1353: 287–297

92    Swinnen JV, Joseph DR, Conti M (1989) Molecular cloning of rat homologues of the drosophila melanogaster dunce cAMP phosphodiesterase: evidence for a family of genes. *Proc Natl Acad Sci* 86: 5325–5329

93    Monaco L, Vicini E, Conti M (1994) Structure of two rat genes coding for closely related rolipram-sensitive cAMP phosphodiesterases. Multiple mRNA variants originate from alternative and multiple start sites. *J Biol Chem* 269: 347–357

94    Conti M, Iona S, Cuomo M, Swinnen J, Odeh J, Svoboda M (1995) Characterization of a hormon-inducible, high affinity adenosine 3'-5'-cyclic monophosphate phosphodiesterase from the rat Sertoli cell. *Biochemistry* 34: 7979–7987

95    Baecker PA, Obernolte R, Bach C, Yee C, Shelton ER (1994) Isolation of a cDNA encoding a human rolipram-sensitive cyclic AMP phosphodiesterase (PDE IVD). *Gene* 138: 253–256

96    Nemoz G, Zhang R, Sette C, Conti M (1996) Identification of cyclic AMP-phosphodiesterase variants from the PDE4D gene expressed in human peripheral mononuclear cells. *FEBS Lett* 384: 97–102

97    Truong V, Muller T (1994) Isolation, biochemical characterization and N-terminal sequence of rolipram-sensitive cAMP phosphodiesterase from human mononuclear leukocytes. *FEBS Lett* 353: 113–118

98    Giembycz MA, Corrigan CJ, Seybold J, Newton R, Barnes PJ (1996) Identification of cyclic AMP phosphodiesterases 3, 4 and 7 in human CD4[+] and CD8[+] T-lymphocytes: role in regulating proliferation and the biosynthesis of interleukin-2. *Br J Pharmacol* 118: 1945–1958

99    Essayan DM, Kagey-Sobotka A, Lichtenstein LM, Huang SK (1997) Differential regulation of human antigen-specific Th1 and Th2 lymphocyte responses by isoenzyme selective cyclic nucleotide phosphodiesterase inhibitors. *J Pharmacol Exp Ther* 282: 505–512

100   Erdogan S, Houslay MD (1997) Challenge of human Jurkat T-cells with the adenylate cyclase activator forskolin elicits major changes in cAMP phosphodiesterase (PDE) expression by up-regulating PDE3 and inducing PDE4D1 and PDE4D2 splice variants as well as down-regulating a novel PDE4A splice variant. *Biochem J* 321: 165–175

101   Bolger GB, Erdogan S, Jones R, Loughney K, Scotland G, Hoffmann R, Wilkinson I, Farrell S, Houslay MD (1997) Characterization of five different proteins produced by

alternatively spliced mRNAs from the human cAMP-specific phosphodiesterase PDE4D gene. *Biochem J* 328: 539–548

102 Kovala R, Sanwal BD, Ball EH (1997) Recombinant expression of a type IV, cAMP-specific phosphodiesterase: characterization and structure-function studies of deletion mutants. *Biochemistry* 36: 2968–76

103 Torphy TJ, Stadel JM, Burman M, Cieslinski LB, McLaughlin MM, White JR, Livi GP (1992) Coexpression of human cAMP-specific phosphodiesterase activity and high affinity rolipram binding in yeast. *J Biol Chem* 267: 1798–1804

104 Conti M, Geremia R, Adamo S, Stefanini M (1981) Regulation of Sertoli cell cyclic adenosine 3': 5'-monophosphate phosphodiesterase activity by follicle stimulating hormone and dibutyryl cyclic AMP. *Biochem Biophys Res Commun* 98: 1044–1050

105 Torphy TJ, Zhou HL, Cieslinski LB (1992) Stimulation of beta adrenoceptors in a human monocyte cell line (U937) up-regulates cyclic AMP-specific phosphodiesterase activity. *J Pharmacol Exp Ther* 263: 1195–1205

106 Haider S, Smith C, Cui Y, Ding J, Bentley-Hibbert S, Kmal G, Moggio R, Stemerman M (1995) Cyclic AMP-mediated induction of low $K_m$ cyclic AMP phosphodiesterase in rat aortic smooth muscle. *FASEB J* 9 A678

107 Rose R, Liu H, Palmer D, Maurice D (1997) Cyclic AMP-mediated regulation of vascular smooth muscle cell cyclic AMP phosphodiesterase activity. *Br J Pharmacol* 122: 233–240

108 Kochetkova M, Burns F, Souness J (1995) Isoprenaline induction of cAMP-phosphodiesterase in guinea pig macrophages occurs in the presence, but not in the absence, of the phosphodiesterase type IV inhibitor rolipram. *Biochem Pharmacol* 50: 2033–2038

109 Tenor H, Hatzelmann A, Wendel A, Schudt C (1995) Identification of phosphodiesterase IV activity and its cyclic adenosine monophosphate-dependent up-regulation in a human keratinocyte cell line (HaCaT). *J Invest Dermatol* 105: 70–74

110 Kovala T, Lorimer I, Brickenden A, Ball E, Sanwal B (1994) Protein kinase A regulation of cAMP phosphodiesterase expression in rat skeletal myoblasts. *J Biol Chem* 269: 8680–8685

111 Chang Y, Conti M, Lee Y, Lai H, Ching Y, Chern Y (1997) Activation of phosphodiesterase IV during desensitization of the A2A adenosine receptor-mediated cyclic AMP response in rat pheochromocytoma (PC12) cells. *J Neurochem* 69: 1300–1309

112 Swinnen J, Joseph D, Conti M (1989) The mRNA encoding a high-affinity cAMP phosphodiesterase is regulated by hormones and cAMP. *Proc Natl Acad Sci* 86: 8197–8201

113 Swinnen J, Tsikalas K, Conti M (1991) Properties and hormonal regulation of two structurally related cAMP phosphodiesterases from the rat Sertoli cell. *J Biol Chem* 266: 18370–18377

114 Sette C, Vicini E, Conti M (1994) The rat PDE3/IVD phosphodiesterase gene codes for multiple proteins differentially activated by cAMP-dependent protein kinase. *J Biol Chem* 269: 18271–18274

115 Torphy T, Zhou H, Foley J, Sarau H, Manning C, Barnette M (1995) Salbutamol up-regulates PDE4 activity and induces a heterologous desensitization of U937 cells to

prostaglandin E2. Implications for the therapeutic use of beta-adrenoceptor agonists. *J Biol Chem* 270: 23598–23604

116 Vicini E, Conti M (1997) Characterization of an intronic promoter of a cyclic adenosine 3', 5'-monophosphate (cAMP)-specific phosphodiesterase gene that confers hormone and cAMP inducibility. *Mol Endocrinol* 11: 839–850

117 McCauley L, Koh A, Beecher C, Rosol T (1997) Proto-oncogene c-fos is transcriptionally regulated by parathyroid hormone (PTH) and PTH-related protein in a cyclic adenosine monophosphate-dependent manner in osteoblastic cells. *Endocrinology* 138: 5427–5433

118 Li X, Hales K, Watanabe G, Lee R, Pestell R, Hales D (1997) The effect of tumor necrosis factor alpha and cAMP on induction of AP-1 activity in MA-10 tumor Leydig cells. *Endocrine* 6: 317–324

119 Zhou J, Wright P, Wong E, Katayoun J, Morand J, Carlson D (1997) Cyclic AMP regulation of mouse proline-rich protein gene expression: isoproterenol induction of AP-1 transcription factors in parotid glands. *Arch Biochem Biophys* 338: 97–103

120 Seybold J, Newton R, Wright L, Finney P, Giembycz M, Adcock I, Suttorp N, Barnes P (1997) Gene regulation of cAMP-specific phosphodiesterase IV isoforms and splice variants in human T-lymphocytes. Evidence for desensitization to β-agonists by PDE-induction. *Am J Resp Crit Car Med* 155: A692

121 Giembycz M (1996) Phosphodiesterase IV and tolerance to beta 2-adrenoceptor agonists in asthma. *Trends Pharmacol Sci* 17: 331–336

122 Bochert G, Bartel S, Beyerdorfer I, Kuttner I, Szekeres L, Krause E (1994) Long lasting anti-adrenergic effect of 7-oxo-prostacyclin in the heart: a cycloheximide sensitive increase of phosphodiesterase isoform I and IV activities. *Mol Cell Biochem* 132: 57–67

123 Kostic M, Erdogan S, Rena G, Borchert G, Hoch B, Bartel S, Scotland G, Huston E, Houslay M, Krause E (1997) Altered expression of PDE1 and PDE4 cyclic nucleotide phosphodiesterase isoforms in 7-oxo-prostacyclin-preconditioned rat heart. *J Mol Cell Cardiol* 29: 3135–3146

124 Ye X, Conti M, Houslay M, Farooqui S, Chen M, O'Donnell J (1997) Noradrenergic activity differentially regulates the expression of rolipram-sensitive, high affinity cyclic AMP phosphodiesterase (PDE4) in rat brain. *J Neurochem* 69: 2397–2404

125 Sette C, Iona S, Conti M (1994) The short-term activation of a rolipram-sensitive, cAMP-specific phosphodiesterase by thyroid-stimulating hormone in thyroid FRTL-5 cells is mediated by a cAMP-dependent phosphorylation. *J Biol Chem* 269: 9245–9252

126 Imai A, Nashida T, Shimomuro H (1995) Regulation of cAMP phosphodiesterases by cyclic nucleotides in rat parotid gland. *Biochem Mol Biol Int* 37: 1029–1036

127 Ahlstrom M, Lamberg-Allardt C (1997) Rapid protein kinase A-mediated activation of cyclic AMP-phosphodiesterase by parathyroid hormone in UMR-106 osteoblast-like cells. *J Bone Miner Res* 12: 172–178

128 Madelian V, La Vigne E (1996) Rapid regulation of a cyclic AMP-specific phosphodiesterase (PDE IV) by forskolin and isoproterenol in LRM55 astroglial cells. *Biochem Pharmacol* 51: 1739–1747

129 Ekholm D, Belfrage P, Manganiello V, Degerman E (1997) Protein kinase A-dependent activation of PDE4 (cAMP-specific cyclic nucleotide phosphodiesterase) in cultured bovine vascular smooth muscle cells. *Biochim Biophys Acta* 1356: 64–70

130 Nemoz G, Sette C, Conti M (1997) Selective activation of rolipram sensitive, cAMP-specific phosphodiesterase isoforms by phosphatidic acid. *Mol Pharmacol* 51: 242–249

131 El Bawab S, Macovschi O, Sette C, Conti M, Lagarde M, Nemoz G, Prigent A (1997) Selective stimulation of a cAMP-specific phosphodiesterase (PDE4A5) isoform by phosphatidic acid molecular species endogenously formed in rat thymocytes. *Eur J Biochem* 247: 1151–1157

132 Barnette M, Christensen S, Essayan D, Grous M, Prabhakar U, Rush J, Kagey-Sobotka A, Torphy T (1998) SB207499 (ariflo), a potent and selective second-generation phosphodiesterase 4 inhibitor: *in vitro* anti-inflammatory actions. *J Pharmacol Exp Ther* 284: 420–426

133 Cohan V, Showell J, Fisher D, Pazoles C, Watson J, Turner C, Cheng J (1996) *In vitro* pharmacology of the novel phosphodiesterase type 4 inhibitor, CP-80633. *J Pharmacol Exp Ther* 278: 1356–1361

134 Holbrook M, Gozzard N, James T, Higgs G, Hughes B (1996) Inhibition of bronchospasm and ozone-induced airway hyperresponsiveness in the guinea-pig by CDP840, a novel phosphodiesterase type 4 inhibitor. *Br J Pharmacol* 118: 1192–1200

135 Gozzard N, El-Hashim A, Herd C, Blake S, Holbrook M, Hughes B, Higgs G, Page C (1996) Effect of glucocorticosteroid budesonide and a novel phosphodiesterase type 4 inhibitor CDP840 on antigen induced airway responses in neonatally immunised rabbits. *Br J Pharmacol* 118 1201–1208

136 Hughes B, Howat D, Lisle H, Holbrook M, James T, Gozzard N, Blease K, Hughes P, Kingaby R, Warrellow G et al.(1996) The inhibition of antigen-induced eosinophilia and bronchoconstriction by CDP840, a novel stereo-selective inhibitor of phosphodiesterase type 4. *Br J Pharmacol* 118: 1183–1191

137 Harbinson P, MacLeod D, Hawksworth R, O'Toole S, Sullivan P, Heath P, Kilfeather S, Page C, Costello J, Holgate S, Lee T (1997) The effect of a novel orally active selective PDE4 isoenzyme inhibitor (CDP840) on allergen-induced responses in asthmatic subjects. *Eur Respir J* 10: 1008–1014

138 Cheng J, Watson J, Pazoles C, Eskra J, Griffiths R, Cohan V, Turner C, Showell H, Pettipher E (1997) The phosphodiesterase type 4 (PDE4) inhibitor CP-80, 633 elevates plasma cyclic AMP levels and decreases tumor necrosis factor-alpha (TNFalpha) production in mice: effect of adrenalectomy. *J Pharmacol Exp Ther* 280: 621–626

139 Karlsson J, Aldous D (1997) Phosphodiesterase 4 inhibitors for the treatment of asthma. *Exp Opin Ther Patents* 7: 989–1003

140 Tenor H, Shute J, Church M, Hatzelmann A, Schudt C (1995) Inhibition of human peripheral blood eosinophil LTC4 production by PDE inhibitors. *Eur Res J* 8 (Supp 9): 152

141 Raeburn D, Underwood S, Lewis S, Woodman V, Battram C, Tomkinson A, Sharma S, Jordan R, Souness J, Webber S et al (1994) Anti-inflammatory and bronchodilator prop-

erties of RP73401, a novel and selective phosphodiesterase type IV inhibitor. *Br J Pharmacol* 133: 1423–1431

142 Packer M, Carver J, Rodeheffer R, Ivanhoe R, DiBianco R, Zeldis S, Hendrix G, Bommer W, Elkayam U, Kukin M et al (1991) Effect of oral milrinone on mortality in severe chronic heart failure. The PROMISE Study Research group. *N Engl J Med* 325: 1468–1475

143 Colucci W, Sonnenblick E, Adams K, Berk M, Brozena S, Cowley A, Grabicki J, Kubo S, LeJemtel T, Littler W et al (1993) Efficacy of phosphodiesterase inhibition with milrinone in combination with converting enzyme inhibitors in patients with heart failure. The Milrinone Multicenter Trials Investigators. J Am Coll Cardiol 22: 113A–118A

144 Cowley A, Skene A (1994) Treatment of severe heart failure: quantity or quality of life? A trial of enoximone. Br Heart J 72: 226–230

145 Degerman E, Belfrage P, Manganiello V (1997) Structure, localization and regulation of cGMP-inhibited phosphodiesterase (PDE3). *J Biol Chem* 272: 6823–6826

146 Sheth SB, Chaganti K, Bastepe M, Ajuria J, Brennan K, Biradavolu R, Colman R (1997) Cyclic AMP phosphodiesterases in human lymphocytes. *Br J Haematol* 9: 784–789

147 Tang K, Jang E, Haslam R (1997) Expression and mutagenesis of the catalytic domain of cGMP-inhibited phosphodiesterase (PDE3) cloned from human platelets. *Biochem J* 323: 217–224

148 Komas N, Movsesian M, Kedev S, Degerman E, Belfrage P, Manganiello C (1996) cGMP-inhibited phosphodiesterases (PDE3). In: C Schudt, G Dent, KF Rabe (eds): *Phosphodiesterase inhibitors*. Academic Press, San Diego, 89–109

149 Kasuya J, Goko H, Fujita-Yamaguchi Y (1995) Multiple transcripts for the human cardiac form of the cGMP-inhibited cAMP phosphodiesterase. *J Biol Chem* 270: 14305–14312

150 Rahn T, Ronnstrand L, Leroy M, Wernstedt C, Tornquist H, Manganiello V, Belfrage P, Degerman E (1996) Identification of the site in the cGMP-inhibited phosphodiesterase phosphorylated in adipocytes in response to insulin and isoproterenol. *J Biol Chem* 271: 11575–11580

151 Wagner R, Smith C, Taylor A, Rhoades R (1997) Phosphodiesterase inhibition improves agonist-induced relaxation of hypertensive pulmonary arteries. *J Pharmacol Exp Ther* 282: 1650–1657

152 Rabe K, Tenor H, Dent G, Schudt C, Liebig S, Magnussen H (1993) Phosphodiesterase isozymes modulating inherent tone in human airways: identification and characterization. *Am J Physiol* 264: L458–464

153 Fujimura M. Kamio Y, Myou S, Hashimoto T, Matsuda T (1997) Effect of a phosphodiesterase 3 inhibitor, cilostazol, on bronchial hyperresponsiveness in elderly patients with asthma. *Int Arch Allergy Immunol* 114: 379–384

154 Robicsek S, Blanchard D, Djeu Y, Krzanowski J, Szentivanyi A, Polson J (1991) Multiple high affinity cAMP-phosphodiesterases in human T-lymphocytes. *Biochem Pharmacol* 42: 869–877

155 Tenor H, Stanciu L, Schudt C, Hatzelmann A, Wendel A, Djukanovic R, Church M,

Shute J (1995) Cyclic nucleotide phosphodiesterases from purified human CD4+ and CD8+ T-lymphocytes. *Clin Exp Allergy* 25: 616–624

156 Schudt C, Tenor H, Loos U, Mallmann P, Szamel M, Resch K (1993) Effect of selective phosphodiesterase (PDE) inhibitors on activation of human macrophages and lymphocytes. *Eur Resp J* 6: 367S

157 Pan X, Arauz E, Krzanowski J, Fitzpatrick D, Polson J (1994) Synergistic interactions between selective pharmalogical inhibitors of phosphodiesterase isoenzyme families PDE III and PDE IV to attenuate proliferation of rat vascular smooth muscle cells. *Biochem Pharmacol* 48: 827–835

158 Rabe K, Tenor H, Dent G, Schudt C, Nakashima M, Magnussen H (1994) Identification of PDE isozymes in human pulmonary artery and effect of selective PDE inhibitors. *Am J Physiol* 266: L536–543

159 Schudt C, Winder S, Forderkunz S, Hatzelmann A, Ullrich V (1991) Influence of selective phosphodiesterase inhibitors on human neutrophil functions and levels of cAMP and Ca. *Naunyn-Schmiedebergs Arch Pharmacol* 344: 682–690

160 Kilian U, Beume R, Eltze M, Schudt C (1989) Is phosphodiesterase inhibition a relevant bronchospasmolytic principle? *Agents Actions* 28: 331–348

161 Hoymann H, Heinrich U, Beume R, Kilian U (1994) Comparative investigation of the effects of zardaverine and theophylline on pulmonary functions in rats. *Exp Lung Res* 20: 235–250

162 Hatzelmann A, Engelstätter R, Morley J, Mazzoni L (1996) Enzymatic and functional aspects of dual-selective PDE3/4 inhibitors. In: C Schudt, G Dent, KF Rabe (eds): *Phosphodiesterase inhibitors*. Academic Press, San Diego, 147–160

163 Suttorp N, Ehreiser P, Hippenstiel S, Fuhrmann M, Krull M, Tenor H, Schudt C (1996) Hypermeability of pulmonary endothelial monolayer: protective role of phosphodiesterase isoenzymes 3 and 4. *Lung* 174: 181–194

164 Suttorp N, Weber U, Welsch T, Schudt C (1993) Role of phosphodiesterases in the regulation of endothelial permeability *in vitro*. *J Clin Invest* 9: 1421–1428

165 Houslay M, Milligan G (1997) Tailoring cAMP-signalling responses through isoform multiplicity. *Trends Biochem Sci* 22: 217–224

166 Underwood DC, Matthews JK, Osborn RR, Bochnowicz S, Torphy TJ (1997) The influence of endogeneous catecholamines on the inhibitory effects of rolipram against early- and late-phase response to antigen in the guinea pig. *J Pharmacol Exp Ther* 280: 210–219

167 Iannone M, Wolberg G, Zimmermann T (1989) Chemotactic peptide induces cAMP elevation in human neutrophils by amplification of the adenylate cyclase response to endogenously produced adenosine. *J Biol Chem* 264: 20177–20180

168 Uhlig S, Featherstone R, Held H, Nusing R, Schudt C, Wendel A (1997) Attenuation by phosphodiesterase inhibitors of lipopolysaccharide-induced thromboxane release and bronchochonstriction in rat lungs. *J Pharmacol Exp Ther* 282: 1453–1459

169 Seeger W, Hansen T, Rossig R, Schmehl T, Schutte H, Kramer HJ, Walmrath D, Weissmann N, Grimminger F, Suttorp N (1995) Hydrogen peroxide-induced increase in lung

endothelial and epithelial permeability-effect of adenylate cyclase stimulation and phosphodiesterase inhibition. *Microvasc Res* 50: 1–17

170 Schudt C, Winder S, Eltze M, Kilian U, Beume R (1991). Zardaverine: a cyclic AMP specific PDE III/IV inhibitor. *Agents Actions* (Suppl) 34: 379–402

171 Underwood D, Kotzer C, Bochnowitz S, Osbom R, Luttmann M, Hay D, Torphy T (1994) Comparison of phosphodiesterase III, IV and dual III/IV inhibitors on bronchospasm and pulmonary eosinophil influx in guinea pigs. *J Pharmacol Exp Ther* 270: 250–259

172 Banner, K, Page C (1995) Acute versus chronic administration of phosphodiesterase inhibitors on allergen-induced pulmonary cell influx in sensitized guinea-pigs. *Br J Pharmacol* 114: 93–98

173 Fischer, W, Schudt C, Wendel A (1993) Protection by phosphodiesterase inhibitors against endotoxin-induced liver injury in galactosamine-sensitized mice. *Biochem Pharmacol* 45: 2399–2404

174 Brunnee T, Engelstätter R, Steinijans V, Kunkel G (1992) Bronchodilatory effect of inhaled zardaverine, a phosphodiesterase III and IV inhibitor, in patients with asthma. *Eur J Respir* 5: 982–985

175 Jordan K, Fischer J, Engelstätter R, Steinijans V (1993) Einfluß eines inhalierbaren selektiven Phosphodiesterase-Hemmers (PDEIII/IV-Hemmer Zardaverin) auf die Lungenfunktion von Patienten mit Asthma bronchiale. *Atemw-Lungenkrkh* 19: 358–359

176 Wempe J, Postma D, Diupmans J, Koeter G (1992) Bronchodilating Effect of zardaverine, a selective phosphodiesterase III/IV inhibitor. *Eur Resp J* 5: 213s

177 Schudt C, Tenor H, Wendel A, Eltze M, Magnussen H, Rabe H (1993) Influence of PDE III/IV inhibitor B9004-070 on contraction and PDE activities in airway and vascular smooth muscle. *Am Rev Respir Dis* 147, A183

178 Beume R, Kilian U, Brand U, Haefner D, Eltze M, Flockerzi D (1993) The bronchospasmolytic effect of the PDE III/IV inhibitors B9004-070 and zardaverine-dependency on the route of administration in guinea pigs. *Am Rev Resp Dis* 147, A184

# β₂-Agonists

*Joanna S. Thompson Coon and Anne E. Tattersfield*

Division of Respiratory Medicine, City Hospital, Hucknall Road, Nottingham, NG5 1PB, UK

## Introduction

β₂-Adrenoceptor agonists are widely used as bronchodilators and have been used to treat acute attacks of asthma for decades. They can be divided into the very short acting which last 1 to 2 h (e.g. rimiterol), the short-acting such as salbutamol which produce an effect for 4 to 6 h and the newer longer acting β-agonists such as salmeterol and formoterol which maintain bronchodilatation for at least 12 h [1, 2]. β-Agonists antagonise the effects of a wide variety of bronchoconstrictor agents on airway smooth muscle *in vitro* and *in vivo* and are thus functional antagonists. The main mechanism by which they cause smooth muscle relaxation involves the cyclic 3'5' adenosine monophosphate (cAMP) second messenger system which is linked to the β₂-adrenoceptor by a coupling G-protein and adenylate cyclase, the effector enzyme [3] (Fig. 1). Cyclic AMP is able to modulate a number of processes which are important in governing the contractile state of the cell [4].

The reason for a long duration of action may differ between salmeterol and formoterol. Salmeterol has a large non-polar N-substituent which is thought to interact with specific sites in the receptor to prolong its action and this may explain why the duration of action appears not to be concentration dependent [5]. Formoterol has a long duration of action when inhaled but not when given orally and its duration of action is concentration dependent. It has been proposed that because it is very lipophilic it enters the membrane depot rapidly and only re-equilibrates gradually with the aqueous phase where it interacts with β₂ adrenoceptors [6].

In addition to being bronchodilators β-agonists may also have anti-inflammatory activity. This article discusses the evidence for this and its clinical relevance. Since short and long acting β-agonists have different roles and functions they will be discussed separately.

Anti-Inflammatory Drugs in Asthma, edited by A.P. Sampson and M.K. Church
© 1999 Birkhäuser Verlag Basel/Switzerland

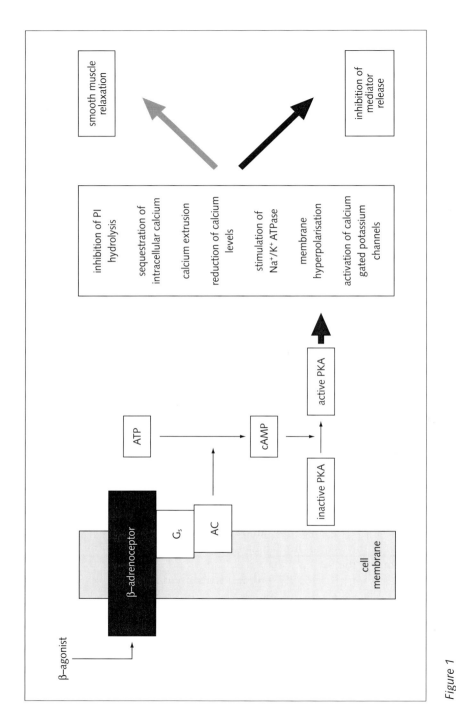

Figure 1

β₂-Receptors are coupled to adenylyl cyclase (AC) via a stimulatory guanine nucleotide regulatory protein (Gs). AC catalyses the conversion of ATP to cyclic AMP which in turn activates protein kinase A (PKA) which phosphorylates several proteins to produce intracellular effects that lead to smooth muscle relaxation and inhibition of mediator release.

## Do β-agonists have anti-inflammatory activity?

The anti-inflammatory effects of β-agonists have been studied *in vitro*, in animal studies, in bronchial biopsies in man and in clinical studies.

## Evidence from studies *in vitro* and in animals

The effect of β-agonists on two aspects of inflammation, plasma exudation and activation and mediator release from inflammatory cells have been studied.

### *Plasma exudation*

Plasma exudation is an important part of airway inflammation and may contribute to the pathophysiology of asthma by increasing airway oedema and thus airflow obstruction and bronchial hyperresponsiveness, and by allowing pro-inflammatory substances into the airways [7].

### Short-acting β-agonists

The short acting β-agonists terbutaline and salbutamol have been shown to inhibit plasma exudation induced by bradykinin and histamine in several animal preparations including hamster cheek pouches [8] and guinea pig airways *in vivo* [9, 10]. The dose of β-agonist required to inhibit the increase in microvascular permeability is generally greater than that required to reverse the increase in airway resistance caused by the same mediators when both are given by the intravenous route but not when given by inhalation [10, 11].

### Long-acting β-agonists

Bronchodilator doses of inhaled salmeterol and formoterol inhibit histamine induced plasma exudation in guinea pig airway [12, 13]. The effect of salmeterol was maintained for 6 h, formoterol for 5 h and salbutamol for 2 to 4 h in one study [14]. The mechanism for the anti-permeability effects of β-agonists is unclear but they are β₂-adrenoceptor mediated [15] and are probably due to a direct action on the endothelial cells of leaky post-capillary venules [16, 17].

### *Effects on inflammatory cells*

β₂-Adrenoceptors coupled to adenylate cyclase are present on several human inflammatory cells including lung mast cells [18], eosinophils [19], alveolar macrophages [20], B and T lymphocytes [21–23] and neutrophils [24]. Many studies have demonstrated effects from both short and long acting β-agonists on these cells (Tab. 1) although tachyphylaxis tends to develop very quickly.

## Short-acting β-agonists

Salbutamol and isoprenaline are potent inhibitors of IgE dependent release of histamine from chopped human lung [25, 26] and of histamine and prostaglandin $D_2$ from dispersed human lung mast cells [27]. Salbutamol inhibited the release of superoxide anions and leukotriene $B_4$ induced hydrogen peroxide release from eosinophils in one study [28], though this has not been seen in all studies possibly due to methodological differences. It appears that longer incubation of eosinophils with a β-agonist results in a loss of its inhibitory effect, presumably due to tachyphylaxis [19]. Salbutamol inhibited the accumulation of neutrophils in guinea pig lung [13] whilst isoprenaline has been shown to inhibit various responses of isolated human neutrophils that are capable of causing tissue inflammation including cell activation, generation of superoxides and release of beta glucuronidase [29]. Although not demonstrated with β-agonists, an increase in intracellular cAMP inhibits interleukin-2 production which in turn has caused a decrease in T lymphocyte proliferation [30–32]. The functional significance of the $\beta_2$ adrenoceptors found on macrophages is unclear since short-acting β-agonists appear not to inhibit mediator release *in vitro* [33–34].

## Long acting β-agonists

Salmeterol and formoterol are also potent inhibitors of IgE dependent histamine release from human lung fragments [6, 35] and dispersed lung mast cells [36]. Salmeterol and formoterol inhibit antigen and platelet activating factor induced eosinophil and neutrophil accumulation in guinea pig airways [13, 37] and the leukotriene $B_4$ induced release of hydrogen peroxide from guinea pig eosinophils was inhibited by formoterol but not salmeterol [28]. The lack of effect of salmeterol in this respect may be due to the low density of $\beta_2$-adrenoceptors on eosinophils, since salmeterol is a partial agonist [28]. Salmeterol has also been shown to reduce *Pseudomonas aeruginosa* damage to both nasal epithelium *in vitro* and cultured nasal epithelial cells, an effect which is attributed to a rise in intracellular cAMP which inhibits various toxins produced by the bacteria [33]. Most of the effects described above are $\beta_2$-adrenoceptor mediated and inhibited by $\beta_2$-adrenoceptor antagonists; salmeterol may however have effects which are not $\beta_2$-adrenoceptor mediated, possibly due to its membrane stabilising properties. Examples include a potent inhibitory effect of salmeterol on TNFα production in a human monocytic cell line (THP-1) [39], inhibition of T lymphocyte activation in mice [39] and modification of thromboxane $B_2$ release from human alveolar macrophages [34, 40].

*Table 1 - Examples of the inhibitory effects of β-agonists on inflammatory cells*

*a) short acting β-agonists*

| Cell type | Drug | Inhibition of | Ref. |
|---|---|---|---|
| Chopped lung | salbutamol | IgE dependent histamine release | [25] |
| | isoprenaline | | [26] |
| Dispersed lung mast cells | salbutamol | IgE dependent histamine and PGD$_2$ release | [27] |
| Guinea pig eosinophils | salbutamol | release of superoxide anions and LTB$_4$ induced H$_2$O$_2$ release | [28] |
| Neutrophils | isoprenaline | release of human neutrophil beta glucuronidase generation of superoxides cell activation | [29] |
| Guinea pig neutrophils | salbutamol | accumulation | [13] |
| Macrophages | isoprenaline | no effect on mediator release | [33] |
| | salbutamol | | [34] |
| Lymphocytes | intracellular cAMP raising agents | increase in T lymphocyte proliferation | [32] [30, 31] |

*b) long acting β-agonists*

| Cell type | Drug | Inhibition of | Ref. |
|---|---|---|---|
| Chopped lung | salmeterol | IgE dependent histamine, LTC$_4$ and PGD$_2$ release | [6] |
| | formoterol | | [35] |
| Dispersed lung mast cells | salmeterol | IgE dependent histamine release | [36] |
| | formoterol | | |
| Eosinophils | salmeterol | H$_2$O$_2$ release and eosinophil accumulation | [28] |
| | formoterol | | [37] |
| Neutrophils | salmeterol | antigen and PAF induced neutrophil accumulation | [13] |
| | formoterol | | |
| Alveolar macrophages | salmeterol | modification of TXB$_2$ release | [34, 40] |
| Cell lines | salmeterol | TNFα production | [39] |
| Murine lymphocytes | salmeterol | cell activation | [39] |

*IgE, immunoglobulin E; PGD$_2$, prostaglandin D$_2$; LTB$_4$, leukotriene B$_4$; H$_2$O$_2$, hydrogen peroxide; LTC$_4$, leukotriene C$_4$; PAF, platelet activating factor; TXB$_2$, thromboxane B$_2$; TNFα, tumour necrosis factor alpha.*

## Evidence from bronchial biopsy, bronchoalveolar lavage, induced sputum and peripheral blood studies in man

Bronchial biopsy and bronchoalveolar lavage have been used to establish the nature of the inflammatory response within asthmatic airways and to investigate the effects of various challenges and treatment regimens on the inflammatory response. More recently sputum induced by hypertonic saline has been developed as a less-invasive method of studying airway inflammation, with sputum being analysed for various constituents including total and differential cell counts and inflammatory mediators [41]. Eosinophils and their activation markers in peripheral blood have also been measured.

### Short-acting β-agonists

Several studies have looked at bronchial biopsies or bronchoalveolar lavage before and after a period of regular treatment with short-acting β-agonists. Study details are given in Table 2 and the main findings in Table 3. In the first study, a small, 3-month, double-blind parallel group study by Laitinen et al. [42], bronchial biopsies were performed in seven patients with mild asthma before and after regular terbu- taline treatment. They found a decrease in lymphocytes in the epithelium, a decrease in lymphocytes, mast cells and plasma cells in the lamina propria but no change in eosinophils, neutrophils, macrophages or monocytes. However two patients re- ceived a 6-day course of prednisolone during the treatment period which may have influenced the results. Manolitsas et al. [43] using bronchial biopsies and bron- choalveolar lavage found an increase in both total and activated eosinophils com- pared with baseline following 16 weeks treatment with regular salbutamol in 13 patients with mild asthma, but no change in mast cell or lymphocyte numbers. When comparisons were made with placebo there were no statistically significant differences in cell number or activation. Two shorter studies found no changes in inflammatory cell number or activation. Evans et al. [44] found no changes in eosinophil numbers, eosinophil cationic protein (ECP) levels or mast cell numbers in induced sputum from 30 rhinitic non-asthmatic subjects before and after 4 weeks' therapy with salbutamol, whilst Di Lorenzo et al. [45] found no change in eosino- phil counts in blood or in serum ECP levels after 1-weeks' therapy with salbutamol. An alternative to looking at inflammatory markers in the basal state is to study the inflammatory response to an antigen challenge. Twentyman et al. found a reduction in the antigen induced increase in neutrophils at 8 h post challenge and in neu- trophils and basophils at 24 h post challenge following a single dose of salbutamol in nine subjects with mild asthma [46], whilst Howarth et al. [47] showed that pre- treatment with a single dose of salbutamol reduced the antigen induced rise in plas- ma histamine and neutrophil chemotactic factor levels for up to 30 minutes in eight subjects with mild asthma.

*Table 2 - Bronchial biopsy, BAL, induced sputum and peripheral blood studies*

*a) short acting β-agonists*

| Method (Ref.) | Sample size | Study type and duration | Treatment |
|---|---|---|---|
| Biopsy [42] | 14 | R, DB, PG, 12 weeks | 375 µg bd terb |
| Biopsy and BAL [43] | 48 | R, DB, PG, 16 weeks | 200 µg qds salb |
| Peripheral blood [45] | 20 | R, O, CO, 1 week | 200 µg qds salb |
| Induced sputum [44] | 30 | R, DB, PG, PC, 4 weeks | 200 µg qds salb |
| ▲ peripheral blood [46] | 9 | R, DB, PC, CO, SD | 200 µg salb |
| ▲ peripheral blood [47] | 8 | PC, CO, SD | 200 µg salb |

*b) long acting β-agonists*

| Method (ref) | Sample size | Study type and duration | Treatment |
|---|---|---|---|
| BAL [48] | 12 | R, DB, CO, PC, 4 weeks | 50 µg bd salm |
| BAL [49] | 23 | R, DB, PG, PC, 6 weeks | 50 µg bd salm |
| biopsy [50] | 23 | R, DB, PG, PC, 6 weeks | 50 µg bd salm |
| BAL [51] | 23 | R, DB, PG, PC, 6 weeks | 50 µg bd salm |
| BAL [52] | 10 | R, DB, CO, PC, 8 weeks | 50 µg bd salm |
| peripheral blood [45] | 20 | R, O, CO, 1 week | 50 µg bd salm |
| ▲ induced sputum and peripheral blood [56] | 8 | R, DB, CO, PC, SD | 100 µg salm |
| ▲ induced sputum and peripheral blood [53] | 6 | SB, CO, PC, SD | 24 µg form |
| ▲ peripheral blood [54] | 12 | R, DB, CO, PC, SD | 50 µg salm |
| ▲ peripheral blood [55] | 19 | R, DB, PG, PC, SD | 50 µg salm |

*BAL, bronchoalveolar lavage; R, randomised; DB, double blind; SB, single blind; CO, cross-over; PG, parallel group; PC, placebo controlled; O, open; SD, single dose; terb, terbutaline; salb, salbutamol; salm, salmeterol; form, formoterol.*

*▲, studies carried out before and after antigen challenge.*

## Long-acting β-agonists

The effect of regular long acting β-agonists on bronchial biopsies in subjects with asthma has also been studied (Tabs. 2 and 3). In 1991, Dahl et al. [46] reported that 4 weeks' treatment with salmeterol produced an improvement in the appearance of

*Table 3 - Effects of β-agonists on inflammatory markers seen in bronchial biopsy, BAL, induced sputum and peripheral blood studies*

*a) short acting β-agonists*

| Study type (ref) | β-Agonist | Eosino-phils | Neutro-phils | Lympho-cytes | Macro-phages | Mast cells | Baso-phils |
|---|---|---|---|---|---|---|---|
| B [42] | terb (375 µg bd) | × | × | ↓ | × | ↓ | – |
| B & BAL [43] | salb (200 µg qds) | ↑ | – | × | – | × | – |
| PB [45] | salb (200 µg qds) | × | – | – | – | – | – |
| IS [44] | salb (200 µg qds) | × | × | × | × | × | – |
| ▲ PB [46] | salb (200 µg) | × | ↓ at 8 h | × | – | – | ↓ at 8 & 24 h |
| ▲ PB [47] | salb (200 µg) | _ | ↓ in NCF | _ | _ | ↓ in histamine | – |

*b) long acting β-agonists*

| Study type (ref) | β-Agonist | Eosino-phils | Neutro-phils | Lympho-cytes | Macro-phages | Mast cells | Baso-phils |
|---|---|---|---|---|---|---|---|
| BAL [48] | salm (50 µg bd) | ↓ in ECP | – | – | ↓ in O$_2$ radical generation | – | – |
| BAL [49] | salm (50 µg bd) | × | – | – | – | × | – |
| B [50] | salm (50 µg bd) | × | _ | × | – | × | – |
| BAL [51] | salm (50 µg bd) | – | – | × | – | – | – |
| BAL [52] | salm (50 µg bd) | × | × | × | × | × | – |
| PB [45] | salm (50 µg bd) | ↓ in ECP | – | – | – | – | – |
| ▲ IS & PB [53] | form (24 µg) | ↓ in ECP | – | × | – | – | – |
| ▲ PB [54] | salm (50 µg) | ↓ in ECP | – | – | – | – | – |
| ▲ PB [55] | salm (50 µg) | × | – | – | – | – | – |
| ▲ IS & PB [56] | salm (100 µg) | × | – | – | – | – | – |

BAL, bronchoalveolar lavage; B, biopsy; IS, induced sputum; PB, peripheral blood; terb, terbutaline; salb, salbutamol; salm, salmeterol; form, formoterol; ECP, eosinophil cationic protein; ×, no effect; –, not measured; ↓, decrease; ↑, increase.
▲, studies carried out before and after antigen challenge.

the mucosa compared with baseline and a reduction in the oxidative metabolism of macrophages, but the differential cell count following bronchoalveolar lavage was unaltered. The authors also reported a statistically significant decrease in ECP levels in lavage. More recently another group found a fall in mean serum ECP concentration with no change in blood eosinophil count following salmeterol treatment for 1 week in 20 patients with mild atopic asthma, suggesting that salmeterol may modify and reduce the release of granular proteins from eosinophils but not total cell numbers [45]. Conversely, several studies have not been able to demonstrate any anti-inflammatory effects of salmeterol. Roberts et al. [49–51] performed detailed analyses of a wide range of inflammatory markers in bronchial biopsies and bronchoalveolar lavage in 23 subjects with mild asthma after six weeks therapy with salmeterol and placebo. Despite improvements in symptoms and morning peak flow after salmeterol there was no difference in differential cell counts, histamine, albumin, prostaglandin D$_2$ or tryptase levels in bronchoalveolar lavage, no difference in T lymphocyte numbers or activation status assessed by flow cytometry and no difference in numbers of mast cells, eosinophils or T lymphocytes on bronchial biopsy. Similarly, a crossover study in nine subjects with mild asthma showed no significant change in BAL cell profile, or in percentages of CD4 and CD8 lymphocytes following 8 weeks' salmeterol treatment compared with placebo [50].

All these studies have looked at patients with stable asthma. Four further studies have looked at the effects of long acting β-agonists on the inflammatory response to an antigen challenge [53–56]. In all four the long acting β-agonist inhibited the early and late response to antigen and provided protection against the subsequent increase in bronchial responsiveness. The effect on inflammatory markers was less clear cut. Formoterol had no effect on the increase in sputum and blood eosinophils and lymphocytes that occurred following antigen challenge in six subjects with mild, atopic asthma studied by Wong et al. [53] although it did inhibit the rise in serum ECP 24 h after the challenge. Similarly, a single dose of salmeterol administered prior to antigen challenge in 12 patients with mild asthma had no effect on the antigen induced rise in blood eosinophils although it again prevented the rise in serum ECP [52]. In two further studies however a single dose of salmeterol administered prior to antigen challenge did not affect the numbers or activation markers of eosinophils in peripheral blood or induced sputum [55, 56].

## Clinical studies

Determining the extent to which the effects of β-agonists in clinical practice can be attributed to an anti-inflammatory effect rather than bronchodilatation is very difficult. Antigen challenge has been used as a model but interpretation of the effects of β-agonists on the response to antigen challenge is not straightforward. β-Agonists are functional antagonists and would be expected to counter the bronchoconstrictive effect of antigen even if they were acting solely on airway smooth muscle.

## Short acting β-agonists

The short acting β-agonists inhibit the early response to antigen [55] and when nebulised salbutamol was given in higher doses (2.5 mg) the late response to antigen and post antigen increase in bronchial responsiveness were also inhibited [57]. High doses of salbutamol have a longer duration of action than smaller doses but the inhibition of the late response lasted for a longer time than the bronchodilatation seen with salbutamol alone on the control day, suggesting that salbutamol might be having effects other than functional antagonism [56] .

## Long acting β-agonists

Salmeterol and formoterol have been shown to inhibit both the early and the late response to antigen [53–56, 58]. The extent of the inhibitory effect of salmeterol on the early and late response to antigen in the study by Twentyman et al. [58] was broadly similar to the bronchodilator effect seen when salmeterol was given alone on the control day, in keeping with functional antagonism. Measurements made 32 h after the antigen challenge when any direct effects of salmeterol had worn off, showed a slightly greater $FEV_1$ and reduced bronchial reactivity following salmeterol than following placebo, suggesting that salmeterol might have had a more specific anti-inflammatory effect during the antigen challenge. However, when inflammatory indices have been compared in blood and sputum following antigen challenges preceded by long acting β-agonists or placebo the differences have been small. The rise in ECP levels following antigen challenge was inhibited by salmeterol in two of the studies [53, 54] but not in the other two [55, 56].

## Conclusion

Both short and long acting β-agonists have actions which can be described as anti-inflammatory. Both reduce plasma exudation *in vitro* and in animal models and both have inhibitory effects on several of the inflammatory cells found in the lung including inhibition of mediator release and cell accumulation. Although these actions would be expected to reduce inflammation in the airways, studies of bronchial biopsies and bronchoalveolar lavage following regular treatment with both short and long acting β-agonists have been largely negative with no consistent increase or decrease in inflammatory cell numbers in the biopsies or bronchoalveolar lavage. Although most of these studies have been small (see Tab. 2), with insufficient power to determine small effects of β-agonists, it is clear that any changes that occur with β-agonists are considerably less than those seen with corticosteroids. It is also important to note that the studies are less able to comment on the functional activity of inflammatory cells.

Determining the extent to which the beneficial effects of β-agonists in patients are due to their anti-inflammatory effect is difficult. It seems likely that the rapid action of short acting bronchodilators in relieving acute asthma is due predominantly to a relaxant effect on smooth muscle. When taken on a regular basis the long acting β-agonists have been shown to provide clinical benefit compared to placebo whereas the effects of regular short acting β-agonists have differed little from placebo [59–62]. The reason for the difference between short and long acting β-agonists in this respect is not clear but it is now apparent that the bronchodilator effect of short acting β-agonists wanes considerably between doses. The same is probably true for their actions on inflammatory cells and this may allow intermittent release of mediators. The more sustained action of a long acting β-agonist would ensure a more continuous inhibitory effect on inflammatory cells and this may explain their greater clinical efficacy.

## References

1    Ullman A and Svedmyr N (1988) Salmeterol, a new long acting inhaled β₂-adrenoceptor agonist: comparisons with salbutamol in adult asthmatic patients. *Thorax* 43: 674–678

2    Ringdal N, Derom E, Pauwels R (1995) Onset and duration of action of single doses of formoterol inhaled via Turbuhaler in mild to moderate asthma. *Eur Respir J* 8: 68S

3    Caron M G, Cerione R A, Benovic J L, Strulovici C, Lefkowitz R J, Codina-Salada J, Birnbaumer L (1985) Biochemical characterization of the adrenergic receptors: Affinity labelling, purification and reconstitution studies. *Adv Cyclic Nucleotide Protein Phosphorylation Res* 19: 1–12

4    Knox AJ, Tattersfield AE (1995) Airway smooth muscle relaxation. Thorax 50: 894–901

5    Green SA, Spasoff AP, Coleman RA, Johnson M, Liggett SB (1996) Sustained activation of a G protein coupled receptor via "anchored" agonist binding. Molecular localization of the salmeterol exosite within the β₂ adrenergic receptor. *J Biol Chem* 271: 24029–24035

6    Nials AT, Ball DI, Butchers PR, Coleman RA, Humbles AA, Johnson M, Vardey CJ (1994) Formoterol on airway smooth muscle and human lung mast cells: a comparison with salbutamol and salmeterol. *Eur J Pharmacol* 251: 127–135

7    Persson CGA (1993) The action of β-receptors on microvascular endothelium or: Is airways plasma exudation inhibited by β-agonists? *Life Sci* 52: 2111–2121

8    Svensjo E, Persson CGA, Rutili G (1977) Inhibition of bradykinin induced macromole-

cular leakage from post capillary venules by a $\beta_2$ adrenoceptor stimulant, terbutaline. *Acta Physiol Scand* 101: 504–506

9    Erjefalt I (1986) Anti-asthma drugs attenuate inflammatory leakage of plasma into airway lumen. *Acta Physiol Scand* 128: 653–654

10   Advenier C, Qian Y, Law Koune J-D, Molimard M, Candenas M-L, Naline E (1992) Formoterol and salbutamol inhibit bradykinin and histamine induced airway microvascular leakage in guinea-pig. *Br J Pharmacol* 105: 792–798

11   Tokuyama K, Lotvall JO, Lofdahl C-G, Barnes PJ, Chung KF (1991) Inhaled formoterol inhibits histamine-induce airflow obstruction and airway microvascular leakage. *Eur J Pharmacol* 193: 35–39

12   Erjefalt I, Persson CGA (1991) Long duration and high potency of anti-exudative effects of formoterol in guinea pig tracheobronchial airways. *Am Rev Resp Dis* 144: 788–791

13   Whelan CJ and Johnson M (1992) Inhibition by salmeterol of increased vascular permeability and granulocyte accumulation in guinea pig lung and skin. *Br J Pharmacol* 105: 831–838

14   Whelan CJ, Johnson M, Vardey CJ (1993) Comparison of the anti-inflammatory properties of formoterol, salbutamol and salmeterol in guinea pig lung and skin. *Br J Pharmacol* 110: 613–618

15   Beets JL and Paul W (1980) Actions of locally administered adrenoceptor agonists on increased plasma protein extravasation and blood flow in guinea-pig skin. *Br J Pharmacol* 70: 461–467

16   Duffey ME, Hainau B, Ho S, Bentzel CJ (1981) Regulation of epithelial tight junction permeability by cyclic AMP. *Nature* 294: 451–453

17   Sulakvelidze I, McDonald DM (1994) Anti-edema action of formoterol in rat trachea does not depend on capsaicin sensitive sensory nerves. *Am J Resp Crit Care Med* 149: 232–238

18   Butchers PR, Skidmore IF, Vardey CJ, Wheldon A (1980) Characterisation of the receptor mediating the anti-analphylactic effects of $\beta$-adrenoceptor agonists in human lung tissue *in vitro*. *Br J Pharmacol* 71: 663–667

19   Yukawa T, Ukena D, Kroegel C, Chanez P, Dent G, Chung KF, Barnes PJ (1990) Beta-adrenergic receptors on eosinophils. *Am Rev Resp Dis* 141: 1446–1452

20   Liggett SB (1989) Identification and characterisation of a homogenous population of $\beta_2$ adrenergic receptors on human alveolar macrophages. *Am Rev Resp Dis* 139: 552–555

21   Williams LT, Snyderman R, Lefkowitz RJ (1976) Identification of $\beta$-adrenergic receptors in human lymphocytes by $(-)[^3H]$ alprenolol binding. *J Allergy Clin Immunol* 57: 149–155

22   Conolly ME, Greenacre JK (1977) The $\beta$-adrenoceptor of the human lymphocyte and human lung parenchyma. *Br J Pharmacol* 59: 17–23

23   Bishopric NH, Cohen HJ, Lefkowitz RJ (1980) Beta-adrenergic receptors in lymphocyte sub-populations. *J Allergy Clin Immunol* 65: 29–33

24   Galant S P and Allred S J (1980) Demonstration of beta-2 adrenergic receptors of high coupling efficiency in human neutrophil sonicates. *J Lab Clin Med* 96: 15–23

25  Assem ESK, Richter AM (1971) Comparison of *in vitro* and *in vivo* inhibition of the anaphylactic mechanism by β-adrenergic stimulants and disodium cromoglycate. *Immunology* 21: 729–739

26  Church MK, Young KD (1983) The characteristics of inhibition of histamine release from human lung fragments by sodium cromoglycate, salbutamol and chlorpromazine. *Br J Pharmacol* 78: 671–679

27  Church MK, Hiroi J (1987) Inhibition of IgE-dependent histamine release from human dispersed lung mast cells by anti-allergic drugs and salbutamol. *Br J Pharmacol* 90: 421–429

28  Rabe KF, Giembycz MA, Dent G, Perkins RS, Evans P, Barnes PJ (1993) Salmeterol is a competitive antagonist at β-adrenoceptors mediating inhibition of respiratory burst in guinea pig eosinophils. *Eur J Pharmacol* 231: 305–308

29  Busse WW, Sosman JM (1984) Isoproteronol inhibition of isolated human neutrophil function. *J Allergy Clin Immunol* 73: 404–410

30  Mary D, Aussel C, Ferrua B, Fehlmann M (1987) Regulation of interleukin 2 synthesis by cAMP in human T cells. *J Immunol* 139: 1179–1184

31  Averill LE, Stein RL, Kammer GM (1988) Control of human T-lymphocyte interleukin-2 production by a cAMP dependent pathway. *Cell Immunology* 115: 88–99

32  Carlson SL, Trauth K, Brooks WH, Roszman TL (1994) Enhancement of beta-adrenergic-induced cAMP accumulation in activated T-cells. *J Cell Physiol* 161: 39–48

33  Fuller RW, O'Malley G, Baker AJ, Macdermot J (1988) Human alveolar macrophage activation: Inhibition by forskolin but not β-adrenoceptor stimulation or phosphodiesterase inhibition. *Pulm Pharmacol* 1: 101–106

34  Baker A J, Palmer J, Johnson M, Fuller R W (1994) Inhibitory actions of salmeterol on human airway macrophages and blood monocytes. *Eur J Pharmacol* 264: 301–306

35  Butchers PR, Vardey CJ, Johnson M (1991) Salmeterol a potent and long acting inhibitor of inflammatory mediator release from human lung. *Br J Clin Pharmacol* 104: 672–676

36  Lau HY, Wong PL, Lai CK, Ho JK (1994) Effects of long acting β₂ adrenoceptor agonists on mast cells of rat, guinea pig and human. *Int Arch Allergy Immunol* 105: 177–180

37  Sanjar S, McCabe PJ, Humbles AH (1991) Inhibition by salmeterol of antigen-induced eosinophil accumulation in guinea pig lung. *Eur Respir J* 4: 200s

38  Dowling RB, Rayner CFJ, Rutman A, Jackson AD, Kanthakumar K, Dewar A, Taylor GW, Cole PJ, Johnson M, Wilson R (1997) Effect of salmeterol on *Pseudomonas aeruginosa* infection of respiratory mucosa. *Am J Resp Crit Care Med* 155: 327–336

39  Sekut L, Champion B R, Page K, Menius J A, Connolly K M (1995) Anti-inflammatory activity of salmeterol; down regulation of cytokine production. Clin Exp Immunol 99: 461–466

40  Baker AJ, Fuller RW (1990) Anti-inflammatory effect of salmeterol on human alveolar macrophages. *Am Rev Resp Dis* 141: A394

41  Pin I, Gibson PG, Kolendowicz R, Girgis-Garbado A, Denburg JA, Hargreave FE,

Dolovich J (1992) Use of induced sputum cell counts to investigate airway inflammation in asthma. *Thorax* 47: 25–29

42   Laitinen LA, Laitinen A, Haahtela T (1992) A comparative study of the effects of an inhaled corticosteroid, budesonide, and a β2-agonist, terbutaline, on airway inflammation in newly diagnosed asthma: A randomised, double-blind, parallel-group controlled trial. *J Allergy Clin Immunol* 90: 32–42

43   Manolitsas ND, Wang J, Devalia JL, Trigg CJ, McAulay AE, Davies RJ (1995) Regular albuterol, nedocromil sodium and bronchial inflammation in asthma. *Am J Resp Crit Care Med* 151: 1925–1930

44   Evans DW, Salome CM, King GG, Rimmer SJ, Seale JP, Woolcock AJ (1997) Effect of regular inhaled salbutamol on airway responsiveness and airway inflammation in rhinitic non-asthmatic subjects. *Thorax* 52: 136–142

45   Di Lorenzo G, Morici G, Norrito F, Mansueto P, Melluso M, D'Ambrosio FP, Sangiorgi GB (1995) Comparison of the effects of salmeterol and salbutamol on clinical activity and eosinophil cationic protein serum levels during the pollen season in atopic asthmatics. *Clin Exp Allergy* 25: 951–956

46   Twentyman OP, Sams VR, Holgate ST (1993) Albuterol and nedocromil sodium affect airway and leukocyte responses to allergen. *Am Rev Respir Dis* 147: 1425–1430

47   Howarth PH, Durham SR, Lee TH, Kay AB, Church MK, Holgate ST (1985) Influence of albuterol, cromolyn sodium and ipratropium bromide on the airway and circulating mediator responses to allergen bronchial provocation in asthma. *Am Rev Resp Dis* 132: 986–992

48   Dahl R, Pedersen B, Venge P (1991) Bronchoalveolar lavage studies. *Eur Resp Rev* 1: 272–275

49   Roberts JA, Bradding P, Walls AF, Holgate ST, Howarth PH (1992) The effect of salmeterol xinafoate therapy on lavage findings in asthma. *Am Rev Resp Dis* 145: A413

50   Roberts JA, Bradding P, Walls AF, Britten KM, Wilson S, Holgate ST, Howarth PH (1992) The influence of salmeterol xinafoate on mucosal inflammation in asthma. *Am Rev Resp Dis* 145: A418

51   Gratziou C, Roberts J A, Bradding P, Holgate S T, Howarth P H (1992) The influence of the long acting β-agonist salmeterol xinafoate on T-lymphocyte lavage populations and activation status in asthma. *Am Rev Resp Dis* 145: A67

52   Gardiner PV, Ward C, Booth H, Allison A, Hendrick DJ, Walters EH (1994) Effect of eight weeks of treatment with salmeterol on bronchoalveolar lavage inflammatory indices in asthmatics. *Am J Resp Crit Care Med* 150: 1006–1011

53   Wong BJO, Dolovich J, Ramsdale HE, O'Byrne PM, Gontovnick L, Denburg JA, Hargreave FE (1992) Formoterol compared with beclomethasone and placebo on allergen-induced asthmatic responses. *Am Rev Resp Dis* 146: 1156–1160

54   Pedersen B, Dahl R, Larsen BB, Venge P (1993) The effect of salmeterol on the early and late phase reaction to bronchial allergen and postchallenge variation in bronchial reactivity, blood eosinophils, serum eosinophil cationic protein and serum eosinophil protein X. *Allergy* 48: 377–382

55 Weersink E J M, Postma D S, Aalbers R, De Monchy J G R (1994) Early and late asthmatic reaction after allergen challenge. *Resp Med* 88: 103–114

56 Pizzichini M M M, Kidney J C, Wong B J O, Morris M M, Efthimiadis A, Dolovich J, Hargreave F E (1996) Effect of salmeterol compared with beclomethasone on allergen-induced asthmatic and inflammatory responses. *Eur Respir J* 9: 449–455

57 Twentyman O P, Finnerty J P, Holgate S T (1991) The inhibitory effect of nebulized albuterol on the early and late asthmatic reactions and increase in airway responsiveness provoked by inhaled allergen in asthma. *Am Rev Resp Dis* 144: 782–787

58 Twentyman OP, Finnerty JP, Harris A, Palmer J, Holgate ST (1990) Protection against allergen induced asthma by salmeterol. *Lancet* 336: 1338–1342

59 Sears M, Taylor DR, Print CG, Lake DC, Li Q, Flannery EM, Yates DM, Lucas MK, Herbison GP (1990) Regular inhaled β-agonist treatment in bronchial asthma. *Lancet* 336: 1391–1396

60 Pearlman DS, Chervinsky P, LaForce C, Seltzer JM, Southern DL, Kemp JP, Dockhorn RJ, Grossman J, Liddle RF, Yancey SW, Cocchetto DM, Alexander WJ, Van As A (1992) A comparison of salmeterol with albuterol in the treatment of mild-to-moderate asthma. *New Engl J Med* 327: 1420–1425

61 D'Alonzo GE, Nathan RA, Henochowicz S, Morris RJ, Ratner P, Rennard SI (1994) Salmeterol xinafoate as maintenance therapy with albuterol in patients with asthma. *JAMA* 271: 1412–1416

62 Drazen JM, Israel E, Boushey HA, Chinchilli VM, Fahy JV, Fish JE, Lazarus SC, Lemanske RF, Martin RJ, Peters SP, Sorkness C, Szefler SJ (1996) Comparison with regularly scheduled with as-needed use of albuterol in mild asthma. *New Engl J Med* 335: 841–847

# Mast cell stabilizing drugs

Guy F. Joos, Renaat A. Peleman, Romain A. Pauwels

Department of Respiratory Diseases, University Hospital Ghent, De Pintelaan 185,
B-9000 Ghent, Belgium

## Introduction

Currently available medication for treating airway inflammation is limited to only a few proven antiinflammatory agents. Cromolyn sodium (sodium cromoglycate, SCG) and nedocromil sodium, traditionally referred to as mast cell stabilizing agents, comprise an important group of mild to moderate anti-inflammatory drugs [1].

## Sodium cromoglycate (Cromolyn sodium)

Sodium cromoglycate (SCG) has been developed from derivatives of khellin and found to inhibit allergen-induced bronchoconstriction in man [2]. It is believed to prevent degranulation of mast cells via a membrane stabilizing effect brought about by the phosphorylation of a protein that results in blocking ionic calcium transport across the cell membrane.

### Cellular effects of sodium cromoglycate

Prevention of the release of mast cell products such as histamine, $PGD_2$ and $LTC_4$ accounts for the action of this drug on the early asthmatic reaction (EAR) which is IgE and mast cell-dependent. Cox demonstrated that SCG inhibits the release of mediators from mast cells triggered by the interaction between antigen and IgE [3]. Sodium cromoglycate inhibited histamine release from passively sensitized human lung fragments in a concentration range of 0.2–200 µM, producing a maximum inhibition of 33% (compared to a maximum inhibition of 72% produced by the $\beta_2$-agonist salbutamol) [4]. Sodium cromoglycate was more effective in inhibiting release of $PGD_2$ (compared to histamine) from human dispersed lung mast cells [5].

The origin of the mast cells is important for the inhibitory activity of cromoglycate. Flint and colleagues demonstrated that mast cells recovered by bronchoalveolar lavage in man were more sensitive to the inhibitory activity of SCG than mast cells obtained by digesting human lung fragments [6]. SCG also inhibits the activation of mast cells by other stimuli [7].

Besides mast cells, other inflammatory cells are sensitive to the inhibitory activity of SCG. Human neutrophils, eosinophils, platelets and macrophages have been used to demonstrate the broad inhibitory activity of SCG on the *in vitro* activation of inflammatory cells [8]. This wide variety of activity of SCG may account for the suppressive activity of this drug on the late asthmatic reaction (LAR). Finally, it was demonstrated that SCG inhibits, in a dose-dependent manner, IL-4-driven T cell-dependent IgE synthesis by PBMC from the majority (65%) of normal human subjects as well as IgE synthesis by B cells stimulated with anti-CD40 plus IL-4 or with hydrocortisone plus IL-4. SCG acts directly on B cells and the inhibition resides at the level of deletional switch recombination. SCG has a minimal effect on B cells that have already undergone isotype switching [9]. These new findings suggest a novel potential mechanism for the prevention of allergic disease.

Cromoglycate may also interfere with neural mechanisms. Dixon et al. demonstrated that SCG inhibited the activation of autonomic C fibre nerves stimulated by capsaicin in dogs *in vivo*, resulting in an inhibition of reflex bronchoconstriction [10]. These and other experiments suggest that SCG also inhibits the activation of certain types of nerves [11].

## Clinical pharmacology: protective effect of SCG in bronchial challenges

### Effect of SCG on airway reactions following allergen challenge
Altounyan and others have demonstrated that SCG, inhaled before allergen challenge, significantly inhibited the immediate bronchoconstriction that developed following the inhalation of allergen [2]. In addition, SCG given before allergen challenge also inhibits the development of the late asthmatic reaction [12] and prevents the increase in airway responsiveness observed following the last asthmatic reaction [13].

### Effect of SCG on airway reactions following challenge with non-allergic stimuli
Immediate pretreatment with SCG has no protective effect on the bronchoconstriction induced by agonists that act directly on airway smooth muscle such as histamine, methacholine, prostaglandins or leukotrienes. In contrast, therapeutic doses of SCG significantly inhibit the bronchoconstriction induced by exercise, cold air, adenosine, substance P, bradykinin, sulphur dioxide and distilled water [14].

Silverman and Andrea demonstrated that SCG only inhibits exercise-induced asthma (EIA) when inhaled before exercise. SCG given after exercise but before the bronchoconstriction developed was not effective [15]. Deal et al. [16] showed that SCG inhibits the bronchoconstriction induced by isocapnic hyperventilation. The airway narrowing induced by hyperventilation of cold air was also inhibited by cromoglycate [17]. The role of mast cells in EIA and in the airway reaction to cold air is still a matter of debate and therefore no uniformly accepted hypothesis on the mechanism responsible for the protective activity of SCG in these clinical pharmacology models is available.

The airway reaction to inhaled adenosine is at least partially due to the activation of mast cells, since $H_1$-antagonists significantly inhibit the bronchoconstriction following the inhalation of adenosine [18]. SCG has a significant protective activity on the adenosine-induced bronchoconstriction. The protective activity of SCG in this model can be explained at least partially by a mast cell stabilizing activity.

Dixon and Barnes observed a significant protective effect of SCG on the bradykinin- induced bronchoconstriction in mild asthmatics [19]. SCG also inhibits the bronchoconstriction in asthmatics induced by the inhalation of sulphur dioxide [20] or metabisulphite [21]. The airway reaction induced by sulphur dioxide or metabisulphite is significantly inhibited by anticholinergics. The bronchoconstriction induced by these agonists is however not inhibited by high doses of the presently available $H_1$-antagonists and the role of mast cells in these types of airway reactions is therefore less likely. The inhibitory effect of SCG on the activation of some autonomic nerve fibres may play a role [14].

### Effect of chronic treatment with SCG on long-term changes in non-allergic airway responsiveness

Although the administration of SCG immediately before challenge does not inhibit the bronchial response to methacholine or histamine, Löwhagen and Rak observed that treatment with SCG prevented the seasonal increase in bronchial responsiveness to histamine in pollen-allergic asthmatics [22]. The effect of SCG on airway responsiveness in non-allergic asthmatics is rather controversial. Löwhagen and Rak did not observe a significant change in histamine responsiveness in non-allergic asthma following treatment with SCG during 8 weeks [23]. In contrast, in the study of Petty et al. the histamine responsiveness decreased significantly over 12 weeks in the SCG-treated group, although the final degree of bronchial responsiveness did not differ significantly from the placebo-treated group [24].

## Clinical use

The drug is particularly active in prevention of seasonal allergic asthma in children and young adults. SCG seems less effective in older patients or in patients whose asthma is not allergic. However, other studies have demonstrated the clinical efficacy of SCG in chronic asthmatics, with a decrease of concomitant medication used, an increase in pulmonary function and significantly fewer exacerbations (reviewed in [25]). On the other hand, long-term prophylactic inhalation therapy with inhaled SCG with a spacer device in 1–4 year old children with moderate asthma was not more effective than placebo [26].

Inhaled sodium cromoglycate may be effective in cough induced by treatment with an ACE-inhibitor. In a double-blind crossover study, 9 of 10 patients reported a reduction in cough after treatment with sodium cromoglycate. Moreover, the cough sensitivity to capsaicin was significantly reduced by treatment with cromoglycate [27].

SCG has to be taken by inhalation and has a relatively short duration of action, requiring administration every 3 to 4 h. SCG is a safe drug. Long-term follow-up studies have shown no serious side-effects [28]. Local irritation of the throat or an occasional mild bronchospasm are more often seen with the dry powder preparation than with the nebulizer and the metered dose inhaler.

## Nedocromil sodium

Nedocromil sodium is a pyranoquinoline dicarboxylic acid that has been developed for the treatment of bronchial asthma. Several clinical trials have demonstrated the therapeutic efficacy of this relatively new prophylactic agent in the treatment of asthma.

## Cellular effects of nedocromil sodium

*In vitro* studies of human eosinophils, neutrophils, mast cells, and bronchoalveolar cells demonstrate that nedocromil sodium exerts its anti-inflammatory effects through regulation of mediator production and release from these cells as well as modulation of inflammatory cell migration. Nedocromil sodium inhibits chemotaxis of human eosinophils and neutrophils induced by platelet activating factor (PAF), zymosan activated serum (ZAS), leukotriene $B_4$ ($LTB_4$), or N-formyl-methionyl-leucylphenylalanine (fMLP) in healthy adults. Both nedocromil and cromoglycate are similarly effective in inhibiting neutrophil chemotaxis induced by PAF, ZAS, $LTB_4$, and fMLP. *In vitro* neutrophil migration was inhibited by 35% after incubation with nedocromil sodium $10^{-6}$ mol/l. Nedocromil sodium also affects the release of a wide variety of inflammatory mediators from various cells (reviewed in [29]). Nedocromil sodium inhibits IgE and IgG4 production in human B cells stimulated with IL-4, presumably at the level of switching, as does SCG. The same authors also demonstrated that nedocromil sodium inhibits the production of IgM, IgG1, IgG2, IgG3, IgG4, IgA, and IgA2 by tonsillar B cells stimulated with *S. aureus* Cowan strain I and IL-6 without affecting proliferation, suggesting that nedocromil sodium may act as a B cell regulatory reagent, thus modulating allergic inflammation [9].

Interleukin (IL)-6 production by alveolar macrophages obtained from patients with asthma, and stimulated by allergen and anti-IgE [30] and IL-1 induced production of IL-8 by cultured human bronchial epithelial cells from normal bronchi [31] was inhibited *in vitro* by nedocromil sodium. However, no effect was observed on the ozone-induced synthesis of IL-8 by bronchial epithelial cells *in vitro*, whereas nedocromil sodium clearly inhibited release of GM-CSF, TNFα and sICAM by these cells [32]. The increased release of GM-CSF induced by IL-1 in bronchial epithelium obtained from patients undergoing surgery was inhibited by nedocromil sodium $10^{-6}$ mol/l, although the constitutive production was not affected [33]. The effect of nedocromil sodium on leakage of plasma proteins into the airway lumen – a feature of chronic inflammation – was assessed by Schoonbrood et al. [34]. There was a very limited effect of treatment on PEF and $FEV_1$, and no effect on symptom score. However, a decrease was noted for the plasma protein leakage as measured in the sputum sol phase. The maximal effect occurred after 4 weeks of treatment. This reduction of protein exudation suggests that nedocromil sodium has anti-inflammatory properties, the mechanism of which is not known [34].

It appears that nedocromil sodium may not be able to alter the resident airway inflammatory cells in mild to moderate asthmatics [35]. Recently, the effect of nedocromil sodium was compared with regular albuterol and albuterol as required, on inflammatory changes in bronchial mucosal biopsies and BAL, obtained before and 4 months after treatment. No significant alteration in the number of inflammatory cells was observed, but there was a decrease in the number of eosinophils with nedocromil sodium and an increase with albuterol [36]. Contradictory results have been reported with regard to inhibitory effects of nedocromil sodium on the release of $LTC_4$ from stimulated eosinophils and on the release of superoxide anion and $LTB_4$ by stimulated neutrophils. Histamine release from mast cells obtained by bronchoalveolar lavage from healthy volunteers and asthmatic patients was inhibited more readily by nedocromil sodium than by cromoglycate [37]. Nedocromil sodium also inhibits histamine release within asthmatic airways following hyperosmolar saline challenge [38].

The neurogenic component of asthmatic inflammation is also inhibited by nedocromil sodium. In guinea pigs, noncholinergic, tachykinin-mediated airway contraction was found to be inhibited by pretreatment with nedocromil [39].

It is apparent from these studies that the mechanism of action of nedocromil sodium in the treatment of asthma is broad. The precise mechanism by which this drug exerts its antiinflammatory effect in man remains unclear.

# Clinical pharmacology: protective effect of nedocromil sodium in bronchial challenges

## *Effect of nedocromil on airway reactions following allergen challenge*

Pretreatment with nedocromil significantly inhibits the immediate reaction and the late reaction following allergen challenge. The inhalation of nedocromil following the immediate reaction partially but significantly reduced the magnitude of the late asthmatic reaction [40]. Inhalation of nedocromil sodium 15 min before house dust mite challenge inhibited the early and late reactions, with a greater protective effect against the late reaction, in 11 of 14 patients with asthma and positive skin tests for *Dermatophagoides pteronyssinus* allergen. There was also a significant improvement in bronchial hyperresponsiveness 3 and 24 h after challenge [41]. However, when given after the occurrence of the early-phase asthmatic reaction, nedocromil sodium was not able to prevent the development of the late reaction: it delayed the onset by 1.5 h. The allergen-induced increase of bronchial responsiveness was not prevented [42].

## *Effect of nedocromil on airway reactions following challenge with non-allergic stimuli*

Pretreatment with nedocromil immediately before challenge does not modify the airway responsiveness to histamine or methacholine [14]. However, the inhalation of 2 or 4 mg of nedocromil significantly inhibits the airway response to almost all indirect stimuli. Nedocromil shares this protective activity with cromoglycate but is more potent in protecting against non-allergic stimuli involving neuronal activation such as metabisulphite and bradykinin.

Crimi et al. have compared the protective effect of 4 mg of nedocromil, 10 mg of cromoglycate and placebo against adenosine challenge [43]. Both agents had a significant protective effect and nedocromil was significantly better than cromoglycate at the doses used. This study confirmed an investigation by Altounyan et al. [44].

Joos et al. investigated the protective effect of nedocromil against neurokinin A-induced bronchoconstriction: 4 mg of nedocromil almost completely prevented the dose-dependent bronchoconstriction induced in asthmatics by the inhalation of neurokinin A [45]. Crimi et al. confirmed the protective activity of nedocromil against neuropeptide-induced bronchoconstriction. The inhalation of 4 mg of nedocromil 30 min before inhalation challenge with substance P significantly increased the dose of substance P necessary to decrease the $FEV_1$ by 20% [46].

Dixon et al. studied the effect of nedocromil on the bronchospasm induced by sulphur dioxide in a group of six asthmatics [20]. Both 2 and 4 mg of nedocromil significantly inhibited the bronchoconstriction and dyspnoea, but using metabisulphite instead of sulphur dioxide, Dixon and Ind investigated in two double-blind, placebo-controlled studies the protective effect of 4 mg of nedocromil, 200 μg of ipratropium bromide or 180 mg of terfenadine [21]. Both ipratropium and nedocromil were protective and nedocromil almost completely prevented any bronchoconstrictive reaction to metabisulphite. The fact that terfenadine had no protective activity attests to the negligible role of the mast cell in this airway reaction. Wright et al. compared the protective effect of 8 mg of nedocromil with that of 4 mg of cromoglycate against metabisulphite challenge in a larger group of asthmatics. Nedocromil blocked the response to metabisulphite in 15 out of 20 asthmatics, whilst this dose of cromoglycate was only protective in three out of 20 subjects [47].

Dixon and Barnes compared the protective effect of 4 mg of nedocromil, 10 mg of cromoglycate and placebo against bradykinin challenge in eight asthmatics. Both drugs had significant protective activity, nedocromil being slightly better than cromoglycate [19].

Robuschi et al. compared 4 mg of nedocromil to placebo in a study using challenge with distilled water. Nedocromil significantly inhibited the fog-induced bronchoconstriction [48]. Along the same line, Roberts and Thomson demonstrated that 2 and 4 mg of nedocromil, inhaled 25 min before exercise, significantly protected against EIA [49].

Juniper et al. studied the effect of 1, 2 and 4 mg of nedocromil on the bronchospasm induced by the hyperventilation of cold air in a placebo-controlled study in 12 asthmatics. The response to cold air was measured at 20, 90 and 300 min after inhalation of the drug. All three doses has a significant protective effect at 20 min, but later on the protective effect of nedocromil was no longer significant [50].

## Effect of prolonged treatment with nedocromil on airway responsiveness

Dorward et al. compared nedocromil to placebo in a double-blind cross-over study in pollen-sensitive asthmatics. The active treatment period had a duration of 2 weeks and nedocromil was inhaled at a dose of 4 mg bid. Nedocromil significantly prevented the seasonal increase in airway responsiveness to histamine [51].

Orefice et al. investigated the effect of chronic treatment with nedocromil on methacholine responsiveness in asthmatics [52]. Patients were treated with 4 mg of nedocromil q.d.s. or placebo, and this was added to their usual antiasthma treatment. A significant decrease in the airway responsiveness to methacholine was observed at 8 and 12 weeks of nedrocromil treatment.

In a parallel-group study design, Bel et al. compared the effect of 4 mg of nedocromil, 100 µg of beclomethasone dipropionate and placebo, given four times per day for 4 months, on methacholine responsiveness in non-steroid-dependent non-atopic asthmatics. Both nedocromil and beclomethasone diproprionate significantly decreased the airway responsiveness to methacholine after 8 weeks of treatment [53]. In contrast, beclomethasone 200 µg twice or 4 times daily for 6 to 8 weeks was more effective than nedocromil sodium 4 mg twice or 4 times daily for the same period in reducing bronchial hyperreactivity to histamine and distilled water [54].

## Nedocromil-sodium: therapeutic efficacy in asthma

Two double-blind, double-placebo, randomized cross-over studies compared the effects of nedocromil sodium with continuous $\beta_2$-agonist treatment [55, 56]. Effects of nedocromil sodium and salbutamol (sal) treatment were investigated in allergic, mild to moderately severe asthmatics. Both studies showed a significant decrease in symptom scores and diurnal PEF variation during nedocromil sodium compared with sal treatment. In addition, de Jong et al. also showed a significant increase in $PC_{20}$ propranolol (0.5 doubling concentrations) and morning PEF (16 L/Min) and a decrease in day-to-day PEF variation and rescue ipratropium bromide use (0.6 puffs/day) [56]. Wasserman et al. showed that regular treatment with nedocromil sodium provided a greater level of asthma symptom control than regular treatment with albuterol with a significantly greater improvement in daytime and nighttime asthma and morning chest tightness [57]. Quality of life was evaluated in a year long, double-blind, placebo-controlled comparative study with nedocromil sodium. The impacts component of the St.George's Respiratory Questionnaire was significantly improved in patients receiving nedocromil sodium (4 mg), as were night-time asthma, asthma severity at clinic and daytime inhaled bronchodilator use [58].

The effects of nedocromil sodium added to treatment with bronchodilators were investigated in seven placebo-controlled, group comparative studies in adults with mild to moderate, mostly allergic asthma (reviewed in [29]). Patients were maintained on oral and/or inhaled bronchodilator therapy and received nedocromil sodium or placebo after a baseline period of 2 to 4 weeks. Most of the studies showed a significant increase in $FEV_1$ (0.2–0.5 L) and PEF (10–75 L/min), a decrease in $\beta_2$-agonist use (1–3 puffs/day), and an improvement of total symptom scores during nedocromil sodium compared with placebo treatment. The morning PEF values during nedocromil sodium therapy continued to increase over the period of treatment [59].

## Nedocromil sodium versus corticosteroids

Inhaled corticosteroids are very effective anti-inflammatory agents in the treatment of asthma. Investigations into the effects of nedocromil sodium compared with corticosteroids can be classified into three categories: (1) Nedocromil sodium compared with inhaled corticosteroids; (2) the addition of nedocromil sodium and the ability of patients to reduce their concomitant corticosteroid therapy without further deterioration of their asthma; and (3) the effects of nedocromil sodium added to corticosteroid inhalation.

## The effects of nedocromil sodium compared with inhaled corticosteroid therapy

In two placebo-controlled studies both nedocromil sodium (16 mg/d) and beclomethasone (400 µg/d) significantly improved symptom scores when compared with placebo. $FEV_1$ also improved during both treatments, but significantly more with beclomethasone than with nedocromil sodium treatment. Bel et al. demonstrated a significant improvement in airway hyperresponsiveness, as measured by the $PC_{20}$ methacholine, both during nedocromil sodium and beclomethasone (1.5 and 1.7 doubling concentrations, respectively) compared with placebo treatment, in nonatopic patients [53]. In three crossover studies in mostly allergic asthmatics both beclomethasone and nedocromil sodium were significantly better at improving $PC_{20}$ histamine (1 to 3 doubling concentrations) but beclomethasone improved the $PC_{20}$ values significantly more compared with nedocromil sodium (reviewed in [29]).

## Addition of nedocromil sodium to corticosteroid therapy: steroid sparing effect?

In six placebo-controlled studies (reviewed in [29]) attempts were made to reduce the doses of inhaled or oral corticosteroids. About half of the patients were allergic, with mild to severe asthma. Paananen et al. stopped inhaled corticosteroids after 3 weeks of active treatment. The results showed a general impairment in PEF values and symptom scores, an increase in $\beta_2$-agonist use and a high number of dropouts during both nedocromil sodium and placebo treatment. Ruffin et al. and Bone et al. halved the amount of inhaled corticosteroids during the baseline period, to make asthma unstable. During nedocromil sodium treatment, PEF values (20 L/min) and symptom scores and $\beta_2$-agonist use improved significantly compared to placebo.

In a group of steroid-dependent chronic asthmatic patients, with a mean oral prednisolone use of > 8 mg/day, it was not possible to reduce the amount of prednisolone significantly more during nedocromil sodium compared with placebo treatment. None of the clinical outcome parameters ($FEV_1$, PEF values, $\beta_2$-agonist use and symptoms scores) changed in either treatment group [60]. In another study [61] a significantly greater reduction of the oral steroid dose during nedocromil sodium treatment was achieved, compared with placebo treatment. However, there was no change in $FEV_1$, PEF or symptom scores. During nedocromil sodium treatment the $\beta_2$-agonist use was increased, as was the use in the placebo group.

In a placebo-controlled study, Orefice et al. compared the effects of treatment with nedocromil sodium (16 mg/day) with cromoglycate (40 mg/day) and beclomethasone (1500 µg/day) [62]. Compared with placebo, all patients managed to improve $FEV_1$ (0.2 l) and $PC_{20}$ methacholine (1.2 doubling doses). $\beta_2$-agonist use and symptom scores decreased significantly during beclomethasone, compared with beclomethasone and placebo treatment, but not in comparison with nedocromil sodium treatment. However the four treatment groups are difficult to compare because all patients, with the exception of the beclomethasone group, received the oral corticosteroid daflazacort.

## The effects of nedocromil sodium when added to the treatment of patients already inhaling corticosteroids

The effects of nedocromil sodium (8–16 mg/day), added to the therapy of subjects who were mostly steroid-dependent with stable, moderate to severe asthma were investigated in five placebo-controlled studies (reviewed in [29]). Most of the studies showed significant improvements in PEF values (14–30 L/min) and symptom scores, and decreases in $\beta_2$-agonist use (about 1 puff/day) in patients treated with nedocromil sodium, compared with placebo. In contrast to patients not receiving corticosteroids, the addition of nedocromil sodium to corticosteroids leads only to an improvement in PEF during the first 4 to 8 weeks, reaching a plateau at that time without further improvement.

In spite of these confounding factors, many studies have demonstrated the non-steroidal anti-inflammatory drug nedocromil sodium to be effective. To summarize:

(i) Nedocromil sodium treatment is clearly superior to placebo and in some studies it provides better clinical improvement compared to continuous bronchodilator therapy.

(ii) Several studies demonstrate that the effects of nedocromil sodium (16 mg/day) are equal to these of beclomethasone (400 μg/day) for some outcome parameters. For changes in symptom score and $\beta_2$-agonist use beclomethasone gives significantly better results.

(iii) No conclusive data can be drawn from studies replacing corticosteroid treatment with nedocromil sodium, because the withdrawal of corticosteroids was too rapid and the amounts used too great.

(iv) Nedocromil sodium seems to be effective especially in mild to moderate allergic and nonallergic asthma.

(v) There may be an important role for nedocromil sodium as an additional therapy in patients already using high doses of inhaled corticosteroids.

(iv) Compared with inhaled cromoglycate (4 × 10 mg/day), nedocromil sodium (4 × 4 mg/day) is more effective in reducing asthma symptoms and extra bronchodilator use. In patients more than 50 years old, there seems to be no difference in the efficacy of the two drugs.

(vii) It is still not clear whether nedocromil sodium can be used as a steroid sparing agent.

## Nedocromil sodium and steroid-resistant asthma

Some patients with asthma respond poorly to corticosteroids and have persistent airway inflammation and daily clinical symptoms. Marin et al. demonstrated that inhaled nedocromil sodium improves pulmonary function and decreased asthma severity in steroid-resistent asthma [63].

## Nedocromil sodium and COPD

The effect of 10 weeks of treatment with nedocromil sodium in non-allergic subjects with COPD was reported. Nedocromil sodium failed to improve clinical parameters (airway responsiveness to histamine, methacholine, AMP, pulmonary function and symptom scores). The only difference with placebo was seen in the lower number of dropouts (because of exacerbations). Also both patients and clinicians favoured treatment with nedocromil sodium [64].

## Safety

No major side-effects have been noted during the therapeutic evaluation with nedocromil. The drug has an excellent safety profile up to the present. The most frequent side-effect is unpleasant taste and occasionally local irritation of the throat and the airways. Some patients treated with nedocromil may also experience headache.

## Summary and conclusion

Cromoglycate and nedocromil work through a number of different mechanisms. Their original designation as "mast cell stabilizing agents" is an oversimplification of their multiple pharmacological activities. According to the international guidelines [1] cromolyn sodium and nedocromil are considered to be long-term-control medications. They have a mild to moderate anti-inflammatory effect and can be the initial choice for long-term-control therapy in children. They can also be used as preventive treatment prior to exercise or unavoidable exposure to known allergens. Safety is one of the primary advantages of these agents. A therapeutic response often occurs within 2 weeks, but a 4-to-6 week trial may be needed to determine the maximum benefit.

## References

1   National Institutes of Health (1997) NIH publication nr. 97-4051A.: Guidelines for the diagnosis and management of asthma. May, 21
2   Altounyan REC (1967) Inhibition of experimental asthma by a new compound, disodium cromoglycate. *Acta Allergol* 22: 487–492

3    Cox JCG (1967) Cromoglycate (FPL 670)('Intal): a specific inhibitor of reaginic anti-body-antigen mechanisms. *Nature* 216: 1328–1329

4    Church MK, Young KD (1983) The characteristics of inhibition of histamine release from human lung fragments by sodium cromoglycate, salbutamol and chlorpromazine *Br J Pharmacol* 78: 671–679

5    Church MK, Hiroi J (1987) Inhibition of IgE-dependent histamine release from human dispersed lung mast cells by anti-allergic drugs and salbutamol. *Br J Pharmacol* 90: 421–429

6    Flint KC, Leung KBP, Pearce FL, Hudspith BN, Brostoff J, Mc Johnson I(1985) Human mast cells recovered by bronchoalveolar lavage: their morphology, histamine release and the effects of sodium cromoglycate. *Clin Science* 68:427–432

7    Orr TSC (1973) Mast cells and allergic asthma. *Br J Dis Chest* 67: 87–106

8    Kay AB (1987) The mode of action of anti-allergic drugs. *Clin Allergy* 17: 153–164

9    Kimata H, Fujimoto M, Mikawa H (1994) Nedocromil sodium acts directly on human B cells to inhibit immunoglobulin production without affecting cell growth. *Immunology* 81: 47–52

10   Dixon CM, Jackson DM, Richards IM (1979) The effects of sodium cromoglycate on lung irritant receptors and left ventricular cardiac receptors in the anaesthetized dog. *Br J Pharmacol* 67: 569–574

11   Biggs DF, Goel N (1985) Mechanisms of action of sodium cromoglycate. *Can J Physiol Pharmacol* 63: 760–765

12   Booij-Noord H, Orie NGM, de Vries K (1971) Immediate and late bronchial obstructive reactions to inhalation of house dust and protective effects of disodium cromoglycate and prednisolone. *J Allergy* 48: 344–354

13   Cockcroft DW, Murdock KY (1987) Comparative effects of inhaled salbutamol, sodium cromoglycate and beclomethasone dipropionate on allergen-induced early asthmatic responses, late asthmatic responses, and increased bronchial responsiveness to histamine. *J Allergy Clin Immunol* 79: 734–740

14   Pauwels RA, Joos GF, Van Der Straeten ME (1988) Bronchial hyperresponsiveness is not bronchial asthma. *Clin Allergy* 18: 317–332

15   Silverman M, Andrea T (1972) Time course of effect of disodium cromoglycate on exercise-induced asthma. *Arch Dis Child* 47: 419–422

16   Deal EC, Wasserman SI, Soter NA, Ingram RH, McFadden ER (1980) Evaluation of role played by mediators of immediate hypersensitivity in exercise-induced asthma. *J Clin Invest* 65: 659–665

17   Breslin FJ, McFadden ER Jr, Ingram RH Jr (1980) The effect of cromolyn sodium on the airway response to hyperpnea and cold air in asthma. *Am Rev Respir Dis* 122: 11–16

18   Holgate ST (1989) Reflections on the mechanisms of action of sodium cromoglycate (Intal) and the role of mast cells in asthma. *Respir Med* 83: 25–31

19   Dixon CM, Barnes PJ (1989) Bradykinin-induced bronchoconstriction: inhibition by nedocromil sodium and sodium cromoglycate. *Br J Clin Pharmacol* 27: 831–836

20   Dixon CM, Fuller RW, Barnes PJ (1987) Effect of nedocromil sodium on sulphur dioxide induced bronchoconstriction. *Thorax* 42: 462–465

21   Dixon CM, Ind PW (1988) Metabisulfite induced bronchoconstriction:mechanisms. *Am Rev Respir Dis* 137: 238

22   Löwhagen O, Rak S (1985) Modification of bronchial hyperreactivity after treatment with sodium cromoglycate during pollen season. *J Allergy Clin Immunol* 75: 460–467

23   Löwhagen O, Rak S (1985) Bronchial hyperreactivity after treatment with sodium cromoglycate in atopic asthmatics not exposed to relevant allergens. *J Allergy Clin Immunol* 75: 343–347

24   Petty TL, Rollins DR, Christopher K, Good JT, Oakley R (1989) Cromolyn sodium is effective in adult chronic asthmatics. *Am Rev Respir Dis* 139: 694–701

25   Edwards AM (1994) Sodium cromoglycate (Intal) as an anti-inflammatory agent for the treatment of chronic asthma. *Clin Exper Allergy* 24: 612–623

26   Tasche MJA, van der Wouden JC, Uijen JHJM, Ponsioen BP, Bernsen RMD, van Suijlekom-Smit LWA, de Jongste JC (1997) Randomised placebo-controlled trial of inhaled sodium cromoglycate in 1–4-year old children with moderate asthma. *Lancet* 350: 1060–1064

27   Hargreaves MR, Benson MK (1995) Inhaled sodium cromoglycate in angiotensin- converting enzyme inhibitor cough. *Lancet* 345: 13–16

28   Morrison-Smith J (1979) Prolonged use of disodium cromoglycate in children and young persons – ten years experience. In: J Pepys, AM Edwards (eds): The mast cell – Its role in health and disease. Pitman Medical, Davos, London, 280–282

29   de Jong JW, Postma DS, de Monchy JGR, Koeter GH (1993) A review of nedocromil sodium in asthma therapy. *Eur Respir J* 3: 511–519

30   Borish L, Williams J, Johnson S, Mascali JJ, Miller R et al (1992) Anti-inflammatory effects of nedocromil sodium: inhibition of alveolar macrophage function. *Clin Exper Allergy* 62: 38–41

31   Vittori E, Sciacca F, Colotta F, Mantovani A, Mattoli S (1992) Protective effect of nedocromil sodium on the interleukin-1-induced production of interleukin-8 in human bronchial epithelial cells. *J Allergy Clin Immunol* 90: 76–84

32   Devalia JL, Rusznak C, Calderon, Sapsford RJ, Davis R (1994) The effect of nedocromil sodium on ozone-induced synthesis of cytokines by human bronchial epithelial cell cultures *in vitro*. *Am J Respir Crit Care Med* 149: A317

33   Marini M, Soloperto M, Zheng Y, Mezzetti M, Mattoli S (1992) Protective effect of nedocromil sodium on the IL-1-induced release of GM-CSF from cultured human bronchial epithelial cells. *Pulmonary Pharmacology* 5: 61–65

34   Schoonbrood DFM, Out TA, Hart AAM, Habets FJM, Roos CM, Jansen H (1997) Nedocromil sodium in obstructive airways disease: effect on symptoms and plasma protein leakage in sputum. *Eur Respir J* 10: 1500–1506

35   Gilbert IA, Logan LS, Hassan MO, Abdul-Karim F, Kenner KA, Nelson JA, McFadden ER (1994) Influence of nedocromil sodium on airway inflammation in asthmatics. *Am J Respir Crit Care Med* 149: A941

36    Manolitsas ND, Wang J, Devalia JL et al (1995) Regular albuterol, nedocromil sodium and bronchial inflammation in asthma. Am J Respir Crit Care Med 151: 1925–1930

37    Leung KBP, Flint KC, Brostoff J (1988) Effects of sodium cromoglycate and nedocromil sodium on histamine secretion from human lung mast cells. Thorax 43: 756–761

38    Maxwell DL, Hawksworth RJ, Lee TH (1993) Inhaled nedocromil sodium reduces histamine release from isolated large airway segments of asthmatic subjects in vivo. Eur Respir J 6: 1145–1150

39    Verleden GM, Belvisi MG, Stretton CD, Barnes PJ (1991) Nedocromil sodium modulates nonadrenergic, noncholinergic bronchoconstrictor nerves in guinea pig airways in vitro. Am Rev Respir Dis 143: 114–118

40    Dahl R, Pedersen B (1986) Influence of nedocromil sodium on the dual asthmatic reactions after allergen challenge: a double blind, placebo-controlled study. Eur J Respir Dis 69 (suppl 147): 263–265

41    Aalbers R, Kauffman HF, Groen H, Koeter GH, de Monchy JGR (1991) The effect of nedocromil sodium on the early and late reaction and allergen-induced bronchial hyperresponsiveness. J Allergy Clin Immunol 87: 993–1001

42    Crimi N, Violante B, Pellegrino R, Brusasco V (1993) Effect of multiple doses of nedrocromil sodium given after inhalation in asthma. J Allergy Clin Immunol 92: 777–783

43    Crimi N, Palermo F, Oliveri R, Vancheri C, Polosa R, Palermo B, Maccarrone C, Mistretta A (1988) Comparative study of the effects of nedocromil sodium (4 mg) and sodium cromoglycate (10 mg) on adenosine-induced bronchoconstriction in asthmatic subjects. Clin Allergy 18: 367–374

44    Altounyan REC, Lee TB, Rocchicciolo KMS, Shaw CL (1986) A comparison of the inhibitory effects of nedocromil sodium and sodium cromoglycate on adenosine monophosphate-induced bronchoconstriction in atopic subjects. Eur J Respir Dis 69 (suppl 147): 277–279

45    Joos GF, Pauwels RA, Van Der Straeten ME (1989) The effect of nedocromil sodium on the bronchoconstrictor effect of neurokinin A in subjects with asthma. J Allergy Clin Immunol 83: 663–668

46    Crimi N, Palermo F, Oliveri R, Palermo B, Vancheri C, Polosa R, Mestretta A (1988) Effect of nedocromil on bronchospasm induced by inhalation of substance P in asthmatic subjects. Clin Allergy 18: 375–382

47    Wright W, Zhang YFG, Salme, CM, Woolcock AJ (1990) Effect of inhaled preservatives on asthmatic subjects. I. Sodium metabisulfite. Am Rev Respir Dis 141: 1400–1404

48    Robuschi M, Vaghi A, Simone P, Bianco S (1987) Prevention of fog-induced bronchospasm by nedocromil sodium. Clin Allergy 17: 69–74

49    Roberts JA, Thomson NC (1985) Attenuation of exercise-induced asthma by pretreatment with nedocromil sodium and minocromil. Clin Allergy 15: 377–381

50    Juniper EF, Kline PA, Morris MM, Hargreave FE (1987) Airway constriction by isocapnic hyperventilation of cold, dry air: comparison of magnitude and duration of protection by nedocromil sodium and sodium cromoglycate. Clin Allergy 17: 523–528

51    Dorward AJ, Roberts JA, Thomson NC (1986) Effect of nedocromil sodium on hista-

mine airway responsiveness in grass-pollen sensitive asthmatics during the pollen season. *Clin Allergy* 16: 309–315

52    Orefice U, Struzzo PL, Pitzalis G, Dei D (1989) A double-blind multicenter group comparative study of the efficacy and safety of nedocromil sodium in the management of asthma. *Chest* 97: 1299–1306

53    Bel EH, Timmers MC, Hermans J, Dijkman JH, Sterk PJ (1990) The long-term effects of nedocromil sodium and beclomethasone dipropionate on bronchial responsiveness to methacholine in nonatopic asthmatic subjects. *Am Rev Respir Dis* 141: 21–28

54    Groot CAR, Lammers JWJ, Molema J, Festen J, Van Herwaarden CLA (1992) Effects of inhaled beclomethasone and nedocromil sodium on bronchial hyperresponsiveness to histamine and distilled water. *Eur Respir J* 5: 1075–1082

55    Marcoux JP, Findlay SR, Furukaway CT (1992) A placebo-controlled comparison of nedocromil sodium (Tilade) and salbutamol in mild to moderate asthma. *Eur Respir J* 5:83s (abstract)

56    de Jong JW, Teengs JP, Postma DS, van der Mark TW, Koeter GH, de Monchy JGR (1994) Nedocromil sodium versus albuterol in the management of allergic asthma. *Am J Respir Crit Care Med* 149: 91–7

57    Wasserman SI, Furukawa CT, Henochowicz SI et al (1995) Asthma symptoms and airway hyperresponsiveness are lower during treatment with nedocromil sodium than during treatment with regular inhaled albuterol. *J Allergy Clin Immunol* 95: 541–547

58    Jones PW (1994) Nedocromil sodium quality of life study group. Quality of life, symptoms and pulmonary function in asthma: long-term treatment with nedocromil sodium examined in a controlled multicentre trial. *Eur Respir J* 7: 55–62

59    Fink J, Forman S, Silvers SS, Soifer MM, Tashkin DP, Wilson AF (1994) A double-blind study of the efficacy of nedocromil sodium in the management of asthma in patients using high doses of bronchodilators. *J Allergy Clin Immunol* 94: 473–481

60    Goldin JG, Bateman ED (1988) Does nedocromil sodium have a steroid sparing effect in adult asthmatic patients requiring maintenance oral corticosteroids? *Thorax* 43: 982–9866.

61    Boulet LP, Cartier A, Cockcroft DW et al (1990) Tolerance to reduction of oral steroid dosage in severely asthmatic patients receiving nedocromil sodium. *Respir Med* 84: 317–323

62    Orefice U, Struzzo P, Dorigo R, Peratoner A (1990) Long-term effects of nedocromil sodium and beclomethasone diproprionate on bronchial responsiveness to methacholine in nonatopic asthmatic subjects. *Am Rev Respir Dis* 141: 21–28

63    Marin JS, Carrizo SJ, Garcia R, Ejea MV (1996) Effects of nedocromil sodium in steroidresistant asthma: a randomized controlled trial. *J Allergy Clin Immunol* 97: 602–610

64    de Jong JW, Postma DS, van der Mark TW, Koeter GH (1994) Effects of nedocromil sodium in the treatment of non-allergic subjects with chronic obstructive pulmonary disease. *Thorax* 49: 1022–1024

# Anti-leukotriene therapy for asthma

*Zuzana Diamant[1] and Anthony P. Sampson[2]*

[1]Erasmus University Medical Centre Rotterdam, Department of Respiratory Diseases, Dr Molewaterplein 40, NL-3015 GD Rotterdam, The Netherlands; [2]Immunopharmacology Group, Level F, Centre Block (825), Southampton General Hospital, Tremona Road, Southampton, SO16 6YD, UK

## Introduction

Human bronchial asthma is a chronic disorder of the airways, associated in most cases with atopy (i.e. specific immunoglobulin E responses to allergens), and characterised by a range of abnormalities on various levels. Early definitions of asthma stressed the aspects of variable lung function, reversible spontaneously or with treatment, but more recent definitions also place emphasis on the underlying airway inflammation that is thought to promote bronchial hyperresponsiveness [1]. The asthma syndrome comprises firstly, clinical symptoms, such as chest tightness, dyspnoea, coughing, and/or wheeze, secondly, pathophysiological features, such as variable airway obstruction and bronchial hyperresponsiveness (BHR) to a variety of stimuli which may be physical (e.g. cold dry air, hyper/hypotonic saline), pharmacological (e.g. histamine, methacholine), chemical (e.g. $SO_2$), or physiological (e.g. exercise), and thirdly, pathohistological parameters, particularly eosinophilic airway inflammation, resulting in structural changes within the airways ("airway remodelling") [2, 3]. Asthma may occur in varying degrees of severity ranging from intermittent to severe persistent forms [1].

Airway inflammation plays a central role in the pathogenesis of asthma [2]. Hence, in recent asthma management guidelines, anti-inflammatory therapy ("controller" medication, mostly inhaled corticosteroids) is advocated as first-line treatment of persistent asthma, in combination with "reliever" medication (specific $\beta_2$-bronchodilators) as required for rescue medication [1]. Despite the well-documented effectiveness and relative safety of these drugs, too many asthmatic patients are still being treated suboptimally, resulting in a poor quality of life [4]. The reasons for suboptimal treatment include poor compliance with treatment, sometimes due to misunderstanding by patients of the different roles of anti-inflammatory prophylaxis and bronchodilator "rescue" drugs, and sometimes due to largely misplaced anxiety about adverse drug effects, particularly with corticosteroids. In addition, a world-wide trend of increasing prevalence, morbidity, and mortality of asthma has been observed in the last decade [1]. Therefore, many research groups have sought

Anti-Inflammatory Drugs in Asthma, edited by A.P. Sampson and M.K. Church
© 1999 Birkhäuser Verlag Basel/Switzerland

alternative anti-inflammatory drugs, preferably to be combined with bronchodilator activity. The anti-leukotriene (anti-LT) drugs seem to comply with this profile.

## Experimental models of asthma

In preclinical studies, exacerbations of asthma can be mimicked in appropriate patients by a number of well-documented models including exercise and aspirin challenge, inhalation of allergen or ozone, experimental virus infections, or even withdrawal of regular anti-asthma controller treatment [5].

The characteristics of the allergen challenge model make it one of the most suitable systems for intervention studies with experimental anti-asthma drugs. Inhalation of a specific allergen by a sensitive asthmatic patient induces acute airway narrowing, the so-called early asthmatic response (EAR), usually defined as a fall in forced expiratory volume in 1 s ($FEV_1$) of at least 20% from baseline [6]. The EAR involves IgE-triggered mast cell mediator release, predominantly causing acute airway smooth muscle contraction, occurring within 10 min after allergen inhalation and mostly recovering within 3 h [6, 7]. In approximately 50% of cases, the EAR is followed by a late asthmatic response (LAR) at 3–7 h, defined as a fall in $FEV_1$ of at least 15% from baseline [6]. The LAR is characterised by inflammatory events within the airways in which activated eosinophils are thought to play a key role. In particular, airway oedema and mucus hypersecretion, as well as airway smooth muscle contraction, may make significant contributions to airflow obstruction in the LAR. Eosinophil release of pro-inflammatory mediators and basic proteins may induce the subsequent BHR which may last for several days or weeks following the LAR [7–9], perhaps due to damage to the airway epithelium which allows greater access of airborne irritants to the bronchial submucosa. The LAR is thus thought to mimic the underlying pathophysiological changes in the asthmatic airway.

Despite many advantages for the investigator, experimental models of asthma can only reflect the acute inflammatory processes occurring within the airways during exacerbations of asthma. Inflammatory changes in clinical asthma may occur in response to persistent exposure to low levels of airborne allergens or sensitising chemicals, rather than the large bolus doses of allergens and stimuli administered in the laboratory. Long-term follow-up studies in patients with persistent asthma are therefore essential to evaluate the possible effects of novel anti-asthma therapies on the chronic, structural changes which determine clinical outcome. Both types of intervention have been applied with anti-LT drugs [10]. Although airway inflammation and remodelling involve complex networks of inflammatory cells and mediators, the central role of the leukotriene family of mediators in these processes has been amply demonstrated by the surprising effectiveness of anti-LT drugs.

## Leukotrienes and human lung cells

### The leukotriene synthetic pathway

The eicosanoids are a heterogeneous group of biologically-active mediators derived from the 20-carbon fatty acid arachidonic acid, and include leukotrienes (LTs), prostaglandins (PGs), thromboxane (TX), lipoxins (LX), and hydroxylated derivatives (HETEs)[11]. Leukotrienes are derived from arachidonic acid via the 5-lipoxygenase (5-LO) pathway (Fig. 1) [11, 12]. 5-LO is a 78 kDa haem protein found in the cytosol of a limited number of resting cells of myeloid origin [13, 14]. 5-LO activating protein (FLAP), an 18 kDa nuclear membrane-bound protein, is essential for translation and activation of 5-LO, together with Ca$^{2+}$ and ATP [15, 16]. First, free arachidonic acid cleaved from membrane phospholipids by cytosolic phospholipase A$_2$ or other phospholipases, is donated by FLAP to 5-LO, which converts it to 5-

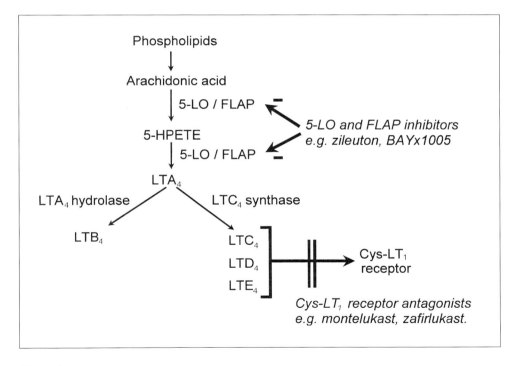

*Figure 1*
*Arachidonic acid metabolism: 5-lipoxygenase pathway with sites of action of leukotriene receptor antagonists and leukotriene biosynthesis inhibitors.*
*Abbreviations: 5-LO, 5-lipoxygenase; FLAP, 5-lipoxygenase activating protein; (cys-)LT, (cysteinyl-) leukotriene; 5-HPETE, 5-hydroperoxy-eicosatetraenoic acid*

hydroperoxy-eicosatetraenoic acid (5-HPETE) and thence to the unstable epoxide $LTA_4$. Subsequently, depending on cell-type, $LTA_4$ is converted either to $LTB_4$ by $LTA_4$ hydrolase [17], or to the first of the cysteinyl-leukotrienes (cys-LTs), $LTC_4$, by $LTC_4$ synthase [18]. $LTC_4$ synthase, a homodimer of 16.6 kDa subunits, is an integral membrane protein with striking sequence homology to FLAP [19]. Following carrier-mediated export from the cell [20], $LTC_4$ is metabolized via $LTD_4$ to the relatively stable $LTE_4$ by extracellular enzymes found in lung tissue and plasma [21, 22]. Both $LTE_4$ and $LTB_4$ are then degraded by $\omega$- and $\beta$-oxidation in the liver [23]. $LTB_4$ may also be rapidly degraded by $\omega$-oxidation within activated neutrophils at the inflammatory site [24]. A small proportion (about 5%) of total systemic $LTC_4$ is excreted unchanged as $LTE_4$ in the urine [25].

## Actions of leukotrienes on human lung cells

While $LTB_4$ is predominantly synthesized by monocytes, macrophages, and neutrophils, cys-LTs are mainly produced by mast cells, basophils, and eosinophils [11, 12, 26–31]. Monocyte-macrophages may also contribute to cys-LT formation. Both subfamilies of leukotrienes possess distinct biologic properties which may account for many of the features of asthma, as well as of other inflammatory diseases [11, 12, 32, 33]. $LTB_4$ is a potent chemoattractant and activator of neutrophils, monocytes, and eosinophils in several species *in vitro* and *in vivo* [11, 12, 34, 35], but does not contract human airway smooth muscle [36]. In contrast, cys-LTs are exquisitely potent in contracting airway smooth muscle in normals and asthmatics [37–40]. They are also potent enhancers of airway microvascular permeability, resulting in oedema, and they stimulate mucus secretion [41, 42]. Furthermore, recent evidence shows that cys-LTs also possess potent and specific chemoattractant activity for eosinophils in animals and humans both *in vitro* and *in vivo* [35, 43–45]. This is in contrast to other chemoattractant lipids such as platelet-activating factor (PAF) and $LTB_4$ which also attract neutrophils.

## Leukotriene receptors

The pro-inflammatory effects of leukotrienes are mediated by stimulation of specific receptors [46]. Although bronchoconstriction of isolated human airways by cys-LTs is mediated by a direct effect at specific receptors on airway smooth muscle [36], such effects may be supplemented or modulated in whole lung *in vivo* by secondary release of other pro-inflammatory mediators, such as neuropeptides [47]. While $LTB_4$ is likely to occupy a distinct receptor, the BLT receptor [11], many details of cys-LT receptor pharmacology remain to be clarified. In guinea-pig airways, distinct receptor subtypes have been isolated for $LTC_4$ and $LTD_4$, termed $LTR_c$ and $LTR_d$

respectively [48, 49]. The latter has been characterised as a 45 kDa membrane protein [50]. Conflicting data exist on possible receptor heterogeneity in human airways. Investigations with an early leukotriene receptor antagonist (FPL-55712) in isolated human airways suggested that all cys-LTs interact with a single receptor [51], whereas binding studies with [$^3$H]-leukotriene radioligands pointed to the existence of two distinct cys-LT receptors: one for $LTD_4$ and $LTE_4$, and a second for $LTC_4$ [46]. Such experiments may be confounded by non-specific binding of $^3$H-$LTC_4$ to cell-associated enzymes including $LTC_4$ synthase, or to the γ-glutamyl transpeptidase which converts $LTC_4$ to $LTD_4$. Recent evidence however suggests heterogeneity of cys-LT receptors in different tissues; $LTC_4$ and $LTD_4$ are regarded as full agonists, and $LTE_4$ as a partial agonist at cys-$LT_1$ receptors located on airway smooth muscle, which mediate airway smooth muscle contraction, while cys-$LT_2$ receptors, located in the smooth muscle of pulmonary arteries and veins, mediate relaxation [46, 52]. Among the cys-LT receptor antagonists, all of which block the cys-$LT_1$ receptor, only Bay u9773 also blocks the cys-$LT_2$ receptor [52]. In addition, evidence has been provided for similar (auxiliary?) receptors located on human pulmonary vein endothelial cells, which are likely to bear both cys-$LT_1$ receptors, associated with contraction, and cys-$LT_2$ receptors, which mediate relaxation [46]. The further development of potent, selective antagonists for each receptor subtype should clarify the role and mechanism of action of these receptors subsets in the pathophysiology of asthma.

## Detection of endogenous leukotriene production

A number of studies have detected the release of cys-LTs into relevant body compartments in clinical asthma and in various challenge models of asthma. Inhaled allergen challenge of atopic asthmatics causes significant rises in BAL fluid $LTC_4$ levels 5 min after challenge [53] and in urinary $LTE_4$ levels within 4 h [54]. The former is accompanied by rises in BAL fluid histamine, tryptase, and $PGD_2$, suggesting that all four mediators are released by degranulating mast cells. In symptomatic patients with atopic asthma, increased levels of $LTB_4$ and/or cys-LTs have been demonstrated in the exhaled breath condensate, and in biological fluids including blood, urine, sputum, and bronchoalveolar lavage fluid [54–64]. This generation of leukotrienes may either result from direct activation of inflammatory cells [7, 28], or from secondary release by other mediators, such as platelet activating factor (PAF) [65], or bradykinin [66]. Despite conflicting data on cys-LT production following exercise or isocapnic hyperventilation of cold and/or dry air [67–72], several intervention studies using anti-LT drugs have attested that leukotrienes are likely to be involved in the bronchoconstriction induced by these challenges [10, 73].

In aspirin-sensitive asthmatic patients, who are mostly non-atopic [74], basal production of cys-LTs is particularly exaggerated, as reflected by increased urinary

$LTE_4$ levels as compared to aspirin-tolerant asthmatics or normals [75]. Challenge with oral aspirin or inhaled lysine-aspirin produces significant increases in BAL fluid and urinary cys-LTs only in aspirin-intolerant asthmatics [76, 77], probably because NSAIDs remove the chronic suppression of cys-LT synthesis by endogenous $PGE_2$ [78]. The increased basal cys-LT synthesis in aspirin-intolerant asthmatics, and the BHR to inhaled NSAIDs, are closely related to markedly higher expression of $LTC_4$ synthase, the terminal enzyme for cys-LT synthesis, in the bronchial wall of these patients [79]. This is due partly to chronically increased numbers of bronchial mucosal eosinophils in aspirin-intolerant asthmatics [79, 80], and partly to the higher proportion of eosinophils expressing the enzyme, compared to aspirin-tolerant asthmatics [79]. In addition, evidence exists for a selective target organ hypersensitivity to $LTE_4$ in patients with aspirin-induced asthma [81].

## Effects of inhaled leukotrienes in man

Upon inhalation, cys-LTs induce clinical symptoms of asthma, including bronchoconstriction [82, 83]. The cys-LTs are several orders of magnitude more potent than other bronchoconstrictors such as histamine and $PGD_2$, and the bronchoconstriction is longer-lived, lasting 30–40 min compared to the 5–10 min response to histamine. Inhaled cys-LTs also cause increased bronchial responsiveness both in normal and asthmatic individuals [82, 85–87], although late phase responses to inhaled cys-LTs are not reported [88]. In addition, recent studies in asthmatic patients have shown selective influx of eosinophils into the airway in bronchial biopsies [44], and in hypertonic saline-induced sputum [45], 4 h after inhalation of $LTE_4$ and $LTD_4$, respectively. Furthermore, strong evidence exists from animal studies that cys-LTs may contribute to the development of structural changes within the airways, particularly by increasing the airway smooth muscle mass [89–91]. Apart from airway smooth muscle hypertrophy/hyperplasia, this airway remodelling is characterised by loss of airway epithelium and thickening of the airway wall through deposition of fibronectin and collagen [2, 92], and, from the pathophysiological point of view, it is a major determinant of excessive airway narrowing which may cause serious clinical symptoms [93]. In contrast to the cys-LTs, inhalation of $LTB_4$ by normal or atopic asthmatic subjects does not cause acute bronchoconstriction and does not change bronchial responsiveness to histamine [94].

## Anti-leukotriene drugs

Despite the possible involvement of other pro-inflammatory mediators such as histamine, prostanoids, and platelet activating factor in asthma [56–58], therapy with experimental drugs directed against single mediators have mostly shown disappointing results in the treatment of asthma, especially in the case of PAF antagonists [95]. The anti-LT drugs are exceptions to this rule. Two categories of anti-LT agents have been developed. Firstly, the leukotriene receptor antagonists (LTRA) block either cys-LT receptors (cys-LT$_1$) or LTB$_4$ receptors (BLT), and secondly, the leukotriene synthesis inhibitors (LTSIs) which block either 5-LO activity or FLAP activity (Fig. 1), and hence prevent the synthesis both of cys-LTs and of LTB$_4$ [10]. Little evidence exists of any meaningful differences in the therapeutic benefits of LTSIs compared to cysLTRAs .

## Leukotriene B$_4$ receptor (BLT) antagonists

LTB$_4$ has potent chemotactic activity on neutrophils and eosinophils both *in vitro* [33] and *in vivo* [34], and increased LTB$_4$ levels have been reported in body fluids of symptomatic asthmatics [60, 61, 63]. Both neutrophils and eosinophils recruited to the airways of asthmatics by segmental allergen challenge show decreased migratory responses to LTB$_4$ *in vitro* [96, 97], suggesting desensitisation following exposure to endogenous LTB$_4$ *in vivo*. Similarly, in normals, inhalation of LTB$_4$ causes a rapid blood neutropaenia due to margination of circulating neutrophils within the lung vasculature, but patients with stable mild persistent asthma show an attenuated response [98], again suggesting neutrophil desensitisation due to prior exposure to excess endogenous LTB$_4$. Potent (but non-selective) chemoattractants such as LTB$_4$ may cause specific eosinophil migration in atopic subjects, whose eosinophils may be primed by specific (but weak) chemokines such as interleukin-5 [99].

Specific BLT receptor antagonists have been developed. So far, few such compounds have been applied in human studies of asthma. In sensitized guinea-pigs, the BLT antagonist U-75302 considerably reduced peribronchial eosinophil infiltration following antigen challenge, without affecting neutrophil migration [100]. However, this was not confirmed in humans *in vivo* with the BLT receptor antagonist LY-293111 [101]. In the latter study, LY-293111 failed to protect against allergen-induced bronchoconstriction, and had no effect on bronchial responsiveness to histamine, despite significant decreases in neutrophil counts and in myeloperoxidase levels in BAL fluid 24 h after challenge [101]. The role of neutrophils and of LTB$_4$ in allergen-induced airway responses is still under debate [7, 8, 102, 103]. Hence, BLT receptor antagonists may have greater effects in models in which neutrophils are likely to play a more prominent role, such as ozone inhalation, occupational asthma, or experimental virus infections [103]. Evidence for the involvement of neutrophils in sudden-onset fatal asthma [104] and in nocturnal asthma [105] reinforces the need to examine anti-LT drugs in clinically-relevant models other than allergen challenge.

## Cysteinyl-leukotriene receptor (cys-LT$_1$) antagonists (cysLTRAs)

The cys-LT receptor antagonists (cysLTRAs) antagonize the effects of cys-LTs at the cys-LT$_1$ receptor [51]. The first drugs in this category to be evaluated in humans *in vivo* included FPL-55712, L-648051, L-649923, LY-171883 (tomelukast), LY-170680 (sulukast), RG-12525 and SKF-104353 (pobilukast) [106–112]. These compounds had relatively low potency, producing a rightward shift in the LTD$_4$ dose-response curve of only three to 12-fold. Lack of potency, and in some cases undesirable side effects, led to the development of most of these compounds being suspended. In the past 6–7 years, more potent and/or selective cysLTRAs have been developed, among which pranlukast (SB-205312; Ultair or Onon), zafirlukast (ICI 204219; Accolate) and montelukast (MK-0476; Singulair) have been registered, or are close to registration, in a number of countries including the USA, Japan, and several countries in Europe [10]. These compounds are administered orally at a recommended rate of once or twice daily.

The cysLTRAs have a dual mechanism of action. Firstly, these agents have bronchodilator activity, which is additive to $\beta_2$-agonists in patients with mild to moderate persistent asthma [113, 114]. This suggests that part of their efficacy relies on blockade of LT-induced airway oedema and/or mucus hypersecretion, as well as on blocking LT-induced airway smooth muscle contraction. In the inhaled allergen challenge model, potent cysLTRAs inhibit 75–88% of the early response (EAR) and 54–63% of the late response (LAR) [10]. Furthermore, cysLTRAs provide clinically significant protection against bronchoconstriction induced by inhaled lysine-aspirin [115] or exercise challenge [116] in susceptible patients (Tab. 1). Secondly, strong evidence exists for anti-inflammatory activity of cysLTRA [117–122], in that they reduce airway inflammatory cell counts and mediator levels, reduce bronchial hyperresponsiveness, and allow reductions in steroid dosage, suggesting modulation of the underlying disease processes (Tab. 2).

## Clinical effects of cysLTRAs

An increasing number of long-term follow-up studies investigating cysLTRAs in clinical asthma are currently being performed. Consequently, many results are not yet published in full. Several studies in patients with different gradations of asthma have been reported, showing that pranlukast, zafirlukast and montelukast, alone or in combination with anti-inflammatory anti-asthma therapy (mostly theophylline or corticosteroids), are capable of improving both clinical criteria and lung function parameters (Tab. 2). In these studies, more or less comparable increases in lung function parameters (FEV$_1$ and peak flow) have been measured, which are dose- and duration-dependent, and often accompanied by clinically signif cant decreases in daytime and nighttime symptom scores, and in $\beta_2$-agonist use in patients with mild to moderate, or with moderate to severe persistent asthma (Tab. 2) [122–125].

Apart from bronchodilation, cysLTRAs possess anti-inflammatory properties, also dependent on the dose and duration of treatment [117–122, 126–128]. In studies in patients with moderate to severe persistent asthma, 6 to 12 weeks of treatment with various cysLTRAs had a steroid-sparing effect [120–122]. Moreover, oral pranlukast produced small but significant decreases in baseline bronchial responsiveness to methacholine after only 1 week of treatment in patients with stable asthma [121], and this was sustained for up to 24 weeks [128]. Two- to five-fold reductions in baseline bronchial responsiveness to methacholine are obtained with 2–12 weeks of treatment with oral zafirlukast in mild to moderate atopic asthmatics [129]. One week of treatment with oral zafirlukast also produces a significant decrease in basophils and eosinophils in the BAL fluid of patients with mild to moderate atopic asthma 48 h following segmental allergen challenge [117]. Similarly, 4 weeks of treatment with oral montelukast provided a significant reduction in sputum eosinophils in patients with mild to moderate persistent asthma [127]. These studies clearly indicate that cysLTRAs are capable of reducing airway eosinophilia and the associated BHR in clinical asthma.

## Leukotriene synthesis inhibitors

Since $LTB_4$, as well as cys-LTs, may contribute to chronic airway inflammation in asthma, pharmacological agents have been developed (LTSIs) which block the synthesis of both leukotriene subfamilies, by inhibiting 5-lipoxygenase activity (5-LO inhibitors) or 5-LO activating protein activity (FLAP antagonists) (Fig. 1). Fewer long-term clinical studies of LTSIs have been published compared to cysLTRA trials and direct comparison is complicated by the trend for LTSI in slightly more severe asthma patient groups than those investigated in cysLTRA trials. However, LTSIs appear to provide improvements in clinical and lung function parameters in asthma comparable to those obtained with the cysLTRAs (Tabs. 1 and 2).

## Clinical effects of LTSIs

In repeated-dose studies in asthma, most experience has been accumulated with the first generation 5-LO inhibitor zileuton, mostly at oral doses of either 400 or 600 mg q.i.d. [130] (Tab. 2). Zileuton (formally Leutrol™, Zyflo) has recently been registered for treatment of asthma in the United States. Besides, the FLAP antagonists MK-0591 and BAY-x1005 have also shown improvements in clinical and lung function parameters after 4 to 6 weeks of treatment [131, 132].

Table 1 - Effects of cys-LT$_1$ receptor antagonists and leukotriene biosynthesis inhibitors on various bronchoprovocation tests in asthma

| Compound | Type | Stimulus | Dose, route | Effect (% mean inhibition) | Ref. |
|---|---|---|---|---|---|
| ICI-204, 219 (zafirlukast*; Accolate#) | cysLTRA | allergen | 40 mg, p.o. | EAR (max) ↓88%<br>LAR (max) ↓54% | [151] |
| | | exercise | 0.4 mg, I | ↓52% | [152] |
| | | | 20 mg, p.o. | ↓40% | [153] |
| | | eosinophils$<br>basophils$$ | 7 (2 × 160 mg), p.o. | ↓45%<br>↓57% | [117] |
| MK-571 | cysLTRA | allergen | 450 mg, i.v. | EAR (AUC$_{0-3}$) ↓88%<br>LAR (AUC$_{3-10}$) ↓63% | [154] |
| | | exercise | 160 mg, i.v. | ↓68% | [155] |
| MK-0476 (montelukast*; Singulair#) | cysLTRA | allergen | 2 × 10 mg, p.o. | EAR (AUC$_{0-3}$) ↓75%<br>EAR (max) ↓54%<br>LAR (AUC$_{3-8}$) ↓57%<br>LAR (max) ↓36% | [156] |
| | | exercise | 10 mg, p.o. | ↓41% | [157] |
| SK&F104, 353 (pobilukast*) | cysLTRA | aspirin | 893 µg, I | ↓47% | [158] |
| | | exercise | 800 µg, I | ↓33% | [148] |
| MK-0679 (verlukast*) | cysLTRA | aspirin | 750 mg, p.o. | ↑4.4-fold aspirin dose | [115] |
| ONO-1078 = SB205, 312 (pranlukast*; Ultair/Onon#) | cysLTRA | dipyrone | 225 mg, p.o. | ↑14-fold dipyrone dose | [159] |
| | | exercise | 14 (1 × 450 mg), p.o. | ↓45% | [160] |

178

Table 1 (continued)

| Compound | Type | Stimulus | Dose, route | Effect (% mean inhibition) | Ref. |
|---|---|---|---|---|---|
| A-64077 (zileuton*, Leutrol = Zyflo#) | 5-LO inhibitor | cold, dry air | 800 mg, p.o. | ↑47% cold, dry air extra for ↓10% $FEV_1$ | [161] |
| | | exercise | 4 × 600 mg, p.o. | ↓41% | [162] |
| | | aspirin | 6–8 (4 × 600 mg), p.o. | ↓76% | [146] |
| | | eosinophils | 8 (4 × 600 mg), p.o. | ↓66% | [138] |
| ZD2138 | 5-LO inhibitor | aspirin | 2(1 × 350 mg), p.o. | ↓76% | [163] |
| MK-886 | FLAP-antagonist | allergen | 500+250 mg, p.o. | EAR ($AUC_{0-3}$) ↓58% LAR ($AUC_{3-7}$) ↓44% | [164] |
| MK-0591 | FLAP-antagonist | allergen | 3 × 250 mg, p.o. | EAR ($AUC_{0-3}$) ↓79% LAR ($AUC_{3-8}$) ↓39% | [165] |
| BAY-x1005 | FLAP-antagonist | allergen | 3.5 (2 × 500 mg), p.o. | EAR ($AUC_{0-3}$) ↓87% EAR (max) ↓57% LAR ($AUC_{3-7}$) ↓60% LAR (max) ↓46% | [166] |

cysLTRA, cysteinyl leukotriene receptor antagonist; EAR, early asthmatic response; LAR, late asthmatic response; AUC, area under the time-response curve over an indicated time-interval; 5-LO, 5-lipoxygenase; FLAP, 5-lipoxygenase activating protein; p.o., per os; i.v., intravenous; I, inhaled; *, generic name; #, trade name; $/$$, airway eosinophils and basophils, respectively, after a segmental allergen provocation test; dipyrone, a pyrazolone derivate.

*Table 2 - Effect of Cys-LT$_1$ receptor antagonists and leukotriene synthesis inhibitors in clinical asthma*

| Compound | Asthma (n = no. of patients) | Dose, route | Effect | Ref. |
|---|---|---|---|---|
| MK-571 | mild-moderate (n = 43) | 2 wk (3 × 75 mg), p.o.+<br>4 wk (3 × 150 mg), p.o. | ↑8–14% FEV$_1$<br>↓30% symptom scores<br>↓30% β$_2$-agonist use | [167] |
| pranlukast | moderate-severe (n = 42) | 8 wk (2 × 450 mg) | ↑16% morning/evening PEF<br>↓40% daytime symptom scores<br>↓60% nighttime symptom scores | [168] |
| pranlukast | moderate-severe (n = 586) | 12 wk (2 × 150/300/450 mg) | ↑8–12% FEV$_1$<br>↓34% symptom scores<br>↓36% rescue medication | [169] |
| pranlukast | moderate-severe (n = 79;<br>BDP ≥ 1500 μg/day) | 6 wk (2 × 450 mg) | steroidsparing effect: ↓50% BDP | [118] |
| zafirlukast | moderate-severe (n = 276) | 6 wk (2 × 5/10/20 mg) | ↑11% FEV$_1$<br>↓26% daytime symptom scores<br>↓46% nighttime symptom scores<br>↓30% β$_2$-agonist use | [123] |
| zafirlukast | moderate (n = 9; BDP 1500 μg/day) | 12 wk (1 × 20 mg) | steroidsparing effect: ↓BDP | [119] |
| montelukast | moderate-severe (n = 29) | 10.3 days (3 × 200 mg) | ↑9–14% FEV$_1$<br>↓day/nighttime symptom scores<br>↓β$_2$-agonist use | [170] |
| montelukast | moderate-severe (n = 681) | 12 wk (1 × 10 mg) | ↓31% asthma exacerbations<br>↑37% asthma-free days | [171] |
| montelukast | moderate (n = 226;<br>ICS 300–3000 μg/day) | 12 wk (1 × 10 mg) | 40% (M) vs 29% (P) tapering of ICS | [120] |
| montelukast | mild-moderate (n = 40) | 4 wk (1 × 10 mg) | ↓48% sputum eosinophils | [127] |

*Table 2 (continued)*

| Compound | Asthma (n = no. of patients) | Dose, route | Effect | Ref. |
|---|---|---|---|---|
| zileuton | moderate (n = 10) | 13 wk (4 × 400/600 mg) | ↑58% cold, dry air extra for ↓15% $FEV_1$ upto 10 days after cessation of therapy | [136] |
| zileuton | moderate-severe (n = 401) | 13 wk (4 × 400/600 mg) | 6% (Z) vs 16% (P) need for corticosteroids during treatment period<br>↑16% $FEV_1$<br>↓26% $\beta_2$-agonist use<br>↓28% daytime symptom scores<br>↓33% nighttime symptom scores | [172] |
| zileuton | mild-moderate (n = 373) | 26 wk (4 × 400/600 mg) | ↑16% $FEV_1$<br>↑7–10% PEF<br>↓37% daytime symptom scores<br>↓31% nighttime symptom scores<br>↓31% $\beta_2$-agonist use<br>↓62% need for steroids<br>↓ blood eosinophils | [133] |

BDP, beclomethasone; ICS, inhalational corticosteroids; M, montelukast; P, placebo

Considerable dose-dependent improvements in clinical symptoms and in lung function, together with a steroid-sparing effect, have been reported in patients with mild to moderate persistent asthma after 6 months of treatment with oral zileuton [133]. Using a similar treatment protocol, a steroid-sparing effect of zileuton was also demonstrated after 13 weeks treatment in patients with moderate to severe persistent asthma [134]. Further evidence for anti-inflammatory activity of this LTSI has been provided by other long-term studies [135–139]. In aspirin-intolerant asthmatics using corticosteroids, 6 weeks of treatment with oral zileuton produced a significant, additional improvement in clinical symptoms, lung function, and non-specific BHR [135]. In patients with mild to moderate persistent asthma, 13 weeks of treatment with oral zileuton provided adequate protection against bronchoconstriction induced by cold, dry air [136]. Unexpectedly, this protection persisted for up to 10 days after discontinuation of treatment, long after the end of the washout period of this short-lived drug (half life: 2.3 h), suggesting a modulatory effect of leukotriene inhibition on airway inflammation. The ability of zileuton to reduce BHR was comparable to that achieved with high-dose inhaled corticosteroid (budesonide), and better than that achievable with theophylline, cromoglycate, or a $\beta_2$-agonist [136]. In another study in asthmatic patients treated with inhaled corticosteroids for at least 6 months, a single oral dose of zileuton (400 mg) significantly reduced BHR to inhaled histamine (2.1 doubling doses) and to distilled water (1.3 doubling doses), without affecting baseline $FEV_1$ [137]. Furthermore, in atopic asthmatic patients, 8 days of pretreatment with oral zileuton not only reduced BAL fluid and urinary $LTE_4$ levels (by about 85%) 24 h after segmental allergen challenge, but also significantly reduced BAL eosinophil counts by over 60%, with trends to lower basophil and macrophage counts and to reduced BAL fluid levels of eosinophil cationic protein (ECP) [138]. In patients with mild to moderate persistent asthma, 7 days of treatment with zileuton significantly reduced baseline $LTB_4$ and cys-LT levels in BAL fluid and reduced urinary $LTE_4$ excretion, and showed a trend for improvement in nocturnal $FEV_1$ [139]. Moreover, these effects were accompanied by a significant decrease in the percentage of eosinophils both in the BAL fluid and in peripheral blood [139]. Among the group of drugs capable of reducing eosinophilia in asthma, which includes corticosteroids and cromones, only anti-LT agents have a clearly-defined and specific mechanism of action, proving that blood and airway eosinophilia in asthma are due, to a significant degree, to endogenous leukotriene production.

## Adverse effects of anti-leukotriene drugs

Anti-leukotriene drugs are generally well-tolerated. Most cysLTRAs such as zafirlukast show only a low rate of side-effects including headache, gastrointestinal tract disturbance, incidental infections, and rash, and most of these adverse effects are seen in a similar proportion of patients in the placebo group, suggesting that they are not drug-related [140]. However, about 4.5% of patients receiving the LTSI drug zileuton had elevations in hepatic aminotransferase levels compared to only 1.1% of the placebo group [134]. The elevations in hepatic enzymes were reversible either spontaneously following continued treatment for 2–3 months, or by discontinuation of treatment. In the USA, the FDA recommend regular liver function monitoring in patients receiving zileuton. Caution may also need to be exercised in reducing steroid dosage drastically if asthma symptoms improve with concomitant anti-LT drug therapy, as rare cases of re-emergence of underlying hypereosinophilia (Churg-Strauss syndrome) have been reported.

## The place of anti-leukotriene therapy in current asthma management guidelines

Recently, a consensus has emerged in long-term asthma management, which emphasises the need for a stepwise approach covering the spectrum from intermittent to severe persistent asthma, with early intervention with strenuous anti-inflammatory therapy when required [1, 141]. The guidelines also stress the need for educating health professionals and patients to expect high standards of asthma control, and for self-monitoring of lung function and to allow step-down in medication levels when good control is achieved. In intermittent asthma, occasional $\beta_2$-agonist use may be all that is required. In persistent asthma, anti-inflammatory therapy is recommended in combination with bronchodilators p.r.n., depending on the frequency and severity of the clinical symptoms and pathophysiological parameters (Tab. 3).

The anti-LT agents are an entirely new approach which combines both bronchodilator ("reliever") and anti-inflammatory ("controller") properties in one family of drugs. Their efficacy has been demonstrated across the spectrum of disease severity. However, their efficacy may vary between patients at each level of severity, probably linked to recent observations of a non-responder minority [142, 143], who, although asthmatic, are unable to generate leukotrienes due to polymorphism in the 5-LO gene promoter [144]. The improvements achievable within the majority "responder" group may therefore be commensurately better than anticipated from the average values reported in studies where the two sub-groups are not distinguished. Experience in clinical trials and in clinical practice suggests that anti-LT drug therapy can be discontinued if no response is apparent within the first 2 months of treatment. At the opposite extreme, spectacular improvements in objective and subjective measures of quality of life can sometimes be observed in small numbers of responder patients.

Although anti-LT drugs are very unlikely to replace the corticosteroids, particularly in the treatment of severe persistent asthma, and are likely to be used in conjunction with $\beta_2$-agonist rescue medication, their place in the management of asth-

*Table 3 - Stepwise approach to management of asthma according to modern guidelines [1]*

| Severity of asthma | Anti-asthma therapy | |
|---|---|---|
| | Controller | Reliever |
| intermittent | • mostly none needed*) | short-acting inhalational $\beta_2$-agonists, as needed (max. once a week) |
| mild-persistent | • inhaled corticosteroids (200–500 µg), cromoglycate, nedocromil, or<br>• sustained-release theophylline | short-acting inhalational $\beta_2$-agonists, as needed (max. 3–4 × in one day) |
| moderate-persistent | • inhaled corticosteroids (800–2000 µg), and<br>• long-acting bronchodilator: either long-acting inhaled or oral $\beta_2$-agonist, or sustained-release theophylline | short-acting inhalational $\beta_2$-agonists, as needed (max. 3–4 × in one day) |
| severe-persistent | • inhaled corticosteroids (≥800–2000 µg), and<br>• long-acting bronchodilator: either long-acting inhaled or oral $\beta_2$-agonist, or sustained-release theophylline, and<br>• long-term oral corticosteroids | short-acting inhalational $\beta_2$-agonists, as needed |

*during exacerbations short-term oral corticosteroids may be needed ma seems justified [145]. Revised guidelines for their positioning in asthma management will suggest that they are indicated as first-line treatment in specific asthma phenotypes, including most patients with aspirin-induced asthma [146, 147], and also in patients with intermittent or mild persistent asthma who regularly experience exercise-induced bronchoconstriction [136, 147]. In studies comparing the effects of pobilukast or zafirlukast with cromoglycate, these cysLTRAs provided at least equivalent protection against exercise-induced bronchoconstriction, with a better recovery than cromoglycate [148, 149]. Furthermore, in patients with more severe asthma (moderate to severe persistent), who need daily medication with high doses of inhaled or oral corticosteroids, anti-LT drugs may be useful because of their steroid-sparing effect [119, 120]. Moreover, their beneficial effects both on clinical and pathophysiological parameters, in combination with a relatively good side-effect profile, make anti-LT therapy a promising approach in children and adolescents [149, 150]. An additional advantage is the favourable pharmacokinetic profile of some of these compounds: with some cysLTRAs, a single oral dose may provide protection for 24 h [120, 127, 150]. This is likely to enhance compliance with therapy.

In summary, following years of intensive research into the inflammatory basis of asthma, a novel generation of rationally-targeted drugs has been added to the current armoury of asthma medication. Anti-LT drugs represent the first entirely novel approach to asthma therapy since the introduction of inhaled corticosteroids over 25 years ago. Their ultimate position in asthma management will depend upon their effects on the pathophysiology and histopathology of the asthmatic lung. To realise the full potential of this new development, further long-term studies are required to compare the ability of anti-LT therapy to modulate airway inflammation in asthma with that of adequate doses of corticosteroids and other current asthma therapies.

# References

1   Global initiative for asthma (1995) National Institutes of Health, National Heart, Lung, and Blood Institute

2   Djukanovic R, Roche WR, Wilson JW, Beasley CRW, Twentyman OP, Howarth PH, Holgate ST (1990) Mucosal inflammation in asthma. *Am Rev Respir Dis* 142: 434–457

3   Ebina M, Takahashi T, Chiba T, Motomiya M (1993) Cellular hypertrophy and hyperplasia of airway smooth muscles underlying bronchial asthma. *Am Rev Respir Dis* 148: 720–726

4   Barnes PJ, Jonsson B, Klim JB (1996) The costs of asthma. *Eur Respir J* 9: 636–642

5   Sterk PJ, Fabbri LM, Quanjer PhH, Cockcroft DW, O'Byrne PM, Anderson SD, Juniper EF, Malo J-L (1993) Airway responsiveness. Standardized challenge testing with pharmacological, physical and sensitizing stimuli in adults. *Eur Respir J* 6 (Suppl 16): 53–83

6    Cockcroft DW, Murdock KY, Kirby JG, Hargreave FE (1987) Prediction of airway responsiveness to allergen from skin sensitivity to allergen and airway responsiveness to histamine. *Am Rev Respir Dis* 135: 264–267

7    Weersink EJM, Postma DS, Aalbers R, De Monchy JG (1994) Early and late asthmatic reaction after allergen challenge. *Respir Med* 88: 103–114

8    Diaz P, Gonzalez MC, Galleguillos FR, Ancic P, Cromwell O, Shepherd D, Durham SR Gleich GJ, Kay AB (1989) Leukocytes and mediators in bronchoalveolar lavage during allergen-induced late-phase asthmatic reactions. *Am Rev Respir Dis* 139: 1383–1389

9    Bentley AM, Kay AB, Durham SR (1997) Human late asthmatic reactions. *Clin Exp Allergy* 27 (Suppl 1): 71–86

10   Holgate ST, Bradding P, Sampson AP (1996) Leukotriene antagonists and synthesis inhibitors: new directions in asthma therapy. *J Allergy Clin Immunol* 98: 1–13

11   Holtzman MJ (1991) Arachidonic acid metabolism. *Am Rev Respir Dis* 143: 188–203

12   Lewis RA, Austen KF, Soberman RJ (1990) Leukotrienes and other products of the 5-lipoxygenase pathway: biochemistry and relation to pathobiology in human diseases. *N Engl J Med* 323: 645–655

13   Dixon RA, Jones RE, Diehl RE, Bennett CD, Kargman S, Rouzer CA (1988) Cloning of the cDNA for human 5-lipoxygenase. *Proc Natl Acad Sci USA* 85: 416–420

14   Brock TG, McNish RW, Bailie MB, Peters-Golden M (1997) Rapid import of cytosolic 5-lipoxygenase into the nucleus of neutrophils after *in vivo* recruitment and *in vitro* adherence. *J Biol Chem* 272: 8276–8280

15   Dixon RA, Diehl RE, Opas E, Rands E, Vickers PJ, Evans JF, Gillard JW, Miller DK (1990) Requirement of a 5-lipoxygenase-activating protein for leukotriene synthesis. *Nature* 343: 282–284

16   Miller DK, Gillard JW, Vickers PJ, Sadowski S, Leveille C, Mancini JA, Charleson P, Dixon RA, Ford-Hutchinson AW, Fortin R et al (1990) Identification and isolation of a membrane protein necessary for leukotriene production. *Nature* 343: 278–281

17   Samuelsson B, Funk CD (1989) Enzymes involved in the biosynthesis of leukotriene $B_4$. *J Biol Chem* 264: 19469–19472

18   Yoshimoto T, Soberman RJ, Lewis RA, Austen KF (1985) Isolation and characterization of leukotriene C4 synthetase of rat basophilic leukemia cells. *Proc Natl Acad Sci USA* 82: 8399–8403

19   Lam BK, Penrose JF, Freeman GJ, Austen KF (1994) Expression cloning of a cDNA for human leukotriene $C_4$ synthase, an integral membrane protein conjugating reduced glutathione to leukotriene $A_4$. *Proc Natl Acad Sci USA* 91: 7663–7667

20   Lam BK, Owen WFJ, Austen KF, Soberman RJ (1989) The identification of a distinct export step following the biosynthesis of leukotriene $C_4$ by human eosinophils. *J Biol Chem* 264: 12885–12889

21   Conroy DM, Piper PJ (1991) Metabolism and generation of cysteinyl-containing leukotrienes by human lung preparations. *Ann NY Acad Sci* 629: 455–457.

22   Zakrzewski JT, Sampson AP, Evans JM, Barnes NC, Piper PJ, Costello JF (1989) The

biotransformation *in vitro* of cysteinyl leukotrienes in blood of normal and asthmatic subjects. *Prostaglandins* 37: 425–444

23   Keppler D, Huber M, Hagmann W, Ball HA, Guhlmann A, Kastner S (1988) Metabolism and analysis of endogenous cysteinyl leukotrienes. *Ann NY Acad Sci* 524: 68–74

24   Shak S, Goldstein IM (1984) Omega-oxidation is the major pathway for the catabolism of leukotriene $B_4$ in human polymorphonuclear leukocytes. *J Biol Chem* 259: 10181–10187

25   Maltby NH, Taylor GW, Ritter JM, Moore K, Fuller RW, Dollery CT (1990) $LTC_4$ elimination and metabolism in man. *J Allergy Clin Immunol* 85: 3–9

26   Williams JD, Czop JK, Austen KF (1984) Release of leukotrienes by human monocytes on stimulation on their phagocytic receptor for particulate activators. *J Immunol* 132: 3034–3040

27   Fels AO, Pawlowski NA, Cramer EB, King TKC, Cohn ZA, Scott WA (1982) Human alveolar macrophages produce leukotriene $B_4$. *Proc Natl Acad Sci USA* 79: 7866–7870

28   Bochner BS, Undem BJ, Lichtenstein LM (1994) Immunological aspects of allergic asthma. *Annu Rev Immunol* 12: 295–335

29   Peters SP, MacGlashan DW, Schulman ES, Schulman ES, Schleimer RP, Hayes EC, Rokach J, Adkinson NF, Lichtenstein LM (1984) Arachidonic acid metabolism in purified human lung mast cells. *J Immunol* 132: 1972–1879

30   Shaw RJ, Cromwell O, Kay AB (1984) Preferential generation of leukotriene $C_4$ by human eosinophils. *Clin Exp Immunol* 56: 716–722

31   Borgeat P, Fruteau de Laclos B, Rabinovitch H, Picard S, Braquet P, Hébert J, Laviolette M (1984) Eosinophil-rich human polymorphonuclear leukocyte preparations characteristically release leukotriene $C_4$ on ionophore A-23187 challenge. *J Allergy Clin Immunol* 74: 310–315

32   Sampson AP (1996) The leukotrienes: mediators of chronic inflammation in asthma. *Clin Exp Allergy* 26: 995–1004

33   Drazen JM, Evans JF, Stevens RL, Shipp MA (1995) Inflammatory effector mechanisms in asthma. *Am J Respir Crit Care Med* 152: 403–407

34   Martin TR, Pistorese BP, Chi EY, Goodman RB, Matthay MA (1989) Effects of leukotriene $B_4$ in the human lung. *J Clin Invest* 84: 1609–1619

35   Spada CS, Nieves AL, Krauss AH-P, Woodward DF (1994) Comparison of leukotriene $B_4$ and $D_4$ effects on human eosinophil and neutrophil motility *in vitro*. *J Leukoc Biol* 55: 183–191

36   Gardiner PJ, Cuthbert NJ (1988) Characterisation of the leukotriene receptor(s) on human isolated lung strips. *Agents Actions Suppl* 23: 121–128

37   Weiss JW, Drazen JM, Coles N, McFadden ER, Lewis R, Weller P, Corey EJ, Austen KF (1982) Bronchoconstrictor effects of leukotriene C in humans. *Science* 216: 196–198

38   Barnes NC, Piper PJ, Costello JF (1984) Comparative effects of inhaled leukotriene $C_4$, leukotriene $D_4$, and histamine in normal human subjects. *Thorax* 39: 500–504

39  Holroyde MC, Altounyan REC, Cole M, Dixon M, Elliott EV (1981) Bronchoconstriction produced in man by leukotrienes C and D. *Lancet* ii: 17–18

40  Griffin M, Weiss JW, Leitch AG, McFadden ERJ, Corey EJ, Austen KF, Drazen JM (1983) Effects of leukotriene D on the airways in asthma. *N Engl J Med* 308: 436–439

41  Coles SJ, Neill KH, Reid LM, Austen KF, Nii Y, Corey EJ, Lewis RA (1983) Effects of leukotrienes $C_4$ and $D_4$ on glycoprotein and lysozyme secretion by human bronchial mucosa. *Prostaglandins* 25: 155–170

42  Woodward DF, Weichman BM, Gill CA, Wasserman MA (1983) The effect of synthetic leukotrienes on tracheal microvascular permeability. *Prostaglandins* 25: 131–142

43  Foster A, Chan CC (1991) Peptide leukotriene involvement in pulmonary eosinophil migration upon challenge in the actively sensitized guinea-pig. *Int Arch Allergy Appl Immunol* 96: 279–284.

44  Laitinen LA, Laitinen A, Haahtela T, Vilkka V, Spur B, Lee TH (1993) Leukotriene $E_4$ and granulocytic infiltration into asthmatic airways. *Lancet* 341: 989–990

45  Diamant Z, Hiltermann JT, Van Rensen EL, Callenbach PM, Veselic-Charvat MA, Van der Veen H, Sont JK, Sterk PJ (1997) The effect of inhaled leukotriene $D_4$ and methacholine on cell differentials in sputum from patients with asthma. *Am J Crit Respir Care Med* 155: 1247–1253

46  Gorenne I, Norel X, Brink C (1996) Cysteinyl leukotriene receptors in the human lung: what's new? *Trends Pharmacol Sci* 17: 342–345

47  Diamant Z, Timmers MC, van der Veen H, Booms P, Sont JK, Sterk PJ (1994) Effect of an inhaled neutral endopeptidase inhibitor, thiorphan, on airway responsiveness to leukotriene $D_4$ in normal and asthmatic subjects *in vivo*. *Eur Respir J* 7: 459–466

48  Krell RD, Tsai BS, Berdoulay A, Barone M, Giles RE (1983) Heterogeneity of leukotriene receptors in guinea pig trachea. *Prostaglandins* 25: 171–178

49  Israel E, Robin JL, Drazen JM (1987) Differential effects of calcium channel blockers on leukotriene $C_4$- and $D_4$-induced contractions in guinea pig pulmonary parenchyma strips. *J Pharmacol Exp Ther* 243: 424–429

50  Mong S, Wu HL, Stadel JM, Clark MA, Crooke ST (1986) Solubilisation of [$^3$H]-leukotriene $D_4$ receptor complex from guinea pig lung membranes. *Mol Pharmacol* 29: 235–243.

51  Buckner CK, Krell RD, Laravuso, Coursin DB, Bernstein PR, Will JA (1986) Pharmacological evidence that human intralobar airways do not contain different receptors that mediate contractions to leukotriene $C_4$ and leukotriene $D_4$. *J Pharmacol Exp Ther* 237 558–562

52  Gardiner PJ, Abram TS, Tudhope SR, Cuthbert NJ, Norman P, Brink C (1994) Leukotriene receptors and their selective antagonists. *Adv Prostaglandin Thromboxane Leukot Res* 22: 49–61

53  Wenzel SE, Larsen GL, Johnston K, Voelkel NF, Westcott JY (1990) Elevated levels of leukotriene $C_4$ in bronchoalveolar lavage fluid from atopic asthmatics after endobronchial allergen challenge. *Am Rev Respir Dis* 142: 112–119

54  Taylor G, Taylor I, Black P, Maltbey NH, Turner N, Fuller RW, Dollery CT (1989) Uri-

nary leukotriene $E_4$ after antigen challenge and in acute asthma and allergic rhinitis. *Lancet* i: 584–588

55  Turnbull LS, Turnbull LW, Leitch AG, Crofton JW, Kay AB (1977) Mediators of immediate-type hypersensitivity in sputum from patients with chronic bronchitis and asthma. *Lancet* i: 526–529

55  Jarjour NN, Calhoun WJ, Schwartz LB, Busse WW (1991) Elevated bronchoalveolar lavage fluid histamine levels in allergic asthmatics are associated with increased airway obstruction. *Am Rev Respir Dis* 144: 83–87

57  Liu MC, Bleecker ER, Lichtenstein LM, Kagey-Sobotka A, Niv Y, Mclemore TL, Permutt S, Proud D, Hubbard WC (1990) Evidence for elevated levels of histamine, prostaglandin $D_2$, and other bronchoconstricting prostaglandins in the airway of subjects with mild asthma. *Am Rev Respir Dis* 142: 126–132

53  Stenton SC, Court EN, Kingston WP, Goadby P, Kelly CA, Duddridge M, Ward C, Hendrick DJ, Walters EH (1990) Platelet activating factor in bronchoalveolar lavage fluid from asthmatic subjects. *Eur Respir J* 3: 408–413

59  Lam S, Chan H, LeRiche JC, Chan-Yeung M, Salari H (1988) Release of leukotrienes in patients with bronchial asthma. *J Allergy Clin Immunol* 81: 711–717

60  Sampson AP, Thomas RU, Costello JF, Piper PJ (1992) Enhanced leukotriene synthesis in leukocytes of atopic and asthmatic subjects. *Br J Clin Pharmacol* 33: 423–430

61  Shindo K, Miyakawa K, Fukumura M (1993) Plasma levels of leukotriene $B_4$ in asthmatic patients. *Int J Tissue React* 15: 181–184

62  Okubo T, Takahashi H, Sumitomo M, Shindo K, Suzuki S (1987) Plasma levels of leukotrienes $C_4$ and $D_4$ during wheezing attack in asthmatic patients. *Int Arch Allergy Appl Immunol* 84: 149–155

63  Wardlaw AJ, Hay H, Cromwell O, Collins JV, Kay AB (1989) Leukotrienes $LTC_4$ and $LTB_4$ in bronchoalveolar lavage in bronchial asthma and other respiratory diseases. *J Allergy Clin Immunol* 84: 19–26

64  Becher G, Winsel K, Beck E, Neubauer G, Stresemann E (1997) Breath condensate as a method of noninvasive assessment of inflammation mediators from the lower airways. *Pneumologie* 51(2): 456–459

65  Kidney JC, Ridge SM, Chung KF, Barnes PJ (1993) Inhibition of platelet-activating factor-induced bronchoconstriction by the leukotriene $D_4$ receptor antagonist ICI 204,219. *Am Rev Respir Dis* 147: 215–217

66  Abraham WM, Burch RM, Farmer SG, Sielczak MW, Ahmed A, Cortes A (1991) A bradykinin antagonist modifies allergen-induced mediator release and late bronchial responses in sheep. *Am Rev Respir Dis* 143: 787–796

67  Broide DH, Eisman S, Ramsdell JW, Ferguson P, Schwartz LB, Wasserman SI (1990) Airway levels of mast cell-derived mediators in exercise-induced asthma. *Am Rev Respir Dis* 141: 563–568

68  Pliss LB, Ingenito EP, Ingram RH, Pichurko B (1990) Assessment of bronchoalveolar cell and mediator response to isocapnic hyperpnea in asthma. *Am Rev Respir Dis* 142: 73–78

69    Kikawa Y, Miyanomae T, Inoue Y, Saito M, Nakai A, Shigematsu Y, Hosoi S, Sudo M (1992) Urinary leukotriene $E_4$ after exercise challenge in children with asthma. *J Allergy Clin Immunol* 89: 1111–1119.

70    Smith CM, Christie PE, Hawksworth RJ, Thien F, Lee TH (1991) Urinary leukotriene $E_4$ levels after allergen and exercise challenge in bronchial asthma. *Am Rev Respir Dis* 144: 1411–1413

71    Taylor IK, Wellings R, Taylor GW, Fuller RW (1992) Urinary leukotriene $E_4$ excretion in exercise-induced asthma. *J Appl Physiol* 73: 743–748

72    Hejal RB, Walenga RW, Lenner KA, Nelson JA, McLane ML, Gilbert IA (1995) Urinary leukotriene $E_4$ levels following isocapnic hyperventilation in asthmatics. *Am J Respir Crit Care Med* 151: A678 (Abstract)

73    Diamant Z (1996) *Experimental interventions in leukotriene- and allergen-induced airway responses in asthma in vivo*. PhD thesis, Pasmans Publishers, The Hague, The Netherlands

74    Chafee FH, Settipane GA (1974) Aspirin intolerance. 1. Frequency in an allergic population. *J Allergy Clin Immunol* 3: 193–199

75    Smith CM, Hawksworth RJ, Thien FCK, Christie PE, Lee TH (1992) Urinary leukotriene $E_4$ in bronchial asthma. *Eur Respir J* 5: 693–699

76    Christie PE, Tagari P, Ford-Hutchinson AW, Black C, Markendorf A, Schmitz-Schumann M, Lee TH (1992) Urinary leukotriene $E_4$ after lysine-aspirin inhalation in asthmatic subjects. *Am Rev Respir Dis* 146: 1531–1534

77    Sladek K, Dworski R, Soja J, Sheller JR, Nizankowska E, Oates JA, Szczeklik A (1994) Eicosanoids in bronchoalveolar lavage fluid of aspirin-intolerant patients with asthma after aspirin challenge. *Am J Respir Crit Care Med* 149: 940–946

78    Sestini P, Armetti L, Gambaro G, Pieroni MG, Refini RM, Sala A, Vaghi A, Folco GC, Bianco S, Robuschi M (1996) Inhaled $PGE_2$ prevents aspirin-induced bronchoconstriction and urinary LTE4 excretion in aspirin-sensitive asthma. *Am J Respir Crit Care Med* 153: 572–575

79    Sampson AP, Cowburn AS, Sladek K, Adamek L, Nizankowska E, Szczeklik A, Penrose J, Austen KF, Holgate ST (1997) Profound over-expression of leukotriene $C_4$ synthase in the bronchial biopsies of aspirin-intolerant asthmatics. *Int Arch Allergy Immunol* 113: 355–357

80    Nasser SMS, Pfister R, Christie PE, Sousa AR, Barker J, Schmitz-Schumann M, Lee TH (1996) Inflammatory cell populations in bronchial biopsies from aspirin-sensitive asthmatic subjects. *Am J Respir Crit Care Med* 153: 90–96

81    Arm JP, O'Hickey SP, Spur BW, Lee TH (1989) Airway responsiveness to histamine and leukotriene $E_4$ in subjects with aspirin-induced asthma. *Am Rev Respir Dis* 140: 148–153

82    Adelroth E, Morris MM, Hargreave FE, O'Byrne PM (1986) Airway responsiveness to leukotrienes $C_4$ and $D_4$ and to methacholine in patients with asthma and normal controls. *N Engl J Med* 315: 480–484.

83   Smith LJ, Greenberger PA, Patterson R, Krell RD, Bernstein PR (1985) The effect of inhaled leukotriene $D_4$ in humans. *Am Rev Respir Dis* 131: 368–372

84   Kern R, Smith LJ, Patterson R, Krell RD, Bernstein PR (1986) Characterization of the airway response to inhaled leukotriene D4 in normal subjects. *Am Rev Respir Dis* 133: 1127–1132

85   O'Hickey SP, Hawksworth RJ, Fong CY, Arm JP, Spur BW, Lee TH (1991) Leukotrienes $C_4$, $D_4$ and $E_4$ enhance histamine responsiveness in asthmatic airways. *Am Rev Respir Dis* 144: 1053–1057

86   Arm JP, O'Hickey SP, Hawksworth RJ, Fong CY, Crea AEG, Spur BW, Lee TH (1990) Asthmatic airways have a disproportionate hyperresponsiveness to $LTE_4$, as compared with normal airways, but not to $LTC_4$, $LTD_4$, methacholine, and histamine. *Am Rev Respir Dis* 142: 1112–1118

87   Bel EH, van der Veen H, Kramps JA, Dijkman JH, Sterk PJ (1987) Maximal airway narrowing to inhaled leukotriene $D_4$ in normal subjects: comparison and interaction with methacholine. *Am Rev Respir Dis* 136: 979–984

88   Higgins DA, O'Byrne PM (1987) Inhaled leukotriene $D_4$ does not cause a late response in atopic subjects. *J Allergy Clin Immunol* 79: 141 (Abstract)

89   Wang CG, Du T, Xu LJ, Martin JG (1993) Role of leukotriene $D_4$ in allergen-induced increases in airway smooth muscle in the rat. *Am Rev Respir Dis* 148: 413–417

90   Kurosawa M, Yodonawa S, Tsukagoshi H, Miyachi Y (1994) Inhibition by a novel peptide leukotriene receptor antagonist ONO-1078 of airway wall thickening and airway hyperresponsiveness to histamine induced by leukotriene $C_4$ or leukotriene $D_4$ in guinea-pigs. *Clin Exp Allergy* 24: 960–968

91   Cohen P, Noveral JP, Bhala A, Nunn SE, Herrick DJ, Grunstein MM (1995) Leukotriene $D_4$ facilitates airway smooth muscle cell proliferation via modulation of the IGF axis. Am J Physiol 269: L151–L157

92   Laitinen LA, Laitinen A (1994) Structural and cellular changes in asthma. *Eur Respir Rev* 4: 348–351

93   Lambert RK, Wiggs BR, Kuwano K, Hogg JC, Pare PD (1993) Functional significance of increased airway smooth muscle in asthma and COPD. *J Appl Physiol* 74: 2771–2781

94   Sampson SE, Costello JF, Sampson AP (1997) The effect of inhaled leukotriene $B_4$ in normal and in asthmatic subjects. *Am J Respir Crit Care Med* 155: 1789–1792

95   Kuitert L, Barnes NC (1995) PAF and asthma – time for an appraisal? *Clin Exp Allergy* 25: 1159–1162

96   Koh YY, Dupuis R, Pollice M, Albertine KH, Fish JE, Peters SP (1993) Neutrophils recruited to the lungs of humans by segmental antigen challenge display a reduced chemotactic response to leukotriene $B_4$. *Am J Respir Cell Mol Biol* 8: 493–499

97   Kim CJ, Kane GC, Zangrilli JG, Cho SK, Koh YY, Peters SP (1994) Eosinophils recruited to the lung by segmental antigen challenge show a reduced chemotactic response to leukotriene $B_4$. *Prostaglandins* 47: 393–403

98  Powell WS (1982) Rapid extraction of arachidonic acid metabolites from biological samples using octadecylsilyl silica. *Methods Enzymol* 86: 467–477

99  Sehmi R, Wardlaw AJ, Cromwell O, Kurihara K, Waltmann P, Kay AB (1992) Interleukin-5 selectively enhances the chemotactic response of eosinophils obtained from normal but not eosinophilic subjects. *Blood* 79: 2952–2959

100 Richards IM, Griffin RL, Oostveen JA, Morris J, Whishka DG, Dunn CJ (1989) Effect of the selective leukotriene $B_4$ antagonist U-75302 on antigen-induced bronchopulmonary eosinophilia in sensitized guinea pigs. *Am Rev Respir Dis* 140: 1712–1716

101 Evans DJ, Barnes PJ, Spaethe SM, van Alstyne EL, Mitchell MI, O'Connor BJ (1996) Effect of a leukotriene $B_4$ receptor antagonist, LY-293, 111, on allergen induced responses in asthma. *Thorax* 51: 1178–1184

102 Rossi GA, Crimi E, Lantero S, Gianiorio P, Oddera S, Crimi P, Brusasco V (1991) Late-phase asthmatic reaction to inhaled allergen is associated with early recruitment of eosinophils in the airways. *Am Rev Respir Dis* 144: 379–383

103 Christie PE, Barnes NC (1996) Leukotriene $B_4$ and asthma. *Thorax* 51: 1171–1173

104 Sur S, Crotty TB, Kephart GM, Hyma BA, Colby TV, Reed CE, Hunt LW, Gleich GJ (1993) Sudden-onset fatal asthma: a distinct entity with few eosinophils and relatively more neutrophils in the airway submucosa? *Am Rev Respir Dis* 148: 713–719

105 Wenzel SE, Trudeau JB, Westcott JY, Beam WR, Martin RJ (1994) Single oral dose of prednisone decreases leukotriene $B_4$ production by alveolar macrophages from patients with nocturnal asthma but not control subjects: relationship to changes in cellular influx and $FEV_1$. *J Allergy Clin Immunol* 94: 870–881

106 Holroyde MC, Altounyan RE, Cole M, Dixon M, Elliott EV (1982) Selective inhibition of bronchoconstriction induced by leukotrienes C and D in man. *Adv Prostagland'n Thromboxane Leukot Res* 9: 237–242

107 Jones TR, Guindon Y, Young R, Champion E, Charette L, Denis D, Ethier D, Hamel R, Ford-Hutchinson AW, Fortin R et al (1986) L-648, 051, sodium 4-[3-(4-acetyl-3-hydroxy-2-propyl-phenoxy)-propylsylfonyl]-τ-oxo-benzenebutanoate: a leukotriene $D_4$ receptor antagonist. *Can J Physiol Pharmacol* 64: 1535–1542

108 Barnes NC, Piper PJ, Costello J (1987) The effect of an oral leukotriene antagonist L-649,923 on histamine and leukotriene $D_4$-induced bronchoconstriction in normal man. *J Allergy Clin Immunol* 79: 816–821

109 Phillips GD, Rafferty P, Robinson C, Holgate ST (1988) Dose-related antagonism of leukotriene D4-induced bronchoconstriction by p.o. administration of LY-171883 in nonasthmatic subjects. *J Pharmacol Exp Ther* 246: 732–738

110 Wood-Baker R, Phillips GD, Lucas RA, Turner GA, Holgate ST (1991) The effect of inhaled LY-170680 on leukotriene $D_4$-induced bronchoconstriction in healthy volunteers. *Drug Invest* 3: 239–247

111 Wahedna I, Wisniewski AS, Tattersfield AE (1991) Effect of RG 12525, an oral leukotriene $D_4$ antagonist, on the airway response to inhaled leukotriene $D_4$ in subjects with mild asthma. *Br J Clin Pharmacol* 32: 512–515

112 Joos GF, Kips J C, Pauwels RA, Van der Straeten ME (1991) The effect of aerosolized

SK&F 104353-Z$_2$ on the bronchoconstrictor effect of leukotriene D$_4$ in asthmatics. *Pulmon Pharmacol* 4: 37–42

113 Gaddy JN, Margolskee DJ, Bush RK, Williams VC, Busse WW (1992) Bronchodilation with a potent and selective leukotriene D$_4$ (LTD$_4$) receptor antagonist (MK-571) in patients with asthma. *Am Rev Respir Dis* 146: 358–363

114 Lammers J-WJ, Van Daele P, Van den Elshout FMJ, Decramer M, Buntinx A, De Lepeleire I, Friedman B (1992) Bronchodilator properties of an inhaled leukotriene D$_4$ antagonist (verlukast, MK-0679) in asthmatic patients. *Pulmon Pharmacol* 5: 121–125

115 Dahlen B, Kumlin M, Margolskee DJ, Larsson C, Blomqvist H, Williams VC, Zetterstrom O, Dahlen SE (1993) The leukotriene-receptor antagonist MK-0679 blocks airway obstruction induced by inhaled lysine-aspirin in aspirin-sensitive asthmatics. *Eur Respir J* 6: 1018–1026

116 Adelroth E, Inman MD, Summers E, Pace D, Modi M, O'Byrne PM (1997) Prolonged protection against excercise-induced bronchoconstriction by the leukotriene D$_4$ receptor antagonist cinalukast. *J Allergy Clin Immunol* 99: 210–215

117 Calhoun WJ, Williams KL, Simonson SG, Lavins BJ (1997) Effect of zafirlukast (Accolate) on airway inflammation after segmental allergen challenge in patients with mild asthma. *Am J Respir Crit Care Med* 155: A662

118 Tamaoki J, Kondo M, Tagaya E, Takemura H, Nagai A, Takizawa T, Konno K (1997) Leukotriene antagonist prevents exacerbation of asthma during reduction of high-dose inhaled corticosteroid. *Am J Respir Crit Care Med* 155: 1235–1240

119 Micheletto C, Turco P, Dal Negro R (1997) Accolate 20 mg works as steroid sparing in moderate asthma. *Am J Respir Crit Care Med* 155: A664 (Abstract)

120 Leff JA, Israel E, Noonan MJ, Finn AF, Godard P, Lofdahl CG, Friedman BS, Connors L, Weinland DE, Reiss TF et al (1997) Montelukast (MK-0476) allows tapering of inhaled corticosteroids (ICS) in asthmatic patients while maintaining clinical stability. *Am J Respir Crit Care Med* 155: A976

121 Fujimura M, Sakamoto S, Kamio Y, Matsuda T (1993) Effect of a leukotriene antagonist, ONO-1078, on bronchial hyperresponsiveness in patients with asthma. *Respir Med* 87: 133–138

122 Margolskee DJ (1991) Clinical experience with MK-571, a potent and specific LTD$_4$ receptor antagonist. *Ann NY Acad Sci* 629: 148–156

123 Spector SL, Smith LJ, Glass M (1994) Effects of 6 weeks of therapy with oral doses of ICI204,219, a leukotriene D$_4$ receptor antagonist, in subjects with bronchial asthma. *Am J Respir Crit Care Med* 150: 618–623

124 Reiss TF, Altman LC, Chervinsky P, Bewtra A, Stricker WE, Noonan GP, Kundu S, Zhang J (1996) Effects of montelukast (MK-0476), a new potent cysteinyl leukotriene (LTD$_4$) receptor antagonist, in patients with chronic asthma. *J Allergy Clin Immunol* 98: 528–534

125 Barnes NC, Pujet J-C (1997) Pranlukast, a novel leukotriene receptor antagonist: results of the first European, placebo-controlled, multicentre clinical study in asthma. *Thorax* 52: 523–527

126  Grootendorst DC, Diamant Z, Veselic M, Hiemstra PS, DeSmet M, Leff JA, Peszek I, Sterk PJ (1997) Effect of oral montelukast, a cysLT$_1$-receptor antagonist, on eosinophil counts and ECP in induced sputum before and after allergen challenge in asthmatics. *Am J Respir Crit Care Med* 155: A976

127  Leff JA, Pizzichini E, Efthimiadis A, Boulet LP, Wei LX, Weinland DE, Hendeles L, Hargreave FE (1997) Effect of montelukast (MK-0476) on airway eosinophilic inflammation in mildly uncontrolled asthma: a randomized placebo-controlled trial. *Am J Respir Crit Care Med* 155: A977

128  Taki F, Suzuki R, Torii K, Matsumoto S, Taniguchi H, Takagi K (1994) Reduction of the severity of bronchial hyperresponsiveness by the novel leukotriene antagonist 4-oxo-8-[4-(4-phenyl-butoxy)benzoylamino]-2-(tetrazol-5-yl)-4H-1-benzopyran hemihydrate. *Arzneimittelforschung* 44: 330–333

129  Rosenthal RR, Lavins BJ, Hanby LA (1996) Effect of treatment with zafirlukast ('Accolate') on bronchial hyperresponsiveness in patients with mild-to-moderate asthma. *J Allergy Clin Immunol* 97: 250

130  McGill KA, Busse WW (1996) Zileuton. *Lancet* 348: 519–524

131  Storms W, Friedman BS, Zhang J, Santanello N, Allegar N, Appel D, Beaucher W, Bronsky F, Busse W, Chervinsky P et al (1995) Treating asthma by blocking the lipoxygenase pathway. *Am J Respir Crit Care Med* 151: A377

132  Virchow JC, Noller PS, Wiessmann KJ, Buhl R, Thalhofer S, Dorow G, Kunkel G, Ukena D, Ulbrich E, Sybrecht G, Matthys H (1995) Multicenter trial of BAY-x1005, a new 5-lipoxygenase activating protein (FLAP) inhibitor in the treatment of chronic asthma. *Am J Respir Crit Care Med* 151: A377

133  Liu MC, Dubé LM, Lancaster J, Zileuton Study Group (1996) Acute and chronic effects of a 5-lipoxygenase inhibitor in asthma: a 6-month randomized multicenter trial. *J Allergy Clin Immunol* 98: 859–871

134  Israel E, Cohn J, Dube L, Drazen J (1996) Effect of treatment with zileuton, a 5-lipoxygenase inhibitor, in patients with asthma: a randomized controlled trial. *JAMA* 275: 931–936

135  Dahlén S-E, Nizankowska E, Dahlén B, Bochenek G, Kumlin M, Mastalerz L, Blomqvist H, Pinis G, Rasberg B, Swanson LJ et al (1995) The Swedish-Polish treatment study with the 5-lipoxygenase inhibitor zileuton in aspirin-intolerant asthmatics. *Am J Respir Crit Care Med* 151: A376

136  Fischer AR, McFadden CA, Frantz R, Awni WM, Cohn J, Drazen JM, Israel E (1995) Effect of chronic 5-lipoxygenase inhibition on airway hyperresponsiveness in asthmatic subjects. *Am J Respir Crit Care Med* 152: 1203–1207

137  Dekhuijzen PNR, Bootsma GP, Wielders PLML, Van den Berg LRM, Festen J, Van Meerwaarden CLA (1997) Effects of single-dose zileuton on bronchial hyperresponsiveness in asthmatic patients treated with inhaled corticosteroids. *Eur Respir J* 10: 2749–2753

138  Kane GC, Pollice M, Kim C-J, Cohn J, Dworski RT, Murray JJ, Sheller JR, Fish JE, Peters SP (1996) A controlled trial of the effect of the 5-lipoxygenase inhibitor, zileuton,

on lung inflammation produced by segmental antigen challenge in human beings. *J Allergy Clin Immunol* 97: 646–654

139 Wenzel SE, Trudeau JB, Kaminsky DA, Cohn J, Martin RJ, Westcott JY (1995) Effect of 5-lipoxygenase inhibition on bronchoconstriction and airway inflammation in nocturnal asthma. *Am J Respir Crit Care Med* 152: 897–905

140 Spector SL (1996) Management of asthma with zafirlukast: clinical experience and tolerability profile. *Drugs* 52 Suppl 6: 36–46

141 British Thoracic Society, Research Unit of the Royal College of Physicians of London, King's Fund Centre and National Asthma Campaign (1990) Guidelines for the management of asthma in adults – I. Chronic persistent asthma. *Br Med J* 301: 651–653

142 Drazen JM, Israel E (1991) Asthma: a solution of half the puzzle? *Am Rev Respir Dis* 144: 743–744

143 Ikeda K, Hyashi M, Obata H, Fujita H, Nakanishi T, Izumi T (1997) Two weeks' observation of pranlukast (ONO-1078, leukotriene receptor antagonist) by peak expiratory flow rate (PEFR) was enough to evaluate clinical efficacies in severe chronic adult asthmatics. *Am J Respir Crit Care Med* 155: A664

144 In K, Asano K, Beler D, Grobholz J, Finn PW, Solverman EK, Silverman ES, Collins T, Fischer AR, Keith TP et al (1997) Naturally-ocurring mutations in the human 5-lipoxygenase gene promoter that modify transcription factor binding and reporter gene transcription. *J Clin Invest* 99: 1130–1137

145 Sampson AP, Corne J, Holgate ST (1997) Will the advent of anti-leukotriene therapy lead to changes in asthma treatment guidelines? *BioDrugs* 7: 167–173

146 Israel E, Fischer AR, Rosenberg MA, Lilly CM, Callery JC, Shapiro J, Cohn J, Rubin P, Drazen JM (1993) The pivotal role of 5-lipoxygenase products in the reaction of aspirin-sensitive asthmatics to aspirin. *Am Rev Respir Dis* 148: 1447–1451

147 O'Byrne PM, Israel E, Drazen JM (1997) Antileukotrienes in the treatment of asthma. *Ann Intern Med* 127: 472–480

148 Robuschi M, Riva E, Fuccella LM, Vida E, Barnabe R, Rossi M, Gambaro G, Spagnotto S, Bianco S (1992) Prevention of exercise-induced bronchoconstriction by a new leukotriene antagonist (SK&F 104,353). *Am Rev Respir Dis* 145: 1285–1288

149 Hofstra WB, Sterk PJ, Neijens HJ, Van der Weij AM, Van Zoest JGCM, Duiverman EJ (1997) Two weeks treatment with zafirlukast (Accolate™), sodium cromoglycate or placebo on exercise-induced bronchoconstriction in asthmatic adolescents. *Am J Respir Crit Care Med* 155: A665

150 Knorr B, Matz J, Bernstein JA, Nguyen H, Seidenberg BC, Reiss TF, Becker A (1998) Montelukast for chronic asthma in 6- to 14-year-old children: a randomized, double-blind trial. *JAMA* 279: 1181–1186

151 Taylor IK, O'Shaughnessy KM, Fuller RW, Dollery CT (1991) Effect of cysteinyl-leukotriene receptor antagonist ICI 204,219 on allergen-induced bronchoconstriction and airway hyperreactivity in atopic subjects. *Lancet* 337: 690–694

152 Makker HK, Lau LC, Thomson HW, Binks SM, Holgate ST (1993) The protective effect

of inhaled leukotriene $D_4$ receptor antagonist ICI 204,219 against exercise-induced asthma. *Am Rev Respir Dis* 147: 1413–1418

153 Finnerty JP, Wood-Baker R, Thomson H, Holgate ST (1992) Role of leukotrienes in exercise-induced asthma. *Am Rev Respir Dis* 145: 746–749

154 Rasmussen JB, Eriksson L-O, Margolskee DJ, Tagari P, Williams VC, Andersson K-E (1992) Leukotriene $D_4$ receptor blockade inhibits the immediate and late bronchoconstrictor responses to inhaled antigen in patients with asthma. *J Allergy Clin Immunol* 90: 193–201

155 Manning PJ, Watson RM, Margolskee DJ, Williams VC, Schwartz JI, O'Byrne PM (1990) Inhibition of exercise-induced bronchoconstriction by MK-571, a potent leukotriene $D_4$-receptor antagonist. *N Engl J Med* 323: 1736–1739

156 Diamant Z, Grootendorst DC, Veselic-Charvat M, Timmers MC, De Smet M, Leff JA, Seidenberg BC, Zwinderman AM, Peszek I, Sterk PJ (1999) The effect of montelukast (MK-0476), a cysteinyl leukotriene receptor antagonist, on allergen-induced airway responses and sputum cell counts in asthma. *Clin Exp Allergy* 29: 42–51

157 Reiss TF, Bronsky E, Hendeles L, Hill J, Harman E, Guerreiro D, Zhang J (1995) MK-0476, a potent leukotriene (LT)$D_4$ receptor antagonist, inhibits exercise induced bronchocontriction in asthmatics at the end of a once daily dosing interval. *Am J Respir Crit Care Med* 151: A377

158 Christie PE, Smith CM, Lee TH (1991) The potent and selective sulfidopeptide leukotriene antagonist, SK&F 104353, inhibits aspirin-induced asthma. *Am Rev Respir Dis* 144: 957–958

159 Yamamoto H, Nagata M, Kuramitsu K, Tabe K, Kiuchi H, Sakamoto Y, Yamamoto K, Dohi Y (1994) Inhibition of analgesic-induced asthma by leukotriene receptor antagonist ONO-1078. *Am J Respir Crit Care Med* 150: 254–257

160 Suguro H, Majima T, Ichimura K, Hashimoto N, Koyama S, Horie T (1997) Effect of a leukotriene antagonist, pranlukast hydrate, on exercise-induced bronchoconstriction. *Am J Respir Crit Care Med* 155: A662

161 Israel E, Dermarkarian R, Rosenberg M, Sperling R, Taylor G, Rubin P, Drazen J (1990) The effects of 5-lipoxygenase inhibitor on asthma induced by cold, dry air. *N Engl J Med* 323: 1740–1744

162 Meltzer SS, Hasday JD, Cohn J, Bleecker ER (1996) Inhibition of exercise-induced bronchospasm by zileuton: a 5-lipoxygenase inhibitor. *Am J Respir Crit Care Med* 153: 931–935

163 Nasser SMS, Bell GS, Foster S, Spruce KE, MacMillan R, Williams AJ, Lee TH, Arm JP (1994) Effect of the 5-lipoxygenase inhibitor ZD2138 on aspirin-induced asthma. *Thorax* 49: 749–756

164 Friedman BS, Bel EH, Buntinx A, Tanaka W, Han Y-HR, Shingo S, Spector R, Sterk P (1993) Oral leukotriene inhibitor (MK-886) blocks allergen-induced airway responses. *Am Rev Respir Dis* 147: 839–844

165 Diamant Z, Timmers MC, Van der Veen H, Friedman BS, De Smet M, Depre M, Hilliard D, Bel EH, Sterk PJ (1995) The effect of MK-0591, a novel 5-lipoxygenase activating

protein inhibitor, on leukotriene biosynthesis and allergen-induced subjects *in vivo. J Allergy Clin Immunol* 95: 42–51

166  Hamilton AL, Watson RM, Wyile G, O'Byrne PM (1997) Attenuation of early and late phase allergen-induced bronchoconstriction in asthmatic subjects by a 5-lipoxygenase activating protein antagonist, BAYx1005. *Thorax* 52: 348–354

167  Margolskee D, Bodman S, Dockhorn R, Israel E, Kemp J, Mansmann H, Minotti DA, Spector S, Stricker W, Tinkelman D, Townley R, Winder J, Williams V (1991) The therapeutic effects of MK-571, a potent and selective leukotriene (LT) $D_4$ receptor antagonist, in patients with chronic asthma. *J Allergy Clin Immunol* 87: 309

168  Suzuki N, Kudo K, Sano Y, Adachi M, Kanazawa M, Kudo S, Horie T, Kobayashi H, Konno K, Itoh K, Miyamoto T (1997) Efficacy of oral pranlukast, a leukotriene receptor antagonist, in the treatment of asthma: an open study in Tokyo. *Am J Respir Crit Care Med* 155: A664

169  Sahn S, Galant S, Murray J, Bronsky E, Spector S, Faiferman I, Stober P et al (1997) Pranlukast (UltairTM) improves $FEV_1$ in patients with asthma: results of a 12-week multicenter study vs nedocromil. *Am J Respir Crit Care Med* 155: A665

170  Reiss TF, Altman LC, Chervinsky P, Bewtra A, Stricker WE, Noonan GP et al (1996) Effects of montelukast (MK-0476), a new potent leukotriene ($LTD_4$) receptor antagonist, in patients with chronic asthma. *J Allergy Clin Immunol* 98: 528–534

171  Reiss TF, Chervinsky P, Edwards T, Dockhorn R, Nayak A, Hess J, Zhang J, Shingo S et al (1997) Montelukast (MK-0476), a $CysLT_1$ receptor antagonist, improves asthma outcomes over a 3-month treatment period. *Am J Respir Crit Care Med* 155: A662

172  Israel E, Cohn J, Dube L, Drazen JM (1996) Effect of treatment with zileuton, a 5-lipoxygenase inhibitor, in patients with asthma. A randomized controlled trial. *JAMA* 275: 931–936

# Immunomodulators

*Li Cher Loh and Neil C. Barnes*

Department of Respiratory Medicine, The London Chest Hospital, Bonner Rd,
London E2 9JX, UK

## Introduction

Airway inflammation is fundamental to the disease process in chronic asthma. Different components of the immune system play important roles in perpetuating and orchestrating this inflammatory response. Many types of cells are involved, the airway epithelium is shed; eosinophils, T lymphocytes, polymorphonuclear cells, mast cells, and macrophages are present in an activated state and release proinflammatory mediators, cytokines and growth factors. From inflammation, a process of healing and repair may follow and this has been postulated to lead to remodeling of the airways.

This immunological basis underlying asthma is increasingly recognised and may explain many of the pathophysiological features characteristic of asthma. Recently, considerable interest and emphasis have been put on a subtype of CD4+T lymphocytes, termed type 2 T helper cells (Th2) .These Th2 cells preferentially elaborate and release cytokines such as interleukin-4 and 5 that promote eosinophilic inflammation. Although not all asthmatics are atopic, they all share similar pathologic features, which supports the importance of these CD4+ T lymphocytes in the pathophysiology of chronic asthma [1].

Many of the established therapies in asthma, notably corticosteriods, have their clinical activity because they affect these immunologically important cells. Theophylline, traditionally considered a bronchodilator, has now been shown to have immuno-modulatory effects with evidence for regulation of the expression of CD4+ and CD8+ cells in the airway (see Chapter by Tenor and Schudt, this volume). The concept of modulating or suppressing the immune system using other therapeutic agents forms the theoretical basis for the use of immunosuppressants to treat patients with severe and difficult-to-control asthma.

Patients with severe chronic asthma currently represent a management problem. They may need long-term oral corticosteroids in addition to high doses of inhaled

Anti-Inflammatory Drugs in Asthma, edited by A.P. Sampson and M.K. Church
© 1999 Birkhäuser Verlag Basel/Switzerland

corticosteroids and additional bronchodilators to control their asthma. Many of these individuals become chronically dependent on oral corticosteroids and suffer the side-effects arising from their chronic use. Despite this, they are often symptomatic and their daily activities are severely restricted.

## Modulating the immune system in chronic asthma

Currently, drugs that suppress the immune system may be divided into three categories: first, anti-inflammatory agents such as those of the corticosteroid family and gold; secondly, cytotoxic dugs such as methotrexate and azathioprine; and thirdly, fungal and bacterial derivatives, such as cyclosporin A and tacrolimus (FK506), which inhibit signaling events by T lymphocytes.

Corticosteroids are by far the most effective agent to suppress unwanted immune responses in the airways of chronic asthmatics (see Chapter by Barnes, this volume). The introduction of inhaled steroids has revolutionized the management of asthma worldwide. Nevertheless, these agents are only partially successful in treating the more severe asthmatics, many of whom are dependent on oral corticosteroids. The use of other potent anti-inflammatory/immunosuppressive agents may have particular value in such patients.

Cytotoxic drugs inhibit all proliferating cells indiscriminately, including those of the immune system. Their toxicity and uncertain safety in long-term use would limit their use in treatment of many immune-mediated diseases. Immunosuppressants such as cyclosporin A, however, have a more selective action on immune cells, in particular T lymphocytes, and thus leave other cells relatively unaffected, potentially limiting the extent of unwanted cytotoxic side-effects.

The clinical use of intravenous serum immune globulin (IVIG) in severe asthmatics, has also received some attention in view of its increasingly recognised beneficial effect in treating other immune-mediated diseases, an effect which is distinct from simple replacement of immunoglobulins. Many of these efficacies observed are believed to be related to a variety of "immune-modulatory" activities that IVIG possesses.

Other experimental "immunomodulators" are presently being investigated. They include anti CD4+ lymphocyte monoclonal antibody, anti-IgE agents (see Chapter by Patalano, this volume) and cytokine receptor antagonists (see Chapter by Foster and Hogan, this volume). These new agents represent exciting challenges to our present understanding of the immunopathogenesis of severe asthma and may provide potentially effective alternative treatment for asthma patients. This chapter will focus on the use of immunosuppressants and IVIG as immunomodulators. These agents have primarily been assessed for their potential to reduce the requirements for corticosteroid ("steroid-sparing") on which many patients become dependent.

## Cold

The exact mechanism by which gold salts exert their anti-inflammatory activity is unknown. They have been shown to inhibit IgE-mediated release of histamine and leukotriene $C_4$ from human basophils and mast cells [2]. Gold also interferes with T cell function, which may partly explain its efficacy in rheumatoid arthritis. Otherwise its ability to arrest progression of disease and induce apparent remission ('disease modifying") in rheumatoid arthritis is largely unexplained.

The clinical use of oral gold (auranofin) in corticosteroid-dependent asthmatics has been studied in several trials. The first [3] was an open trial involving 20 recruits who showed an improvement in symptoms and a reduced frequency of asthma attacks. They also had reduced bronchial reactivity to methacholine and a 34% reduction in corticosteroid requirement. Following this, a controlled trial [4] in 32 corticosteroid dependent asthma patients given oral gold (3 mg twice daily) or placebo for 26 weeks also showed promising results. The gold treated group showed a statistically significant reduction in oral corticosteroid use and the number of asthma exacerbations requiring rescue courses of corticosteroid, together with a small improvement in lung function compared to the placebo group. More recently, a double-blind study of the effect of oral gold (3 mg twice daily) or placebo over 12 weeks in 19 mild non-corticosteroid dependent asthma patients showed a greater reduction in bronchial responsiveness to methacholine in those treated with gold [5].

Recently, a large trial of oral gold therapy in corticosteroid-dependent asthmatics has been reported [6]. 275 patients were recruited in this placebo-controlled, double-blind, multicentre U.S. study and patients were followed-up over a 9-month period. On completion, 60% of the gold-treated patients achieved a 50% reduction in oral corticosteroid requirement, while only 32% of the placebo-treated patients reached this end point. This study showed a clear "steroid-sparing" effect with gold therapy, although improvement were not seen until after several weeks of treatment.

Gold salts are associated with side-effects. Problems include dermatitis, stomatitis, proteinuria, blood dyscrasias, deranged liver function and gastrointestinal disturbances. However they usually resolve after reducing or stopping treatment.

## Hydroxychloroquine

Hydroxychloroquine can inhibit phospholipase $A_2$, an enzyme involved in the release of arachidonic acid from membrane phospholipids. This could potentially lead to a reduction in the production of leukotrienes and prostaglandins in the airways, many of which are bronchoconstrictor or proinflammatory. Hydroxychloroquine is mainly used as an antimalarial agent but has been used in rheumatod arthritis and in systemic and discoid lupus erythematosus.

The steroid-sparing effect of hydroxychloroquine was first suggested in a case report in 1983 [7]. However, a placebo-controlled, crossover trial [8] in nine steroid-dependent asthmatics over 9 weeks did not show any steroid-sparing effect nor were there any significant difference in symptom scores, lung function or requirement for β agonists. Another open trial [9] performed in 11 asthmatic patients for 28 weeks with hydrochloroquine (300–400 mg daily) reported improvement in lung function and symptom scores. The dose of corticosteroid was reduced in seven corticosteroid-dependent asthmatics by 50%. The absence of a control group in this study makes any useful interpretation of results difficult. A serious side-effect of irreversible retinal damage caused by hydroxychloroquine is rare except in overdose.

## Methotrexate

Methotrexate is an antimetabolite that acts by causing folate coenzyme deficiency in all cells. When administered in low doses (10 to 15 mg weekly), methotrexate possesses anti-inflammatory properties which can be used to treat chronic inflammatory disorders such as rheumatoid arthritis and severe psoriasis. It can inhibit neutrophil chemotaxis and interleukin-1 (IL-1) production from activated peritoneal macrophages in animal models as well as inhibit histamine release from human basophils.

The results from a number of "steroid-sparing" studies with low dose methotrexate have produced both positive and negative results. The general trend however is of a positive effect. Mullarkey and colleagues [10] performed the first randomised, double-blind, crossover study of 22 steroid-dependent asthmatics, requiring at least 10 mg prednisolone a day. They showed that treatment with oral methotrexate (15 mg/week) for 12 weeks could result in a 36% reduction in oral steroid requirement compared to placebo. There were also subjective improvements in asthma symptoms without deterioration in pulmonary function.

The largest placebo-controlled study was performed by Shiner et al. [11] involving 69 corticosteroid-dependent asthmatics randomised to receive oral methotrexate (15 mg/week) or placebo for 24 weeks. At the end of the study there was a greater reduction in prednisolone dose in the methotrexate treated group than in the placebo treated group (50% versus 14%). However this benefit was not seen in the first 10 weeks after commencing treatment compared to placebo and was not sustainable after cessation of treatment. There were fewer asthma exacerbations during methotrexate treatment while symptom scores and lung function remained stable throughout the study. Recently, in a meta-analysis of 11 controlled trials [12], the author showed that low-dose oral methotrexate used in severe asthmatics has a statistically significant steroid-sparing effect. Overall steroid usage was decreased by 23.7% (4.37 mg prednisolone/ day) from baseline.

The adverse effects reported with the use of low dose methotrexate in these trials include nausea, anorexia, transient liver enzyme elevations, dermatitis and myelosuppression. These effects are dose-related and usually disappear when methotrexate is discontinued or the dose reduced. The more serious side-effects that have been reported with the use of methotrexate are opportunistic infections with *Pneumocystis carinii* [13, 14], varicella-zoster pneumonia [15], pulmonary cryptococcosis [16], nocardiosis [17], and pulmonary as well as hepatic fibrosis.

## Azathioprine

Azathioprine is an antimetabolite which by being incorporated into cellular DNA, prevents cell division. It has been shown to suppress T cell mediated immunity and is therefore useful in prevention of allograft rejection. It is used for patients with severe rheumatoid arthritis and has also been used in chronic inflammatory bowel diseases.

It has been investigated in two short and small scale clinical trials. Asmundsson et al. [18] showed in an open study that on improvement in lung function and a reduction in asthma exacerbations were possible in selected patients with asthma, but not with chronic bronchitis, following 12-week treatment with azathioprine. However in a later study [19] where 20 patients with corticosteroid dependent asthma were randomised to receive placebo or azathioprine, 2 mg/kg or 5 mg/kg/ day for 3 and 4 weeks respectively, there were no improvements in symptoms or lung function in the actively treated group compared to placebo. Corticosteroid dose was held constant throughout the study. The adverse effects experienced included mild dyspepsia and dose-related myelosuppression. Based on its mode of action, azathioprine should be effective but in the absence of controlled trials, it is difficult to advocate its use.

## Cyclosporin A

Cyclosporin A (CsA) is a cyclic undecapeptide produced by the fungus *Tolypocladium inflatum*. It inhibits the activation of T lymphocytes [20], the production of cytokines such as IL-2, IL-4, IL-5 and tumour necrosis factor-$\alpha$ (TNF$\alpha$) and the release of histamine and leukotriene $C_4$ from mast cells and basophils [21].

The introduction of CsA has provided an entirely new approach to immunosuppression in organ transplantion. By virtue of its selective ability to inhibit activation of T cells, it can be used at therapeutic concentrations which do not cause myelosuppression, unlike those of other cytotoxic immunosuppressants. This relatively selective activity has been useful in the treatment of severe psoriasis, atopic dermatitis, anterior uveitis and Crohn's disease with varying degrees of success.

The first study was a placebo-controlled, crossover study in 33 steroid-dependent asthmatics giving low dose oral CsA (5 mg/kg/day) [22]. At the end of 12 weeks, the CsA treated group showed a significant improvement in pulmonary function and a reduction in the number of asthma exacerbations requiring extra prednisolone compared to placebo treated subjects. Corticosteroid doses were kept constant throughout this period apart from when required to treat exacerbations.

Two subsequent controlled studies were performed to address the issue of "steroid-sparing" effect of CsA. Nizankowska et al. [23] in a double-blind, placebo-controlled study of 34 corticosteroid-dependent asthma patients showed that CsA therapy could only confer slight benefit over placebo treatment in terms of oral corticosteroid reduction and subjective parameters of asthma severity. Lung function showed no significant difference between the groups at the end of the study. This result is in contrast to another study [24] in which 39 corticosteroid-dependent asthmatics were randomised to receive either CsA or placebo for 36 weeks. CsA therapy resulted in reduction in median prednisolone dose of 62% (10 to 3.5 mg) compared with a decrease of 25% (10 to 7.5 mg) in placebo-treated patients. This reduction with CsA therapy was most pronounced during the last 12 weeks of treatment. There were improvements in peak expiratory flow rate despite reduction in corticosteroid use following CsA therapy. However upon stopping treatment, steroid requirements returned to baseline values.

The main adverse effect of low-dose CsA is decreased renal function. In studies to date which have been less than 12 months in duration, renal impairment has not been a significant problem especially when whole blood CsA is maintained between 100 and 200 ng/ml. Any decrease in renal function is reversible upon stopping treatment. Other side-effects however have occasionally led to discontinued treatment. These include hypertrichosis, hypertension and neuropathy.

CsA has a more selective action (i.e. to CD4+ helper T lymphocytes) compared to other immunosuppressants which affect all dividing cells. However it also has activity on mast cells and basophils which have recognised roles in the pathogenesis of asthma. In a recent double-blind, placebo-controlled study assessing the effect of CsA on allergen induced bronchoconstriction, it was demonstrated that the late asthmatic response (thought to be mainly T cell mediated) could be abrogated by CsA while the early asthmatic response (mainly mast cell mediated) was unaffected [25]. This lends support to the hypothesis that the effects of CsA in asthma are related to inhibition of T lymphocytes rather than mast cells. With the accumulating evidence to implicate T lymphocytes in "driving" the ongoing airway inflammation in chronic severe asthma, CsA may be of particular value as effective alternative treatment in these difficult patients.

## Intravenous Serum Immune Globulin (IVIG)

Pooled human immunoglobulin has been used to confer broad-based humoral immunity on immunodeficient patients since congenital agammaglobulinaemia was first described by Bruton in the early 1950s. These products are prepared from the blood of thousands of healthy donors and invariably contain a wide variety of antibody specificities.

Intravenous serum immune globulin (IVIG) appears to have therapeutic effects in patients with diseases mediated by immune mechanisms, most notably, autoimmune diseases such as immune thrombocytopaenia [26]. These patients are not necessarily lacking in any classes of immunoglobulins. This observation has now been extended to include other immune-mediated conditions such as myasthenia gravis, bullous pemphigoid and systematic lupus erythematosus. Thus IVIG may possess immune-modulatory properties which may be beneficial in the treatment of refractory asthma.

Two early open clinical trials of IVIG in severe asthma were performed in children and involved small numbers of patients. The first [27] involved eight asthmatic children who required continuous oral corticosteroids. They were treated with IVIG at a dose of 1 g/kg for two consecutive days each month for a total of six months- a dose regime similar to those used for treating autoimmune diseases. At the end of six months treatment, prednisolone was reduced from a mean dose of 32 mg daily to 11 mg alternate-day therapy. Symptom scores and home peak expiratory flow had significantly improved. In the second open study [28], nine asthmatic adolescents who were dependent on moderately high dosage of inhaled corticosteroid alone were treated with IVIG for 5 months at a mean dosage of 0.8 g/kg on a single day each month. Of these nine patients, six were able to reduce dosages of inhaled corticosteroid from a mean of 720 mcg/day to 400 mcg/day. Their asthma symptoms as well as bronchial reactivity to histamine were also reduced. This benefit was not maintained 10 months after completion of scheduled therapy. This study suggested that the effect of IVIG was apparent even in moderately severe asthmatic patients not requiring oral corticosteroids, albeit small and short-lived.

Recently, preliminary results of a multicentre, double-blind, placebo-controlled trial of IVIG in oral corticosteroid-dependent asthmatics has been reported [29]. Forty patients were randomised to receive either placebo (albumin 2 g/kg) or IVIG at dose of 1 g/kg or 2 g/kg , administered once a month for 7 months. At the end of the scheduled therapy, both groups receiving active treatment showed a 41% reduction in their oral corticosteroid requirement, compared to a 30% reduction in placebo-treated group. This difference did not reach statistical significance. Adverse experiences reported were similar in both actively treated groups and were more frequent than in those treated with placebo.

The results from this controlled trial, studying the "steroid-sparing" effect of IVIG in oral corticosteroid-dependent asthmatics do not seem to support its use. The authors however recognised the highly heterogenous nature of the studied population which may be reflected in the marked placebo effect. Nevertheless the effectiveness of IVIG in severe asthmatics should now be treated more cautiously in view of the findings in this controlled trial.

The most common side-effects relating to IVIG were post-infusion headache, fever and rigors. They appear to be temporary and the severity could be overcome by reducing the infusion dose of immunoglobulin. This phenomenon is largely unexplained but may be due to formation of antigen-antibody complexes. IVIG has also been associated with aseptic meningitis [30].

How may IVIG mediate improvement in asthmatics patients? Over 90% of IVIG is monomeric IgG with only a small proportion of other immunoglobulins such as IgA and IgM. Many of the effects of IVIG observed in autoimmune diseases especially in immune cytopaenias appear to be mediated by the Fc portion of IgG through the Fcg receptor on phagocytic and other cells. Binding of these Fc portions to the receptor sites can either inhibit or modulate phagocytic functions resulting in disease control. Such modulation of Fcγ receptor bearing monocytic/phagocytic cells can also affect both T and B lymphocytes, influencing both cellular and humoral immune responses.

We now know that IVIG preparations also contain many other substances such as solubilized membrane components, and possibly important solubilized receptors, as well as specific antibodies to HLA determinants and lymphocyte surface molecules. In fact solubilized CD4, solubilized CD8, HLA class I and class II determinants have been isolated from commercial IVIG preparations [31]. These cell surface molecules could interfere with antigen presentation by blocking the interaction between HLA class II and membrane-bound CD4 on T cells or between HLA class I and CD8 in T cell-mediated cytotoxicity. Specific antibodies to HLA determinants and lymphocyte surface molecules could similarly affect the immune regulation of T cells. This perhaps explains why large amounts of IVIG preparation are required for clinical benefit to be realized.

## Key issues in the use of immunosuppressive therapy

All immunosuppressive therapies have potentially serious adverse effects. Therefore their clinical use should be confined to asthmatic patients who are dependent on unacceptably high maintenance doses of corticosteroids. The side-effects of corticosteroids are usually not troublesome until doses in excess of 7.5 mg prednisolone per day (above the physiologic level) are used over a long period of time.

The first question is how effective immunosuppressive agents are in patients with severe chronic corticosteroid-dependent asthma, whether they are administered as adjunctive or alternative ("steroid-sparing") therapy. Secondly, how does the toxicity of such agents compare to the reduction in unwanted side-effects of corticosteroids? Can short-term administration of these agents provide sustainable benefits, and therefore improve the long-term outlook for these patients?

Many of the activities of these agents are felt to be "additive" to the anti-inflammatory /immunosuppressive actions aimed at by the use of corticosteroids. In doing so, some of the effects of corticosteroids can be "replaced" and their requirement reduced. Most studies primarily aimed at assessing their "steroid-sparing" efficacy. Whether there is any unique benefit conveyed from administration of one agent compared to another, is unclear at the moment until there are studies specifically designed to address this issue.

## ' Steroid-sparing" capability of immunosuppressive agents

Of the agents studied, methotrexate, cyclosporin A and gold provide more consistent evidence of a "steroid-sparing" benefit. At present, hydroxychoroquine have not been adequately assessed in larger, controlled trials for potential "steroid-sparing" effect, nor has azathioprine shown proof of clinical benefit when added to the steroid regime of studied populations of asthmatics. The "steroid-sparing" effect of IVIG appears to be minimal. The administration of IVIG can be costly despite the attractiveness of its relatively "benign" side-effects when compared to those observed with immunosuppressants.

The mean reduction in prednisolone use is possibly in the range of 0–9.5 mg/day with methotrexate and 0–5 mg/day with CsA and gold, as suggested from these trials. This indicates that the mean overall "steroid-sparing" effect of these immunosuppressants is modest. However, it is important to recognise that individual responses to immunosuppressive agents, whether in terms of benefit or side-effects, are unpredictable. This creates the difficulty in trying to equate benefit and risk for any single individual with certainty.

For some asthmatic responders, a small reduction of 5 mg prednisolone/day may perhaps be all that is required to significantly reduce the side-effects caused by corticosteroids whilst experiencing no adverse effects from the use of immunosuppressants. However the converse can also be true in that patients may suffer considerable side-effects from taking these immunosuppressants while experiencing little success in reducing corticosteroid dosage. This consideration may be further compounded by an observation in a recent meta-analysis of low-dose methotrexate [12], that greater steroid sparing benefit occurred in those who took lower doses of oral steroids (≤20 mg/day). This may be because these patients are less intractable than those requiring higher doses of corticosteroids.

## Safety and clinical benefits from short-term use of immunosuppressive agents

Long-term depression of immune surveillance by immunosuppressive agents increases the incidence of malignancy seen in patients after allograft transplant [32]. However the incidence of malignancy with use of these agents in autoimmune diseases is much lower, probably due to the lower doses used and the shorter treatment periods employed. If possible, only a short duration of treatment with immunosuppressants should be used in treating severe asthma.

Unwanted side-effects associated with different immunosuppressants have been discussed earlier. They may be equally or even more unpleasant to those resulting from corticosteroids. Sometimes, they are distressing enough to warrant discontinuing treatment. The increased risk of opportunistic viral, bacterial and fungal infections should always be borne in mind when using immunosuppressants. These can develop rapidly and may on occasion be fatal. It is therefore important for both physicians and patients to be vigilant for any signs of infection and to respond appropriately.

The "steroid-sparing" effect from these immunosuppressive agents is observed to be short-lived. Corticosteroid requirement seems to return to baseline values after immunosuppressive agents are discontinued, although some studies have reported success in stopping all asthma medications or lasting improvements in lung function after gold and CsA treatment [4, 22, 33]. Some observed rebound exacerbations of asthma within 6 weeks following 18 months' treatment with CsA [34]. However it is conceivable that such potent agents could have "reset" the level of airway inflammation and perhaps made airway disease more amenable to subsequent treatment. In fact this has been claimed to occur in patients who responded to relatively long-term therapy (18 to 28 months) of low-dose methotrexate [35]. They responded more rapidly to doses of prednisolone that were ineffective prior to the use of methotrexate and tolerated more rapid reductions in corticosteroids than before methotrexate treatment.

## Practical considerations in the use of immunosuppressive therapy

The clinical use of immunosuppressive therapy should be restricted to physicians familiar with the management of chronic severe asthmatics and the pharmacology of these agents. The oral steroid dose should be reduced to the lowest possible level to maintain symptom control prior to the use of immunosuppressants. In doing so, the benefit/risk ratio of adding immunosuppressants to existing asthma medication can be accurately assessed and treatment adjusted accordingly. Prior to commencing immunosuppressants, it is essential to exclude other factors which may be responsible for poor control such as non-compliance with medication, hyperventilation, occupational factors, continued exposure to specific allergens and significant gastroesophageal reflux disease. Issues concerning the pharmacokinetics of corticosteroids may require consideration especially in an individual who receives high doses of corticosteroids and fails to demonstrate any "anticipated" side-effects. This involves questions of whether there is insufficient corticosteroid absorption from the gastrointestinal tract or accelerated catabolism/elimination from the body. Here, measurement of plasma prednisolone levels may be useful. Close monitoring of routine blood and urine tests is also essential, and investigations will vary, depending on the type of immunosuppressive agents selected.

Potential benefit from immunosuppressive agents should not be dismissed until a reasonable trial period has passed. Obviously if there are unacceptable adverse effects, these agents will have to be discontinued. The steroid-sparing benefit of methotrexate appears to take effect only after prolonged treatment of at least 6 months [12]. Cyclosporin A and gold seem to act more rapidly and steroid reduction may be possible within 3 months.

In patients who respond to immunosuppressive therapy, how long should we continue the treatment? There are reports [35] to suggest that stopping methrotrexate within the first month of discontinuing oral corticosteroids could led to disease exacerbation. Hence it is reasonable to continue treatment for up to 6 months after stopping oral corticosteroids. Using this regime, some patients have managed to stay off continuous oral corticosteroids for over 2 years. Our experience with Cyclosporin A has been that patients generally relapse on stopping treatment. From the existing literature, it is unclear how long gold therapy should continue after stopping oral corticosteroids.

It is also important to remember that improvement with immunosuppressants does not obviate the need for periodic rescue courses of oral steroids during disease exacerbations. Its chief objective is to reduce dependency on oral corticosteroids and may, as earlier stated, "reset" the level of airway inflammation and influence the natural course of disease.

## Future considerations in immunosuppressive/immune-modulatory therapy

### Inhaled route of administration

There is obviously a need for safer immunosuppressive agents. One possibility is to deliver these agents by the inhaled route, thus maximising delivery to the target site of inflammation while reducing systemic uptake. Aerosolized cyclosporin A has been used in lung allograft recipients with some success [36]. Similarly, the development of inhaled formulations for other immunosuppressive agents could represent a way forward for better tolerated therapy.

## Newer immunosuppressive agents

Rapamycin and tacrolimus (FK506) are new immunosuppressive agents presently studied in the field of organ transplantion. They share a molecular structure related to CsA and appear to be more potent, yet less toxic than CsA [37]. Tacrolimus, like CsA, exerts its effects principally through alteration of T cell gene expression, while rapamycin blocks signal transduction mediated by interleukin-2 and other cytokines, therefore inhibiting T cell activation at a later stage. Another immuno-suppressant presently being evaluated is mycophenolate mofetil acid, which acts by inhibiting *de novo* synthesis of pyrimidines and purines. These agents have potential in overcoming the problems of earlier immunosuppressants and may be useful to treat severe asthmatics.

## Experimental immune-modulatory agents

Specifically targeting immunologically important cells/cytokines/immune-mediated inflammatory cascade in asthma may be another way forward. These possibilities are presently being explored in animal models and as yet, their potential therapeutic role in humans is undefined.

As discussed earlier, CD4+ T lymphocytes are implicated in orchestrating ongoing airway inflammation, particularly in chronic asthma. By modulating their function, the airway inflammatory process may be attenuated and disease control improved. Recently we have completed a small, double-blind, placebo-controlled study assessing the effect of a humanised antiCD4 monoclonal antibody in steroid-dependent asthmatics [38]. Our results showed that following a single infusion of 3 mg/kg of the monoclonal antibody keliximab, an improvement in lung function could be observed as early as 24 h which persisted for 14 days when compared to placebo. The effect of repeated dosage and any "steroid-sparing" action were not studied. Larger, longer term trials are now being set up to investigate this further.

## Potential role of immunosuppressants in corticosteroid-resistant asthma

Patients with corticosteroid-resistant asthma are fortunately few. The potential of benefit with the use of immunosuppressive therapy in this group of patients has not been thoroughly studied. The mechanism of steroid resistance is complex and is still poorly understood. Yet it is conceivable that immunosuppressive agents may benefit this group of patients because their mechanisms of action are primarily independent of the glucocorticoid receptor. In fact there is *in vitro* evidence that while stimulated T cell proliferation from corticosteroid-resistant asthmatics was relatively unaffected by corticosteroid, it was inhibited by CsA, tacrolimus and mycophenolate mofetil [39]. A clinical study to specifically address this question will be most interesting.

## Early introduction of immunosuppressants in difficult-to-control asthma

Asthma management has changed significantly over the last few years, in particular with earlier and more aggressive use of anti-inflammatory agents. This is based on the evidence that airway inflammation is present early in the asthma disease process and early introduction of anti-inflammatory agents would be a logical step in improving the prognosis in asthma.

It is still unclear why certain asthmatics appear to have a more aggressive onset of disease. Their airway inflammation continues to be active despite being treated with high doses of corticosteroids. In patients such as these, should we consider bringing our most potent drugs, i.e. immunosuppressive drugs, into action early rather than late? Obviously the risk of potential toxicity should be weighed against the benefit of early and adequate control of airway inflammation and consequently reduction in longer term morbidity and indeed mortality from progressively destructive disease.

Interestingly, some open studies [40] have suggested that early introduction of immunosuppressants in selected groups of patients with severe asthma could reduce the incidence of corticosteroid dependency. Already other chronic autoimmune/ inflammatory diseases have been managed with such an "aggressive" approach with the intention of making long-term prognosis favourable.

## Conclusion

The immunological basis of the disease of asthma is now more clearly defined than before. Clinical studies with existing therapeutic drugs have in fact shown immunosuppressive or immune-modulatory activity relevant to the pathophysiology of chronic asthma. Corticosteroids remain our best "immunosuppressant". Many potent agents have been tried as adjuncts or alternatives to corticosteroids, mostly in situations when side-effects from corticosteroids become unacceptable. Of these, methotrexate, gold salts and cyclosporin A have the best documented "steroid-sparing" effect in severe asthmatics. However, with increased potency comes the "price" of toxicity and the uncertainty of long-term beneficial effect. Their clinical use must therefore be weighed carefully and individually assessed. The clinical efficacy of intravenous serum immune globulin in severe asthma appears to be minimal despite the increasing recognition of its varied immune-modulatory effects and clear benefits in treating some autoimmune/inflammatory diseases. "Safer" and more "effective" immunosuppressive/immune-modulatory agents are always needed because of the clear management problem in patients with severe asthma due to the lack of effective alternative treatment.

## References

1   Corrigan C, Kay AB (1992) T cells and eosinophils in the pathogenesis of asthma. *Immunol Today* 13: 501–507

2   Marone G, Columbo M, Galeone D, Guidi G, Kagey-Sobotka A, Lichtenstein LM et al (1986) Modulation of the release of histamine and arachidonic acid metabolites from human basophils and mast cells by auranofin. *Agents Actions* 18: 100–102

3   Bernstein DI, Bernstein IL, Bodenheimer SS, Pietrusko RG (1988) An open study of auranofin in the treatment of steroid-dependent asthma. *J Allergy Clin Immunol* 81: 6–16

4   Nierop G, Gitjzel WP, Bel EH, Zwinderman AH, Dijkman KH (1992) Auranofin in the treatment of steroid-dependent asthma: a double blind study. *Thorax* 47: 349–354

5   Honma M, Tamura G, Shirato K, Takishima T (1994) Effect of an oral gold compound auranofin, on non-specific bronchial hyper-responsiveness in mild asthma. *Thorax* 49: 649–651

6   Bernstein IL, Bernstein DI, Dubb JW, Faiferman I, Wallin B et al (1996) A placebo-controlled multicentre study of auroanofin in the treatment of patients with corticosteroid-dependent asthma. *J Allergy Clin Immunol* 98: 317–324

7   Goldstein JA (1983) Hydroxychloroquine for asthma (letter). *Am Rev Resp Dis* 128: 1100–1101

8   Roberts JA, Gunneberg A, Elliott JA, Thomson NC (1988) Hydroxychloroquine in steroid dependent asthma. *Pulm Pharmacol* 1: 59–61

9   Charous BL (1990) Open study of hydroxychloroquine in the treatment of severe symptomatic or corticosteroid-dependent asthma. *Ann Allergy* 65: 53–58

10  Mullarkey MF, Blumenstein BA, Pierre Andrade W, Bailey GA, Olason I, Wetzel CE (1988) Methotrexate in the treatment of corticosteroid-dependant asthma. *New Engl J Med* 318: 603–607

11  Shiner RJ, Nunn AL, Fan Chung K, Geddes DM (1990) Randomised, double-blind, placebo-controlled trial of methotrexate in steroid-dependent asthma. *Lancet* 335: 137–140

12  Marin GM (1997) Low-dose methotrexate spares steroid usage in steroid-dependent asthmatic patients. *Chest* 112: 29–33

13  Kuitert LM, Harrison AC (1991) *Pneumocystis carinii* pneumonia as a complication of methotrexate treatment of asthma. *Thorax* 46: 936–937

14  Vallerand H, Cossart C, Milosevic D, Lavaud F, Leone J (1992) Fatal pneumocystis pneumonia in asthmatics patient treated with methotrexate. *Lancet* 339: 1551

15   Gatnash AA, Connolly CK (1995) Fatal chickenpox pneumonia in an asthmatic patient on oral steroids and methotrexate. *Thorax* 50: 422–423

16   Altz-Smith M, Kendall LGJ, Stamm AM (1987) Cryptococcosis associated with low-dose methotrexate for arthritis. *Am J Med* 83: 179–181

17   Keegan JM, Byrd JW (1988) Nocardiosis associated with low dose methotrexate for rheumatoid arthritis (letter). *J Rheumatol* 15: 1585–1586

18   Asmundsson T, Kilburn KH, Lazzlo J, Krock CJ (1971) Immunosuppressive therapy of asthma. *J Allergy* 47: 136–147

19   Hodges NG, Brewis RAL, Howell JBL (1971) An evaluation of azathioprine in severe chronic asthma. *Thorax* 26: 734–739

20   Kahan BD (1989) Cyclosporin. *New Engl J Med* 321: 1725–1738

21   Cirillo R, Triggiani M, Sirih et al (1990) Cyclosporin A rapidly inhibits mediator release from human basophils presumably by interacting with cyclophilin. *J Immunol* 144: 389–397

22   Alexander AG, Barnes NC, Kay AB (1992) Trial of cyclosporin in corticosteroid-dependent chronic severe asthma. *Lancet* 339: 324–328

23   Nizankowska E, Soja J, Pinis G, Bochenek G, Sladek K, Domagala B, Pajak A, Szczeklik A (1995) Treatment of steroid-dependent bronchial asthma with cyclosporin. *Eur Respir J* 8: 1091–1099

24   Lock SH, Kay AB, Barnes NC (1996) Double-blind, placebo-controlled study of cyclosporin A as a corticosteroid-sparing agent in corticosteroid-dependent asthma. *Am J Respir Crit Care Med* 153: 509–514

25   Sihra BS, Kon OM, Durham SR, Walker S, Barnes NC, Kay AB (1997) Effect of cyclosporin A on the allergen-induced late asthmatic reaction. *Thorax* 52: 447–452

26   Bussel JB, Szatrowski TP (1995) Uses of intravenous gammaglobulin in immune haematologic disease. *Immunol Invest* 24: 451–456

27   Mazer BD, Gelfand EW (1991) An open-label study of high-dose intravenous immunoglobulin in severe childhood asthma. *J Allergy Clin Immunol* 87: 976–983

28   Jakobsson T, Croner S, Kjellman N, Pettersson A, Vassella C, Bjorksten B (1994) Slight steroid sparing effect of intravenous immunoglobulin in children and adolescents with moderately severe bronchial asthma. *Allergy* 49: 413–420

29   Valacer DJ, Kishiyama JL, Com B, Richmond GW, Bacot B, Glovsky M, Stiehm R, Stocks J, Rosenberg LA, Tonetta SA (1997) A multi-center, randomized, placebo-controlled trial of high dose intravenous gammaglobulin (IVIG) for oral corticosteroid-dependent asthma. *Am J Respir Crit Care Med* 155: A659

30   Pallares DE, Marshall GS (1992) Acute aseptic meningitis associated with administration of intravenous immunoglobulin. *Am J Paediatr Hematol Oncol* 14: 279–281

31   Blaszcyk R, Westhoff U, Grosse-Wilde M (1993) Soluble CD4, CD8 and HLA molecules in commercial immunoglobulin preparations. *Lancet* 341: 789–790

32   Boitard C, Bach JF (1989) Long-term complications of conventional immunosuppressive treatment. *Adv Nephrol* 18: 335–354

33   Muranaka M, Nakajima K, Suzuki S (1981) Bronchial responsiveness to acetylcholine

in patients with bronchial asthma after long-term treatment with gold salts. *J Allergy Clin Immunol* 67: 350–356

34    Szczeklik A, Nizankowska E, Sladek K (1992) Cyclosporin and asthma (letter). *Lancet* 339: 873

35    Mullarkey MF, Lammart JK, Blumenstein BA (1990) Long-term methotrexate treatment in corticosteroid-dependent asthma. *Ann Intern Med* 112: 577–581

36    O'Riordan TG, Iacono A, Keenan RJ et al (1995) Delivery and distribution of aerosolized cyclosporine in lung allograft recipients. *Am J Respir Crit Care Med* 151: 516–512

37    Chang JY, Seagal SN, Bansdach C (1991) FK506 and rapamycin: novel pharmacological probes of the immune response. *Trends Pharmacol Sci* 12: 218–222

38    Kon OM, Sihra BS, Compton CH, Leonard TB, Kay AB, Barnes NC (1998) Randomised, dose-ranging, placebo-controlled study of chimeric antibody to CD4 (keliximabb) in chronic severe asthma. *Lancet* 352: 1109–1113

39    Corrigan CJ, Bungre JK, Assoufi B, Cooper AE, Seddon H, Kay AB (1996) Glucocorticoid resistant asthma: T-lymphocyte steroid metabolism and sensitivity to glucocorticoids and immunosuppressive agents. *Eur Respir J* 9: 2077–2086

40    Mullarkey MF (1997) Methotrexate revisited. *Chest* 112: 1–2

# Anti-IgE agents

*Francesco Patalano*

Novartis Pharma A.G., Project Management, S-386.12.15, CH-4002 Basel, Switzerland

## Introduction

There is little debate over the essential role of IgE in allergic reactions. During an allergic response, CD4+ T lymphocytes of the Th2 phenotype stimulate allergen-specific B cells to produce IgE molecules via the release of IL-4/IL-13. The receptors for IgE are found on a multitude of different cells and two different types have been identified: the high-affinity receptor (FcεRI) on mast cells, basophils, and antigen-presenting cells, and the low-affinity receptor (FcεRII or CD23) on B lymphocytes, monocytes/macrophages, eosinophils, dendritic cells, and epithelial cells. After interaction with allergens, IgE-armed cells release a number of inflammatory mediators and enhance and redirect antigen presentation. This cascade of events seems to have a crucial role in the generation and persistence of symptoms in allergic diseases. The development of drugs that interfere with IgE production and function may therefore represent a more specific approach to treat these pathological conditions [1, 2].

A number of different strategies have been devised to inhibit IgE synthesis on the basis of studies *in vitro* or in animal models of allergic inflammation. These studies have indicated that it may be possible to inhibit IgE production by using STAT-6 inhibitors, which interfere with the signal transduction of IL-4 and IL-13 in B cells [3], or molecules that interfere with the binding of IL-4 to its receptor on B cells (IL-4 antagonists and neutralizing antibodies to IL-4) [4]. IgE production has also been shown to be partially inhibited by anti-CD23 antibodies [5]. However, no clinical evidence of benefit in allergic conditions has been demonstrated with these strategies.

In 1976, a complete suppression of the IgE-mediated response to *Nippostrongylus Brasiliensis* was reported in mice following treatment with specific polyclonal antibodies [6–8]. This set the stage for studying methods of antibody-mediated IgE inhibition suitable for human use and notable progress has been made since then. At present, the use of monoclonal antibodies that inhibit IgE function by preventing the binding of IgE to effector cells represents the most promising strategy for treatment of allergic diseases. In fact, it has been proven to be effective in asthma and allergic rhinitis, as described in the next sections.

## Development of a non-anaphylactogenic monoclonal antibody (mAb) to human IgE

A therapeutically viable anti-human IgE mAb should have the following character-istics: (1) It should bind specifically to IgE to minimize the unwanted effects on the immune system; (2) it should not bind to IgE attached to the receptors on cell sur-faces to minimize the risk of triggering cell degranulation and mediator release; (3) it should not trigger immune complex diseases.

Anti-human IgE antibodies were first described in 1981 by Hook et al. [9]. Later, anti-mouse IgE antibodies were shown to inhibit IgE binding to the FcεRI, but in so doing they induced mast cell degranulation by receptor cross-linking [10]. This was avoided by producing mAbs that recognized IgE at the same site as FcεRI and FcεRII [11–13]. These mAbs were shown to bind to free IgE. They were unable to bind to IgE attached via IgE receptors to the cell surfaces [2, 13–15].

Antibody 1-5 [12], TES-C21 [14] and MAE 11 [15] were rodent antibodies that recognized IgE at a target structure located within the Fcε3 domain containing the binding site for FcεRI. Six amino acids of the binding site (Arg-408, Ser-411, Lys-414, Glu-452, Arg-465 and Met-468) are critically involved in the binding of IgE to FcεRI and represented the ideal target for these non-anaphylactogenic anti-human IgE mAbs [15]. Since the binding site for FcεRI is contained within the same domain as the site for FcεRII, they also inhibited the binding of IgE to the low-affinity recep-tor [15–17].

A major factor that limited the use of these murine antibodies as therapeutic agents was the fact that an antigenic (anti-antibody) response can occur following repeated administration of xenogenic mAbs. This antigenic response can decrease the efficacy of the antibodies by reducing their half-life through the formation of antibody-anti-antibody complexes, and it carries the danger of anaphylaxis [18–22]. Since the antigenic response against the constant region of a xenogenic mAb comprises as much as 90% of the total response, the potential for an anti-anti-body response was reduced by generating recombinant hybrid mAbs. These mAbs retain the mouse variable regions, and therefore retain specificity for the antigen. The constant regions of the immunoglobulins have been replaced by human con-stant regions. Chimeric and humanized mAbs have been generated by ligation of entire mouse V region genes with human constant region genes or by grafting the murine antigen-binding loops onto a human IgG1 subclass framework, respective-ly. Humanized recombinant mAbs possess little or no expected antigenicity [2, 22–29].

CGP 51901 and E25 are the chimeric and humanized constructs of the murine antibodies TES-C21 and MAE11, respectively. Most of the clinical data available have been obtained with these mAbs.

## Effect of anti-human IgE antibodies in atopic subjects

The humanized antibody E25 and the chimeric antibody CGP 51901 were tested in a series of single and multiple dose clinical trials in subjects with elevated serum IgE. Their administration resulted in a dose-dependent decrease in serum free IgE levels.

In 23 atopic subjects, single doses of 3, 10, 30, and 100 mg i.v. of CGP 51901 induced an immediate fall in the concentration of circulating free IgE. Free serum IgE levels decreased by more than 95% after the highest dose, with a mean recovery to 50% of baseline levels by 39 days. Total IgE (sum of IgE-anti-IgE complexes and free IgE) increased, indicating that clearance of the immune complex is slow [30].

E25 was also shown to induce and maintain extremely low IgE levels for a long period of time. In an open trial, 45 atopic subjects received 0.015 or 0.03 mg of E25/kg/total serum IgE i.v. every 2 weeks. After 182 days of treatment, serum IgE levels were still less than 2% of the baseline value. After reducing the dose, serum IgE levels promptly began to return to pre-treatment values [31].

Antibodies against the anti-IgE mAbs were measured in all the clinical trials performed. A weak antigenic reaction was measured in only one of the subjects treated with the chimeric antibody CGP 51901 [30] and in none of those treated with the humanized mAb E25. Both antibodies were well tolerated.

## Effect of anti-human IgE antibodies in allergic diseases

### Allergic rhinitis

Two trials [32, 33] have been performed to test the efficacy of the anti-IgE mAbs in seasonal allergic rhinitis.

The first trial [32] was designed to evaluate the ability of CGP 51901 to prevent symptoms caused by mountain cedar pollen in subjects with a history of rhinitis upon exposure to this pollen. The administration of CGP 51901 every 2 weeks, at doses of 15, 30, or 60 mg, prevented the development of symptoms during the pollen season in a dose-dependent manner. This effect was achieved in patients whose IgE levels were reduced by at least 85 % from the baseline value. In this trial, approximately 25% of the patients treated with the highest dose did not need additional medication during the season, whereas 35 out of 36 patients in the placebo group needed symptomatic treatment.

One could speculate that repeated administration of these antibodies may allow recovery from chronic mucosal inflammation due to recurrent allergen exposure, thereby preventing or reversing some common complications of the chronic inflammatory process, particularly sinusitis and polyps.

## Models of allergic asthma

Antigen challenge in the laboratory represents a model for mimicking the changes occurring in the airways of subjects with allergic asthma after natural exposure to an allergen. This model has been repeatedly used in the development of antiasthmatic drugs to predict their efficacy before embarking on large and expensive trials. Most of the drugs capable of affecting bronchial responses to allergen inhalation, particularly those affecting the late asthmatic response, have been effective in the clinical setting. This is the case with inhaled corticosteroids which have been shown to inhibit the late reaction by interfering with several steps of the associated inflammatory response [34, 35].

The role of IgE in the development of the allergen-induced early asthmatic reaction is undisputed, because the early response is the result of the release of mediators triggered by IgE cross-linking on mast cell surfaces [36]. The direct involvement of IgE in the late reaction and in the associated inflammatory and functional changes, such as tissue eosinophil accumulation and increased bronchial hyperresponsiveness, is still unclear [37]. The study of the effect of anti-IgE mAbs on allergen-induced early and late asthmatic reactions can therefore provide important information on the pathogenesis of the inflammatory response that follows allergen exposure, in addition to giving an indication of their therapeutic potential in asthma.

One randomized, double-blind study by Boulet and colleagues [38] tested the ability of E25 to affect the allergen-induced early asthmatic response. After an initial loading dose of 2 mg/kg, E25 was administered i.v. to 10 allergic asthmatic individuals, on study days 7, 14, 28, 42, 56 and 70, at a dose of 1 mg/kg. Nine individuals received placebo. The allergen concentration able of inducing a 15% fall in FEV1 (PC15) was measured on days 1, 27, 55, and 77. E25 administration resulted in a significant increase in the PC15, that was 2.2 to 2.7 doubling doses higher than the baseline value (Fig. 1). The magnitude of this increase exceeds that reported with inhaled corticosteroids [39].

In another randomized double-blind study, Fahy and colleagues [40] tested the effect of E25 on the allergen-induced early and late asthmatic responses and on some inflammatory parameters measurable in induced sputum. Either E25 (0.5 mg/kg) or placebo were administered i.v. every week for 9 weeks. Allergen challenge was carried out before and at the end of the treatment phase. E25 significantly attenuated the early asthmatic response and reduced the magnitude of the late asth-

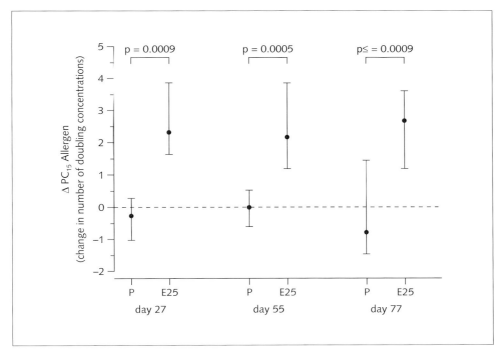

*Figure 1*
*Effect of E25 and placebo (P) on allergen-induced bronchoconstriction measured as PC15. The change in allergen PC15 during treatment is reported as median change in doubling concentrations of allergen and 25th–75th quartiles [38]. Reproduced by permission.*

matic response by more than 60% (Fig. 2). These effects were statistically significant versus placebo (p = 0.01 for the early response and p = 0.047 for the late response). In addition, the airway hyperresponsiveness to inhaled methacholine measured 24 h after allergen inhalation was significantly lower at the end of treatment with E25 than before. E25 administration had a small overall effect on inflammatory parameters as compared to placebo, probably because higher concentrations of the allergen were inhaled after E25 administration than after placebo. However, the allergen-induced increase in the number of eosinophils and the release of eosinophil cationic protein in sputum were lower after treatment with the anti-IgE mAb than before (all p < 0.05).

Taken together, these studies provide the first direct evidence of the involvement of IgE in both the early and late asthmatic reactions that follow allergen inhalation, and predict therapeutic utility of E25 and similar anti-IgE mAbs in asthma.

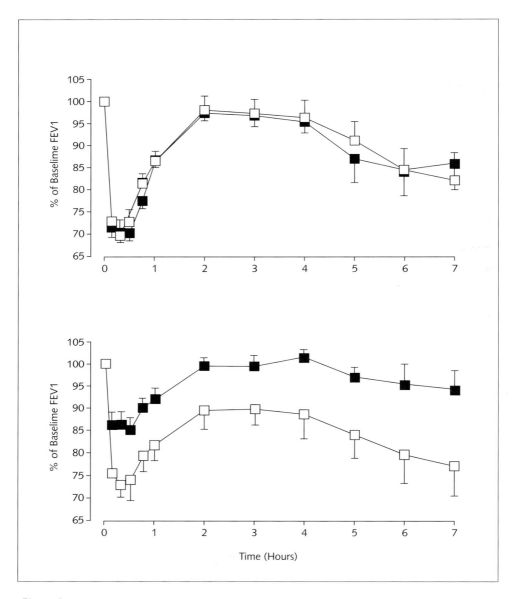

*Figure 2*
*Effect of E25 on the allergen-induced early and late asthmatic responses. Changes in FEV₁*
*in the first hour after allergen challenge (early response) and from 2 to 7 h after allergen*
*challenge (late response) in the placebo (top panel) and E25 (lower panel) treated groups*
*are reported as mean percent of baseline values ± SD before treatment (open squares) and*
*at the end of treatment (closed squares) [40]. Reproduced by permission.*

## Naturally occurring asthma

There is an ongoing debate on the percentage of patients with bronchial asthma who are atopic. In addition, it is difficult to estimate the pathogenetic importance of the atopic status per se. However, several investigators have found significant correlations between total serum IgE concentration, clinical parameters of disease severity [41], bronchial hyperresponsiveness [42, 43] and risk of emergency room admission [44].

E25 has been tested in asthmatic patients with positive skin prick test to at least two allergens known to be associated with bronchial asthma. Those patients were moderate to severe asthmatics treated with a standard dose of inhaled steroids and bronchodilators. A subgroup of them was receiving oral steroids. The study design involved two phases. During the first 12-week phase either E25 or placebo was added at random and double-blind to a standard treatment for moderate to severe bronchial asthma that included inhaled $\beta_2$-receptor agonists and inhaled or oral steroids and was chosen on the basis of the current guidelines [45]. During the second 8-week phase, a forced reduction in the dose of the inhaled and oral steroids was attempted [46].

When E25 was added to the standard treatment, it significantly reduced symptoms and improved PEFR while decreasing simultaneously the use of rescue medications with $\beta_2$-receptor agonists. The most remarkable effect of E25 during this study phase was its ability to reduce the number of asthma exacerbations by approximately 50% [45]. During the second study phase, patients receiving E25 were able to reduce their dose of inhaled and oral steroids by 50%, whereas patients in the placebo group were able to reduce the dose of inhaled steroids by 25% [46]. No reduction in the dose of oral steroids was possible in the placebo group. In spite of the reduction in the dose of steroids, the improvement observed in the patients receiving E25 during the first phase continued during the second phase, and the number of asthma exacerbations was further reduced [46].

These results demonstrate the effectiveness of E25 in chronic asthma and its ability to reduce the use of steroids in patients that otherwise need continuous administration of these agents.

In another randomized, double blind study [38], repeated administration of 1 mg/kg of E25 on study days 7, 14, 28, 42, 56 and 77, after an initial loading dose of 2 mg/kg, induced a significant reduction in the airway hyperresponsiveness to inhaled methacholine in 10 atopic asthmatics (p = 0.048 on day 76). As mentioned in the previous section, this study was designed to assess the effect of E25 on airway response to allergen inhalation test. The subjects recruited were therefore mild asthmatic patients with little or no symptoms and no recent or concurrent natural exposure to the relevant allergen. Since E25 is IgE- specific, it should be able to modify only allergen-induced airway inflammation and airway hyperresponsiveness. Thus, even the minimal effect on airway hyperresponsiveness observed in this study was totally unexpected.

## Effect of anti-human IgE on cutaneous reactivity

As mentioned in the previous sections, the anti-IgE mAbs tested in the studies reported above do not bind to the IgE already attached to their receptors on the cell surfaces. This is the most plausible reason to explain why the administration of these agents for a short period of time does not change skin reactivity. Longer periods of treatment seem to affect allergen-induced cutaneous reactions, and a reduction in the wheal response to skin prick testing after the administration of E25 for 3 and 6 months has been reported recently [31, 47]. The apparent dissociation between the onset of the effect in the lung and in the nose and the onset of the effect in the skin is unclear. It is possible that effective IgE depletion in the skin requires prolonged administration of the mAb, or that cells bearing the receptors for IgE play different roles in the immediate reactions induced by allergens in the airway and in the skin, or that inhibition of allergen-induced immediate reactions like the cutaneous wheal-and-flare response does not represent the mechanism by which anti-IgE mAbs improve allergic rhinitis and asthma. The latter hypothesis would imply that the clinical efficacy of anti-IgE mAbs is not merely due to the inhibition of mast cell degranulation or mediator release from other cells that bind IgE, and that it depends on more complex mechanisms, such as interference with dendritic cell function and antigen presentation or eosinophil trafficking and activation.

## Other effects of long-term treatment with anti-human IgE mAbs

At the time of this writing, the longest period of administration of anti-human IgE mAbs in atopic individuals has been 1 year [31]. No serious unwanted effects have been reported. The virtual absence of an antigenic (anti-antibody) reaction and the absence of any sign of deleterious effect due to the formation of immune complexes predict an excellent tolerability of these agents during longer periods of treatment.

There are many hypotheses on the consequence of prolonged administration of anti-human IgE mAbs in allergic individuals. It has been speculated that long-term treatment with these mAbs may reduce IgE synthesis through interference with a feedback mechanism mediated by IL4 [1]. Furthermore, treatment with E25 has been shown to reduce the expression of IgE receptors on the surfaces of circulating basophils [47]. On the basis of these putative mechanisms, it has been suggested that it may be possible to reduce the dose of the mAbs and achieve a more permanent effect on clinical parameters of disease severity after long-term administration. Data available up to now, however, do not support those theories. When the dose of E25 was reduced in 54 subjects after 6 months of high-dose therapy, IgE levels rose immediately. Treatment withdrawal after 1 year induced a further rise in IgE levels, and the expression of the IgE receptor returned to 80 % of the baseline value [48].

While these observations are reassuring for the long-term safety of the drug, because there is no permanent modification of the immunological characteristics, they also anticipate the necessity of prolonged administration of anti-IgE mAbs for achieving permanent remission of allergic diseases. Longer trials and observational studies will clarify this point.

Another issue concerning the long-term treatment with anti-IgE mAbs is the protection against parasitic diseases. Elevated IgE levels are an important characteristic of the immune response during and after parasitic infections, and are considered to be a host defense against secondary infections [49]. Recent epidemiological studies have also indicated a correlation between schistosome-specific IgE levels and resistance to reinfection [50, 51]. However, protection against parasites is not solely an IgE-dependent phenomenon, as it involves many cellular and humoral factors [52, 53]. In addition, several studies have demonstrated a neutral or beneficial effect of low IgE on the outcome of parasitic infection and resistance to reinfection in mice [52–54].

Some studies have suggested that the atopic status may protect against the development of cancer [55, 56]. This effect has not been related specifically to IgE levels, and other studies have failed to confirm the reduced risk of neoplasia in allergic individuals [57, 58].

Whatever role IgE molecules may play in immunological responses other than allergic reactions, it must be considered that during treatment with anti-human IgE mAbs atopic individuals have circulating levels of IgE similar to those commonly detectable in non-atopic subjects. It is therefore extremely unlikely that a population treated with anti-IgE differs from a normal population in terms of relative risk for diseases not associated with atopy.

## Conclusions

IgE molecules are key mediators in the development and maintenance of allergic reactions. The inhibition of IgE function by preventing the binding of IgE to specific receptors on effector cells represents a valid therapeutic strategy in allergic diseases such as allergic asthma and seasonal allergic rhinitis. The development of chimeric and humanized anti-IgE monoclonal antibodies has provided the first agents capable of obtaining this effect efficiently and safely.

*Acknowledgments*
The author thank Dr. F.M. Davis, Tanox Biosystems, Inc., Houston, TX, Dr. R.B. Fick, Genentech, Inc., South San Francisco, CA, and Dr. P. Rohane, Novartis Pharmaceuticals, Co., Summit, NJ, for helpful comments on this manuscript, and AVAIL GmbH, Biomedical Research, Basel, Switzerland, for expert assistance.

# References

1   Heusser C, Jardieu P (1998) Therapeutic potential of anti-IgE antibodies. *Curr Opin Immunol* 9: 805–814

2   Jardieu P (1995) Anti-IgE therapy. *Curr Opin Immunol* 7: 779–782

3   Shimoda K, van Deuren J, Sangster MY, Sarawar SR, Carson RT, Tripp RA, Chu C, Quelle FW, Nosaka T, Vignali DA et al (1996) Lack of IL-4 induced Th2 responses and IgE class switching in mice with disrupted Stat 6 gene. *Nature* 380: 630–633

4   Paul WE (1997) Interleukin 4: signalling mechanisms and control of T cell differentiation. *Ciba Foundation Symposium* 204: 208–216

5   Flores-Romo L, Shields J, Hubert Y, Graber P, Aubry J-P, Gauchat J-F, Ayala G, Allet B, Gnavaz M, Bazin H et al (1993) Inhibition of an *in vivo* antigen-specific IgE response by antibodies to CD23. *Science* 261: 1036–1041

6   Manning DD, Nanning JK, Reed NR (1976) Suppression of reaginic antibody (IgE) formation in mice by treatment with anti-μ antiserum. *J Exp Med* 144: 288–292

7   Bozelka BE, McCants ML, Salvaggio JE, Lehrer SB (1992) IgE isotype suppression in anti-μ treated mice. *Immunology* 46: 527–532

8   Bozelka BE, McCants ML, Salvaggio JE, Lehrer SB (1885) Effect of anti-IgE on total and specific IgE levels in adult mice. *Int Arch Allergy Appl Immunol* 78: 51–56

9   Hook WA, Berenstein E, Basciano LA, Fox PC, Siraganian RP (1981) Monoclonal antibodies to human IgE. *Fed Proc* 40: 986 A 41777

10  Banyash M, Eshar Z (1984) Inhibition of IgE binding to mast cells and basophils by monoclonal antibodies to murine IgE. *Eur J Immunol* 14: 799–807

11  Chang TW , Davis FM, Sun NC, Sun CRY, MacGlashan DW, Hamilton RG (1990) Monoclonal antibodies specific for human IgE-producing B cells: a potential therapeutic for IgE-mediated allergic diseases. *Bio/Technology* 8: 122–126

12  Heusser CH, Bews J, Brinkmann V, Delespesse G, Kilchnerr E, Ledermann F, LeGros G, Wagner K (1991) New concept of IgE regulation. *Int Archs Allergy Appl Immunol* 94: 87–90

13  Banyash M, Kerhy M, Eshar Z (1988) Anti-IgE monoclonal antibodies directed at the Fcε receptor binding site. *Mol Immunol* 25: 705–711

14  Davis FM, Gossett LA, Pinkston KL, Liou RS, Sun LK, Kim YW, Chang NT, Chang TW, Wagner K, Bews J et al (1993) Can anti-IgE be used to treat allergy? *Springer Seminars in Immunopathology* 15: 51–73

15  Presta L, Shields R, O'Connels L, Lahr S, Porter J, Gorman C, Jardieu P (1994) The binding site of on human Immunoglobulin E for its high affinity receptors. *J Biol Chem* 269 (42): 26368–26373

16  Nissim A, Eshar Z (1991) Localization of the Fcε receptor binding site to the third constant domain of IgE. *Int Arch Allergy Appl Immunol* 94: 93–95

17  Weetal M, Shopes B, Holowka D, Baird B (1990) Mapping the site of interaction between murine IgE and its high affinity receptor with chimeric Ig. *J Immunol* 145(11): 3849–3854

18  Khazaeli MB, Saleh MN, Wheeler RH, Huster WJ, Holden H, Carrano R, LoBuglio AF (1988) Phase I trial of multiple large doses of murine monoclonal antibody CO17-1A. II. Pharmacokinetics and immune response. *J Natl Cancer Inst* 80: 937–947

19  Jaffers GJ, Fuller TC, Cosimi AB, Russel PS, Winn HJ, Colvin RB (1986) Monoclonal antibody therapy: anti-idiotypic and non-anti-idiotypic antibodies to OKT3 arising despite intense immunosuppression. *Transplantation* 41: 572–578

20  Shawler DL, Bartholomew RM, Smith LM, Dillman RO (1985) Human immune response to multiple injection of murine monoclonal IgG. *J Immunol* 135: 1530–1535

21  Sears HF, Herlyn D, Steplewski Z, Koprowski H (1984) Effects of monoclonal antibody immunotherapy on patients with gastrointestinal adenocarcinoma. *J Biol Response Mod* 3: 138–150

22  Miller RA, Oseroff AR, Stratte PT, Levy R (1983) Monoclonal antibody therapeutic trials in seven patients with T-cell lymphoma. *Blood* 62: 988–995

23  Kolbinger F, Saldanha J, Hardman N, Mendig MM (1993) Humanization of a mouse anti-human IgE antibody: a potential therapeutic for IgE-mediated allergies. *Protein Engineering* 6(8): 971–980

24  Presta L, Lahr S, Shields R, Porter J, Gorman C, Fendly B, Jardieu P (1993) Humanization of an antibody directed against Immunoglobulin E. *J Immunol* 151(5): 2623–2632

25  Morrison SL, Johnson MJ, Herzenberg LA, Oi VT (1984) Chimeric human antibody molecules: mouse antigen-binding domains with human constant region domains. *Proc Natl Acad Sci USA* 81: 6851–6855

26  Reichmann L, Clark M, Waldmann H, Winter G (1988) Reshaping human antibodies for therapy. *Nature* 332: 323–327

27  Jones PT, Dear PH, Foote J, Neuberger MS, Winter G (1986) Replacing the complementarity-determining regions in human antibody with those from a mouse. *Nature* 321: 522–525

28  Amit AG, Mariuzza RA, Phillips SEV, Poljak RJ (1986) Three-dimensional structure of an antigen-antibody complex at 2.8 A resolution. *Science* 233:747– 753

29  Carter P, Presta L, Gorman CM, Ridgway JBB, Henner D, Wong WLT, Rowland AM, Kotts C, Carver ME, Shepard MH (1992) Humanization of an anti-p185 HER2 antibody for human cancer therapy. *Proc Natl Acad Sci USA* 89: 4285–4289

30  Corne J, Djukanovic R, Thomas L, Warner J, Botta L, Grandordy B, Gygax D, Huesser C, Patalano F, Richardson W et al (1997) The effect of intravenous administration of a chimeric anti-IgE antibody on serum IgE levels in atopic subjects: Efficacy, safety and pharmacokinetics. *J Clin Invest* 99(5): 879–887

31  Togias A, Corren J, Shapiro G, Reimann JD, von Schlegell A, Wighton TG, Adelmann DC (1998) Anti-IgE treatment reduces Skin Test (ST) reactivity. *J Allergy Clin Immunol* 101 (1 pt 2): s171 Abstract 706

32  Racine-Poon A, Botta L, Chang TW, Davis FM, Gygax D, Liou RS, Rohane P, Stahelin T, Van Steijn A, Frank W (1997) Efficacy, pharmacodynamics and pharamacokinetics of CGP 51901, an anti-immunoglobulin E chimeric monoclonal antibody, in patients with seasonal allergic rhinitis. *Clin Pharmacol Ther* 62: 675–690

33    Casale TB, Bernstein IL, Busse WW, LaForce CF, Tinkelman DG, Stoltz RR, Dockhcrn RJ, Reimann JR, Su JQ, Fick RB, Adelman DC (1997) Use of an anti-IgE humanized monoclonal antibody in ragweed-induced allergic rhinitis. *J Allergy Clin Immunol* 100: 110–121

34    Cockcroft DW, Murdock KY (1987) Comparative effects of inhaled salbutamol, sodium cromoglycate and bechlomethasone dipropionate on allergen-induced early asthmatic responses, late asthmatic responses, and bronchial responsiveness to histamine. *J Allergy Clin Immunol* 79:734–740

35    Cockcroft DW, Swystun VA, Baghat R (1995) Interaction of inhaled β2 agonist and inhaled corticosteroid on airway responsiveness to allergen and methacholine. *Am J Respir Crit Care Med* 152: 1485–1489

36    Holgate ST, Robinson C, Church MK (1993) Mediators of immediate hypersensitivity. In: E Middleton Jr, CE Reed, EF Regis, NF Adkinson Jr, JW Yuninger, Busse WW (eds): *Allergy principle and practice.* 4th ed, Mosby, St Louis, 267–301

37    Zweiman B (1993) The late phase response: role of IgE, its receptor, and cytokines. *Cur Opin Immunol* 5: 950–955

38    Boulet L-P, Chapman KR, Coté J, Kaira S, Bhagat R, Swystun VA, Laviolette M, C e-land LD, Deschesnes F, Su JQ et al (1997) Inhibitory effects of an anti-IgE antibody E25 on allergen-induced early asthmatic response. *Am J Respir Crit Care Med* 155: 1835–1840

39    Cockcroft DW, Swystun VA, Bhagat R (1995) Interaction of β2 agonist and inhaled corticosteroid on airway responsiveness to allergen and methacholine. *Am J Respir Crit Care Med* 152:1485–1489

40    Fahy JV, Flemming HE, Wong HH, Liu JT, Su JQ, Reimann J, Fick RB, Jr, Boushey HA (1997) The effect of an anti-IgE monoclonal antibody on the early- and late-phase responses to allergen inhalation in asthmatic subjects. *Am J Respir Crit Care Med* 155: 1828–1834

41    Burrows B, Martinez FD, Holonen M, Barbee RA, Cline MG (1989) Association of asthma with serum IgE levels and skin test reactivity to allergens. *N Engl J Med* 320: 271–277

42    Sears MR, Burrows B, Flannery EM, Herbison GB, Hewitt CJ, Holdaway MD. (1991) Relation between airway responsiveness and serum IgE in children with asthma and in apparently normal children. *N Engl J Med* 325: 1067–1071

43    Sunyer J, Munoz A and the Spanish Group of the European Asthma Study (1996) Concentration of methacholine for bronchial responsiveness according to symptoms, smoking and immunoglobulin E in a population based study in Spain. *Am J Respir Crit Care Med* 153: 1273–1279

44    Pollart S, Chapman M, Fiocco G, Rose G, Platt-Mills A (1989) Epidemiology of acute asthma: IgE antibodies to common inhalant allergens as a risk factor for emergency room visits. *J Allergy Clin Immunol* 83: 875–882

45    Fick RB, Simon SJ, Su JQ, Zeiger R and the E25 Study Group (1998) Anti-IgE (rhuM-

Ab) treatment of the symptoms of moderate to severe allergic asthma. *Ann Asthma Allergy Immunol* 80 (1): 80 Abstract 8

46 Metzger WJ, Fick RB and the E25 Asthma Study Group (1998) Corticosteroid (CS) withdrawal in a study of recombinant humanized monoclonal antibody to IgE (RhuM-Ab E25). *J Allergy Clin Immunol* 101 (1 pt 2): s231 Abstract 960

47 MacGlashan DW, Jr, Bochner B, Adelman D, Jardieu P, Togias A, McKenzie-White J, Sterbinsky SA. Hamilton R, Lichtenstein LM (1997) Down-regulation of FcεRI expression on human basophils during anti-IgE antibody therapy. *J Immunol* 158: 1438–1445

48 Saini S, MacGlashan DW, Jr, Adelman D, Togias A, Lichtenstein LM, Blochner BS (1998) Discontinuation of anti-IgE infusions restores basophils (BASO) IgE and FcεRIα expression, and IgE-dependent histamine release. *J Allergy Clin Immunol* 101 (1 pt 2): s105 Abstract 437

49 Capron A, Dessaint JP, Haque A, Capron M (1982) Antibody-dependent cell-mediated cytotoxic against parasites. *Progr Allergy* 31: 234–267

50 Rihet P, Demuere C, Bourgois A, Prata A, Dessein A (1991). Evidence for an association between human resistance to *Schistosoma mansoni* and high-larval IgE levels. *Eur J Immunol* 21: 2679–2686

51 Hagan P, Blumenthal UJ, Dunn D, Simpson AJG, Wilkins HA (1991) Human IgE, IgG4 and resistance to reinfection with *Schistosoma haematobium*. *Nature* 349: 243–245

52 Welge-Roussel F, Ariault C, Damonneville M, Capron A.(1991) Functional analysis of a T cell line specific for antiidiotypic antibodies to a *Schistosoma mansoni* protective epitope. II. Induction of protective immunity in experimental rat schistosomiasis. *J Immunol* 147: 3967–3972

53 Watanabe N, Katakura K, Kobayashi A, Okumura K, Ovary Z (1989) Protective immunity and eosinophilia in IgE-deficient SJA/9 mice infected with *Nippostrogylus brasiliensis* and *Trichinella spiralis*. *Proc Natl Acad Sci USA* 85: 4460–4462

54 Amiri P, Haak-Frendscho M, Robbins K, McKerrow J, Stewart T, Jardieu P. (1994) Anti-immunoglobulin E treatment decreases worm burden and egg production in Schistosoma mansoni infected normal and IFNγ knockout mice. *J Exp Med* 180: 43–51

55 Fisherman E (1960) Does the allergic diathesis influence malignancy? *Allergy* 31: 74–78

56 Allegra J, Lipton A, Harvey H, Luderer J, Brenner D, Mortel R, Semers L, Gillin M, White D, Trautlein J (1976) Decreased prevalence of immediate hypersensitivity (atopy) in a cancer population. *Cancer Res* 36: 3225–3226

57 McKee W, Arnold CA, Perlman M (1967) A double blind study of the comparative incidence of malignancy and allergy. *J Allergy Clin Immunol* 39: 294–301

58 Shapiro S, Heinonen O, Siskind V (1971) Cancer and allergy. *Cancer* 29: 386

# Mast cell proteases as new targets for therapeutic intervention in asthma

*Steven J. Compton and Andrew F. Walls*

Immunopharmacology Group, University of Southampton, Southampton General Hospital, Southampton, SO16 6YD, UK

## Introduction

Mast cells have long attracted attention for their potential to contribute to the disease process in asthma [1]. These cells are widely distributed throughout the body, but are particularly prevalent in tissues which form an interface with the external environment. In the lower airways mast cells are numerous in the bronchial mucosa [2], submucosa and alveolar walls [3], and are even found free in the lumen [4]. The activation of mast cells by allergen or by other stimuli is associated with the rapid release of a range of potent mediators of inflammation and bronchoconstriction.

Mast cell products include proteases, histamine, heparin, prostaglandins and a variety of cytokines [5]. Several of these have been the subject of extensive study and have become targets for drug development, but until recently proteases have been relatively little investigated. Over the past few years, however, evidence has been accumulating that these major products of the mast cell may have potent biological actions. Mast cell proteases, and in particular tryptase and chymase, may be important mediators of inflammation and are showing promise as targets for therapeutic intervention in asthma and other allergic conditions.

## The proteases of human mast cells

Neutral proteases are the most abundant components of the mast cell secretory granule on a weight basis. Five distinct proteases have been localised to the human mast cell, of which three have now been purified, tryptase, chymase and carboxypeptidase (Tab. 1). Tryptase is the major protease with approximately 10 pg per lung mast cell and 35 pg per skin mast cell [6]. There are estimated to be 5–16 pg of carboxypeptidase [7] and 4.5 pg of chymase per skin mast cell [6]. A protease with some enzymatic and antigenic properties in common with neutrophil cathepsin G has also been detected [8, 9] and there are conflicting reports on the presence in mast cells of an elastase-like serine protease [8, 9]. The high concentra-

*Table 1 - Human mast cell proteases*

| Enzyme | Molecular weight (kDa) | Subpopulation |
|---|---|---|
| Tryptase | 132 | $MC_T$ and $MC_{TC}$ |
| Chymase | 30 | $MC_{TC}$ |
| Carboxypeptidase | 34.5 | $MC_{TC}$ |
| Cathepsin G | ND | $MC_{TC}$ |
| Elastase | ND | ? |

*ND, not determined for the protease identified in mast cells.*

tions of proteases in mast cell secretory granules would be consistent with these proteases playing a major mediator role in conditions involving mast cell activation.

Tryptase and chymase have assumed importance as biochemical markers of mast cells [10] and of mast cell heterogeneity in humans [11]. Two distinct subpopulations of mast cells have been identified, those containing both tryptase and chymase ($MC_{TC}$), and those possessing tryptase but not chymase ($MC_T$). Carboxypeptidase and the cathepsin G-like enzyme have been localised to the $MC_{TC}$ subset [9, 12]. Mast cells of the $MC_{TC}$ phenotype are the predominant phenotype in the skin and other connective tissues, while $MC_T$ cells appear to be most numerous in the normal mucosal tissues of the lung and gut [11]. The defined mast cell subpopulations may reflect relative rather than absolute differences in protease composition. Thus, the results of histochemical studies with a chymotryptic substrate [13] or immunocytochemistry with a sensitive protocol for chymase detection [14] have indicated the presence of chymase, or perhaps of a new form of chymase, in the majority of cells generally classed as being of the $MC_T$ phenotype in the gastrointestinal mucosa. Nevertheless, utilising immunocytochemistry under carefully standardised conditions, the detection of $MC_T$ and $MC_{TC}$ subsets can offer important information on mast cell heterogeneity and function. There is no simple relationship between mast cell functional heterogeneity and protease composition in terms of susceptibility to activation by basic peptides or control by pharmacological agents [15]. However, in the upper airways it is the $MC_{TC}$ population which appears to be the principle store of interleukin 4 (IL-4), while IL-5 and IL-6 have been localised to the $MC_T$ subset [16].

The relative numbers of each mast cell subset may be altered in disease. In the gastrointestinal mucosa of patients with AIDS and other immunodeficiency syndromes, a selective deficiency in cells of the $MC_T$ phenotype has been noted [17], prompting the suggestion that the growth and survival of this subset are dependent on intact T lymphocyte function. In keeping with this idea, increased numbers of $MC_T$ cells have been associated with inflammatory changes in seasonal allergic rhinitis [18], atopic dermatitis [19], scleroderma [20], conjunctivitis [21] and rheumatoid arthritis [22]. However, $MC_T$ numbers may also be elevated in osteoarthritis [23], a condition in which inflammation is not a prominent feature. In asthmatic airways there have been no detailed investigations of the distribution of $MC_T$ and $MC_{TC}$ cells, but the evidence available from bronchial biopsies suggests that the relative numbers of each of these subpopulations are relatively little altered [16].

## Tryptase

### Biochemical and enzymatic properties

Early studies with tryptase isolated from human mast cells established that it is a tetrameric serine protease with a molecular weight of approximately 130 kDa and with each of the subunits possessing a single active site [24]. Tryptase expresses optimal catalytic activity when in its tetrameric form. Initially detected in mast cells using histochemical substrates [25], tryptase was later purified to homogeneity from pulmonary mast cells [24], human skin [26] and human lung tissue [27]. Subsequently tryptase has been isolated from cells and tissues of the dog [28], rat [29], cow [30], guinea pig [31] and monkey [32]. Studies in different species have revealed major differences in the types of protease present and in their properties. Thus for example, while tryptase in the dog, rat and monkey appears to be tetrameric and with a molecular weight similar to that in humans [24], that purified from bovine tissues has a molecular weight of 360 kDa [30], and that from guinea pigs, 860 kDa, indicative of a very large structure with some 20–22 subunits [31]. On account of such species-related differences, the focus here will be on the human proteases.

Recently the crystal structure of tetrameric human tryptase has been reported [33] as a square flat ring structure composed of four subunits with the active site of each monomer facing a central pore. This arrangement will restrict access to the catalytic site and helps to explain why tryptase appears to cleave few protein substrates, and exhibits little susceptibility to inhibition by endogenous protease inhibitors. Two complementary deoxyribonucleic acid (cDNA) molecules termed α and β have been cloned from a human lung mast cell library and sequenced [34,35], while three cDNA molecules named type I, II & III have been derived from a human skin library [36]. Beta-tryptase shows 98–100% amino acid sequence homology with the three tryptases from human skin and 90% with alpha tryptase. However, although β-tryptase (or type II tryptase) and types I and III tryptase are similar in sequence, some of the differences may affect the catalytic site. While one putative glycosylation site has been identified for β-tryptase/type II tryptase the other forms possess two putative sites.

Much of the size and charge heterogeneity of purified tryptase observed following electrophoresis on SDS polyacrylamide gels can be attributed to the differences in glycosylation. The extent to which heterogeneity in sequence or glycosylation pattern of tryptase may lead to differences in function remain to be determined. However, a major difference between α-tryptase and β-tryptase-like forms has been suggested by the application of immunoassays using antibodies with different affinities for α and β-tryptase. α-Tryptase appears to be released constitutively from mast cells in an inactive form, while β-tryptase appears to represent the form which is stored in the secretory granules and released on anaphylactic degranulation [37, 38]. In biological fluids, the levels of α-tryptase are likely to reflect numbers of mast cells present in nearby tissues, whereas the concentration of β-tryptase should provide an indication of the degree of mast cell activation. It is α-tryptase which predominates in the serum of normal subjects, and it is present at much higher levels in patients with mastocytosis [37]. α-Tryptase also appears to comprise the majority of tryptase which can be detected in the synovial fluid of most patients with rheumatoid arthritis or osteoarthritis [39], conditions associated with increased numbers of mast cells in synovial tissue [23]. In contrast, tryptase in the serum of anaphylactic patients is predominantly of the β form [37].

In the asthmatic bronchi, there is an increased degree of mast cell activation, with little or no evidence of mast cell hyperplasia. This suggests that much of the tryptase released into the airways in this condition will be of the β form, though this has yet to be tested directly. As enzymatically inactive α-tryptase is not stored, there are particular difficulties in isolating and studying this form other than in recombinant expression systems. The function of α-tryptase in health and disease remains a subject for conjecture. Almost all studies to date have been with the stored forms of tryptase which must represent β or β-like tryptase, and therefore all subsequent references will be to these forms.

The detection of tryptase within mast cells using histochemical substrates [25, 40] indicates that tryptase is stored in the secretory granules in a fully-active state. However, inside the granule, tryptase will be tightly bound to heparin proteoglycan, an association which could serve to maintain the tetrameric structure and hence the stability of the enzyme following secretion into the extracellular space [41]. The high negative charge of heparin is primarily responsible for its binding to tryptase, as other proteoglycans of lower negative charge bind less efficiently [41]. Tryptase has been found to cleave chromogenic substrates with a pH optimum of pH 7 to 8 [26]. In contrast, in the acidic conditions of the mast cell granule (estimated to be in the region of pH 5.5 [42]), tryptase is likely to have relatively little activity [43]. In addition, tryptase activity in the granule will be inhibited by the presence of histamine which at high concentrations can act as a reversible inhibitor of this enzyme [44]. The main actions of tryptase are thus likely to be in the neutral pH conditions outside the cell following mast cell activation. Recently, however, fibrinogen has been identified as a substrate which tryptase may cleave more efficiently at pH 5 [45], indicating a possible role for this protease in acidic pH conditions.

The enzymatic activity of tryptase may be inhibited by diisopropylfluorophosphate (DFP) and benzamidine and by certain natural inhibitors of proteases such as, antipain, leupeptin [27] and an inhibitor isolated from the medicinal leech [46]. However, circulating serine protease inhibitors such as $\alpha_1$-antitrypsin and $\alpha_2$-macroglobulin fail to inhibit the enzymatic activity of tryptase [47]. Secretory leukocyte protease inhibitor (SLPI) has been reported to have some inhibitory actions on tryptase [48], but little evidence has been presented to date that an endogenous human protease inhibitor may be effective as an inhibitor of tryptase. Probably of greater importance is the role of heparin in stabilising the tetrameric structure of this unstable molecule. Tryptase in the absence of heparin dissociates rapidly into inactive monomers in physiological buffers [41]. In contrast, when tryptase is in physiological buffer in the presence of heparin, it retains its activity for several hours. Divalent cations [44] or other heparin binding proteins such as antithrombin III [27] or lactoferrin [49] can serve as inhibitors of tryptase by virtue of their ability to destabilise the tryptase/heparin complex. Tryptase is secreted with proteoglycan in a complex of some 200 kDa [50]. The large size of this complex is likely to hinder diffusion away from the site of its release and it is likely that the actions of tryptase will be in the immediate vicinity of degranulating mast cells.

## Extracellular substrates of tryptase

Studies with synthetic substrates have indicated that tryptase cleaves peptide and ester bonds on the carboxyl side of amino acids [26], but relatively few natural substrates have been identified. Peptide substrates of potential relevance in asthma which are efficiently cleaved by tryptase include the neuropeptides vasoactive intestinal peptide (VIP), peptide histidine methionine (PHM) [51] and calcitonin gene-related peptide (CGRP) [52]. VIP and PHM are both potent relaxants of bronchial muscle [53] and the cleavage of these peptides by tryptase has been suggested to contribute to the bronchoconstriction observed in asthmatics. CGRP is a potent vasodilator [54] and cleavage of this by tryptase results in attenuation of vasodilator activity [52].

The ability of tryptase to generate kinins remains controversial. Some workers have reported that tryptase fails to generate kinins from low molecular weight kininogen (LMWK) [55] or high molecular weight kininogen (HMWK) [56], whilst others have demonstrated kininogenase activity for tryptase with these substrates [57, 58]. Fibrinogen may be degraded by tryptase so that it no longer acts as a substrate for thrombin in the clotting cascade [59]. The anticoagulant properties of tryptase may be of particular importance in acidic conditions as the reaction is optimal at acidic pH [45].

A number of extracellular matrix (ECM) components are cleaved to some extent by tryptase. Tryptase can degrade the ECM synthesised *in vitro* by rat heart smooth muscle cells [60] and by a human lung fibroblast cell line [50]. Cleaved substrates include gelatinase/type IV collagenase and fibronectin [61]. In addition, tryptase can activate stromelysin (matrix metalloprotease 3; MMP 3) [62] resulting in the activation of latent collagenase [63], and also urokinase [64]. These actions of tryptase in degrading the ECM could facilitate the entry of cells and plasma proteins into areas of mast cell degranulation, and tryptase could be an important participant in processes of matrix remodelling and repair. Structural alterations and increased epithelial fragility are features in the bronchial tissue of asthmatics and tryptase may contribute to these.

## Cellular targets of tryptase

Cells in the vicinity of a degranulating mast cell are likely to be exposed to high concentrations of tryptase and other mast cell products (Fig. 1). Recent studies have indicated the potential of tryptase to induce profound alterations in cell behaviour (Tab. 2). The early studies involved incubation of purified dog tryptase with cells of non-human origin. Canine tryptase was found to be a potent mitogen for Chinese hamster lung fibroblasts (CHL cells) and Rat-1 fibroblasts, and in both cases the effect was inhibited by protease inhibitors, suggesting dependence on an intact catalytic site [65]. Moreover, tryptase was reported to act synergistically with basic fibroblast growth factor (FGF), epidermal growth factor (EGF), insulin and thrombin on CHL cells [66]. Human tryptase has now been reported to act as potent mitogen for human lung fibroblasts [66, 67], epithelial cells [68], airway smooth muscle cells [69], including those from the dog [70], and human microvascular endothelial cells [71], but not macrovascular endothelial cells [72]. These various actions could be important in the context of tissue remodelling in asthma and other inflammatory conditions. Of particular importance could be the ability of tryptase to stimulate the synthesis and release from fibroblasts of type I collagen as well as of collagenase activity [67, 73]. In addition tryptase can stimulate fibroblast chemotaxis *in vitro* [73]. The release of tryptase into the upper airways of asthmatics could be a major factor in the induction of myofibroblast and smooth muscle cell hyperplasia and in the deposition of collagen beneath the epithelial basement membrane.

The proinflammatory potential of tryptase is becoming quite well recognised. Studies with animal models have demonstrated that the injection of human tryptase into the skin can induce microvascular leakage [74] and accumulation of eosinophils and neutrophils, and also to some extent of macrophages and lymphocytes [75]. The microvascular leakage induced by tryptase may be inhibited by pretreatment with antihistamines, suggesting that the effect is dependent on mast cell activation by tryptase. This has been confirmed by the demonstration that human

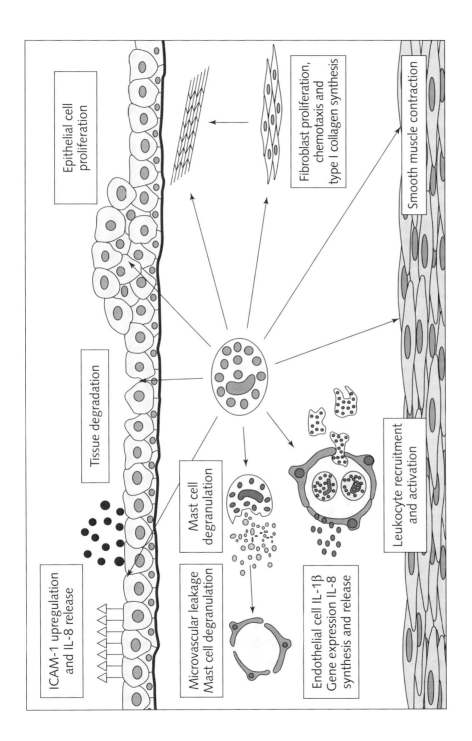

Epithelial cell proliferation

Fibroblast proliferation, chemotaxis and type I collagen synthesis

Smooth muscle contraction

Tissue degradation

ICAM-1 upregulation and IL-8 release

Mast cell degranulation

Microvascular leakage Mast cell degranulation

Endothelial cell IL-1β Gene expression IL-8 synthesis and release

Leukocyte recruitment and activation

Figure 1
Tryptase actions on cell function.

Table 2 - Actions of tryptase on the behaviour of human cells

| Cell type | Effect |
| --- | --- |
| Epithelial cell | Proliferation, IL-8 release and upregulation of ICAM-1 |
| Fibroblast | Proliferation, chemotaxis synthesis and secretion of type I collagen synthesis |
| Endothelial cell | IL-1β gene expression and IL-8 release |
| Airway smooth muscle cell | Proliferation |
| Mast cell | Histamine release |
| Eosinophil | Chemotaxis and ECP release |
| Neutrophil | Chemotaxis |

tryptase can induce histamine release from guinea pig mast cells [74] and from human tonsil mast cells, though this effect has not been found with human skin mast cells [76].

The ability of tryptase to stimulate the accumulation of inflammatory cells *in vivo* is likely to involve a complex interplay between several cell types which are affected by this protease. Tryptase can stimulate the release of the potent granulocyte chemoattractant IL-8 and upregulate expression of intercellular adhesion molecule 1 (ICAM-1) in epithelial cells [68]. In addition, tryptase can induce the secretion of IL-8 and upregulate expression of mRNA for both IL-8 and IL-1β in primary cultures of human umbilical vein endothelial cells (HUVEC) [72] and provoke the release of neutrophil chemotactic activity [77]. Potentiation of IL-6 and IL-8 release from TGFβ or IL-4 stimulated fibroblasts has also been reported in a preliminary study [78]. As well as inducing the release of granulocyte chemoattractants tryptase appears to have direct effects on granulocytes, acting as a chemotactic agent for human eosinophils and neutrophils *in vitro* and provoking the release of eosinophil cationic protein [79]. This latter action is consistent with observations in a guinea pig model in which the presence of partially degranulated eosinophils has been noted at the sites where human tryptase has been injected into skin [75]. There is thus an accumulation of evidence to implicate this major mast cell product as playing a key role in mast cell dependent inflammation.

The precise mechanisms by which tryptase can alter cell function remain to be resolved and this is an issue of considerable interest. The cloning of a receptor for thrombin [80], now termed protease activated receptor-1 (PAR-1), opened the way for the identification of a family of related receptors, and has indicated the potential importance of proteases in regulating cell function. PAR-1 may be activated to some extent by tryptase when expressed in COS-1 cells, but tryptase appears not to activate this receptor on HUVEC [81]. Recently tryptase has been found to cleave PAR-2 [81], a receptor found on human endothelial cells [82], vascular smooth muscle cells [83], keratinocytes [84], rat colonic myocytes [85] and neutrophils [86], but not fibroblasts [84]. The activation of PAR-2 appears to be less efficient with tryptase than with trypsin, a stimulus which is not of physiological importance outside the intestinal tract [87], and there is some uncertainty over the extent to which the actions of tryptase *in vivo* may be dependent on the activation of PAR-2. Thus a peptide agonist for PAR-2 can stimulate a strong proliferative response in HUVEC [82], yet this has not been reproduced using tryptase [72]. The activation of PAR-2 by tryptase may therefore not account for all the actions of this protease observed on cells. Recently the characterisation of a PAR-3 on HUVEC has been described, another receptor which can be cleaved by thrombin [88]. The growing number of PARs suggests that it is possible that other receptors for tryptase are yet to be discovered.

## Chymase

### Biochemical and enzymatic properties

Chymase is a chymotryptic-like protease which has been purified from human skin [89], heart [90] and tonsil [91] with a molecular weight of approximately 30 kDa. Although multiple amino acid sequences have been derived for chymases from rodents [92], to date the sequence of only a single human chymase has been reported from skin, heart and tonsil tissues [91, 93, 94]. This encodes a protein of 25 kDa with a net positive charge of 13. There is evidence from several sources, however, for the presence of more than one type of human chymase. Employing heparin agarose affinity chromatography, at least two distinct forms of chymase-like protease have been identified in high salt extracts of a variety of human tissues [95]. Chymase B eluted with sodium chloride concentrations of 1.0 to 1.2 M, and chymase C at 1.8 to 2.0 M. Both forms exhibited similar enzymatic properties with synthetic substrates and reacted with a range of chymase-specific antibodies, but marked differences were observed in their tissue distribution. Chymase B constitutes the predominant form in extracts of human skin, heart and synovial tissue, while chymase C is the major form in lung tissues. The extent to which differences observed between chymases B and C represent differences in primary sequence or in post-translational modifications remains to be determined. However, the isolation from lung tissue has been reported of a protease with properties similar to chymase, but with an N-terminal sequence which differed at a number of residues [96]. It is possible that as in rodents, there may be quite different chymases expressed in human mucosal and connective tissue compartments.

Understanding of the enzymatic properties of human chymase is based largely on studies with purified preparations in which chymase B is likely to represent the main constituent. This protease exhibits relatively little catalytic activity towards synthetic substrates at pH 5.5 [97], the reported pH of the mast cell granule [42]. Thus, although stored in a catalytically active form in the secretory granules, the principle actions of chymase are likely to be extracellular. Moreover, heparin exerts a further inhibitory effect on chymase activity at pH 5.5, but can enhance activity at pH 7.5, the pH of the extracellular space [97]. The observation that the activation of recombinant prochymase by dipeptidyl peptidase I occurs with a pH optimum in the neutral range and is inhibited by both heparin and histamine [98] would appear to indicate that this process is restricted to the early stages of vesicle formation.

Chymase is released in a complex of 400–560 kDa with proteoglycans and carboxypeptidase, but not with tryptase [99]. Chymase is inhibited by the circulating serine protease inhibitors $\alpha_1$-antichymotrypsin, $\alpha_1$-proteinase inhibitor and $\alpha_2$-macroglobulin [100] and also by SLPI [101].

## Substrates and cellular targets

Compared with tryptase, chymase appears to be much less restricted in substrate specificity. Peptide bonds are cleaved preferentially where there is a phenylalanine residue at the $P_1$ site and hydrophobic residues at $P_2$ and $P_3$ [102]. Angiotensin I is cleaved by chymase in this way to generate angiotensin II, a reaction which is catalysed more efficiently than with angiotensin converting enzyme itself [103]. The ability of chymase to cleave a range of substrates may suggest an important role in tissue degradation and remodelling at sites of mast cell activiation. Addition of chymase to cultures of fresh human skin has been reported to result in extensive degradation of the epidermal-dermal junction [104]. There may be direct actions on components of the extracellular matrix. For example, Type I procollagen is processed by human chymase to initiate the formation of collagen fibrils [105]. A less direct contribution to matrix remodelling may involve the activation of interstitial procollagenase and other proenzymes [106].

The ability of chymase to degrade IL-4 [107], to activate the precursor form of IL-1β [108] and to cleave and release the membrane bound form of stem cell factor (SCF) [109] suggests roles for this protease in the regulation of cytokine bioavailability. Evidence that chymase may exercise a proinflammatory role has come from studies in which the purified enzyme has been injected into laboratory animals. Injection of chymase into the skin of guinea pigs elicits a prolonged increase in microvascular permeability that is still apparent 120 min following injection, and that appears to be dependent on an intact catalytic site [110]. Unlike the skin reactions which may be provoked by tryptase in this model, those induced by chymase are unaffected by antihistamine pretreatment of the animals. This suggests that the mechanism of chymase action does not involve histamine release; a subsequent study with dispersed human lung, tonsil and skin mast cells has failed to demonstrate chymase-induced mast cell activation [111].

238

Several hours following the injection of chymase into guinea pig skin or into the peritoneum of mice a massive accumulation of eosinophils and neutrophils has been observed with significant increases in the numbers of lymphocytes being noted in the mouse model [112]. Quantities of chymase as low as 5ng [$1.7 \times 10^{-13}$ moles] were able to induce an inflammatory infiltrate, and in all cases co-injection with a protease inhibitor, or heat inactivation of the enzyme significantly inhibited the response. Chymase, like tryptase, could thus represent a potent stimulus for the recruitment of inflammatory cells following mast cell activation in bronchial asthma.

In the context of inflammatory conditions of the respiratory tract, the finding that dog chymase can stimulate mucus secretion from glandular cells *in vitro* [113] is of particular interest, and there is a clear need for the potential role of human chymase to be investigated as a stimulus of mucus secretion. The extent to which chymase may alter cell function remains largely unexplored, and it is not known if there are cell surface receptors for chymotryptic proteases.

## Carboxypeptidase

Carboxypeptidase purified from human lung and skin has a molecular weight of 34 to 40 kDa [114, 115]. Sequences for carboxypeptidase cDNA derived from human lung and skin libraries encode a protein with a molecular weight of 36.1 kDa with a net positive charge of 16 [116, 117]. There is little evidence for heterogeneity, with only one sequence being derived.

Mast cell carboxypeptidase possesses a similar substrate profile to pancreatic carboxypeptidase A, although it has greater sequence homology to carboxypeptidase B. Natural substrates include neurotensin, Leu[5]- enkephalin and kinetensin [118]. On mast cell degranulation carboxypeptidase is co-released with tryptase and chymase, and it is bound to the same proteoglycan macromolecular complex as chymase [99]. It seems likely that carboxypeptidase will act in concert with other mast cell proteases.

## Therapeutic potential of inhibitors of mast cell proteases

Mast cell proteases have long been neglected as potential targets for therapeutic intervention. While it has been known for several years that mast cell proteases are released in substantial quantities into the airways of asthmatic subjects, it is only now being recognised that they may possess a range of potent biological activities. The proinflammatory actions of tryptase and chymase implicate these proteases in the genesis of both early and late phase allergic reactions, and they could both play particularly important roles in mediating structural alterations in chronic disease. A consistent finding with *in vitro* and *in vivo* experimental models has been that the biological actions of tryptase and chymase can be inhibited by protease inhibitors. However, information is sparse on the ability of protease inhibitors to modulate processes of allergic disease induced by allergen, and are restricted at present to some relatively small scale studies of the effects of tryptase inhibitors.

The synthetic protease inhibitors APC-366 and BABIM, both of which are relatively selective for tryptase, have been shown to be effective in a sheep model of asthma [119]. Their administration reduced both the early and late phase response to allergen, as well as blocking the acquired airway hyperresponsiveness. Consistent with the findings of purified tryptase in animal models [74, 75], APC-366 was also found to inhibit microvascular leakage and eosinophil accumulation. A subsequent study with the same sheep model has involved administration of a preparation of neutrophil lactoferrin, which has inhibitory activity on human tryptase [49]. While this treatment had little effect on the early reaction to allergen, both the late phase reaction and allergen-induced hyperresponsiveness were abolished.

Recently, the results have been reported of a randomised cross-over study in which APC-366 was administered by aerosol to 16 subjects with mild-to-moderate atopic asthma [120]. Following allergen challenge, administration of APC-366 resulted in a significant reduction in the late phase response compared with placebo, whether assessed as the area under the curve or as the maximum fall in $FEV1$. While there was a trend for APC-366 administration to be associated with a reduced early phase reaction, this did not reach statistical significance and bronchial hyperresponsiveness appeared unaffected.

The studies to date with tryptase inhibitors have been encouraging, and it will be important to determine more precisely their anti-inflammatory properties. Of particular interest must be the ability of tryptase inhibitors to affect processes of tissue remodelling in airways disease. Observations that tryptase is a potent growth factor for fibroblasts [65, 67] and a stimulus for collagen secretion [67, 73] call attention to the potential role of this major mast cell product in inducing the structural alterations which are prominent features of asthmatic bronchi [121]. While experimental evidence with inhibitors of chymase is still lacking, the biological actions described for this protease also suggest that they could prove valuable in modifying processes of both acute inflammation and matrix remodelling in the airways and at other sites. They may also be of benefit in controlling mucus hypersecretion.

Tryptase and chymase represent promising targets for therapeutic intervention in conditions associated with an increased degree of mast cell activation. The design of selective small molecular weight inhibitors of mast cell proteases, or the preparation of certain broad spectrum endogenous protease inhibitors, or even the development of antagonists of protease activated receptors could lead to the provision of some new classes of anti-inflammatory and anti-fibrotic drug.

# References

1   Redington AE, Polosa R, Walls AF, Howarth PH, Holgate ST (1995) The role of mast cells and basophils in bronchial asthma. In: Marone G (ed): *Human basophils and mast cells in health and disease*. Karger, Basel, 22–59

2   Djukanovic R, Wilson JW, Britten KM, Wilson SJ, Walls AF, Roche WR, Howarth PH, Holgate ST (1990) Quantitation of mast cells and eosinophils in the bronchial mucosa of symptomatic atopic asthmatics and healthy control subjects using immunohisto-chemistry. *Am Rev Respir Dis* 142:863–871

3   Fox B, Bull TB, Guz A (1981) Mast cells in the human alveolar wall: an electron micro-scope study. *J Clin Pathol* 34: 1333–1342

4   Walls AF, Roberts JA, Godfrey RC, Church MK, Holgate ST (1990) Histochemical het-erogeneity of human mast cells: disease-related differences in mast cell subsets recovered by bronchoalveolar lavage. *Int Arch Allergy Appl Immunol* 92: 233–241

5   Church MK, Holgate ST, Shute JK, Walls AF, Sampson AP (1998) Mast cell derived mediators. In: Middleton E, Reed CE, Ellis E, Adkinson NF, Yuninger JW, Busse WW (eds): *Allergy: Principles and practice*. Mosby, St Louis, 146–167

6   Schwartz LB, Irani AA, Roller K, Castells MC, Schechter NM (1987) Quantitation of histamine, tryptase and chymase in dispersed human mast cells. *J Immunol* 138: 2611–2615

7   Goldstein SM, Kaempfer CE, Kealey JT, Wintroub BU (1989) Human mast cell car-boxypeptidase: purification and characterisation. *J Clin Invest* 83: 1630–1636

8   Meier HL, Heck LW, Schulman ES, MacGlashan DW (1985) Purified human mast cells and basophils release human elastase and cathepsin G by an IgE-mediated mechanism. *Int Arch Allergy Appl Immunol* 77: 179–183

9   Schechter NM, Irani AA, Soves JL, Abernethy J, Wintroub B, Schwartz LB (1990) Iden-tification of a cathepsin G-like protease in the $MC_{TC}$ type of human mast cell. *J Immunol* 145: 2652–2661

10  Craig SS, DeBlois G, Schwartz LB (1986) Mast cells in human keloid, small intestine and lung by an immunoperoxidase technique using murine monoclonal antibody against tryptase. *Am J Pathol* 124: 427–435

11  Irani AA, Schechter NM, Craig SS, De Blois G, Schwartz LB (1986) Two types of human mast cells that have distinct neutral protease compositions. *Proc Natl Acad Sci USA* 83: 4464–4468

12  Irani AA, Golstein SM, Wintroub BU, Bradford T, Schwartz LB (1991) Human mast cell carboxypeptidase: selective localisation to $MC_{TC}$ cells. *J Immunol* 147: 247–253

13  Huntley JF, Newlands GFJ, Gibson S, Ferguson A, Miller HRP (1985) Histochemical demonstration of chymotrypsin-like serine esterases in mucosal mast cells in four species including man. *J Clin Pathol* 38: 275–382

14  Beil WJ, Schulz M, McEuen AR, Buckley MG, Walls AF (1997) Number, fixation prop-erties, dye-binding and protease expression of duodenal mast cells: comparisons

between healthy subjects and patients with gastritis or Crohn's disease. *Histochemical J* 29: 759–773

15  Church MK, Okayama Y, Bradding P (1995) Functional mast cell heterogeneity. In: Busse WW, Holgate ST (eds): Asthma and rhinitis. Blackwell Scientific Publication, Boston, 209–220

16  Bradding P, Okayama Y, Howarth PH, Church MK, Holgate ST (1995) Heterogeneity of human mast cells based on cytokine content. *J Immunol* 155: 297–307

17  Irani AA, Craig SS, DeBlois G, Elson CO, Schechter NM, Schwartz LB (1987) Deficiency of the tryptase-positive, chymase-negative mast cell type in gastrointestinal mucosa of patients with defective T lymphocyte function. *J Immunol* 138: 4381–4386

18  Bentley AM, Jacobson MR, Cumberworth V, Barkaus JR, Moqbel R, Schwartz LB, Irani AA, Kay AB, Durham SR (1992) Immunohistology of the nasal mucosa in seasonal allergic rhinitis: increases in activated eosinophils and epithelial mast cells. *J Allergy Clin Immunol* 89: 877–883

19  Irani AA, Sampson HA, Schwartz LB (1989) Mast cells in atopic dermatitis. *Allergy* 44: 31–34

20  Irani AA, Gruber BL, Kaufman LD, Kahalch MD, Shwartz LB (1992) Mast cell changes in scleroderma: presence of MCT cells in the skin and evidence of mast cell activation. *Arthritis Rheum* 35: 933–939

21  Irani AA, Butrus SI, Tabbara KF, Schwartz LB (1990) Human conjunctival mast cells: distribution of $MC_T$ and $MC_{TC}$ in vernal conjunctivitis and giant papillary conjunctivitis. *J Allergy Clin Immunol* 86: 34–40

22  Tetlow LC, Woolley DE (1995) Distribution, activation and tryptase/chymase phenotype of mast cells in the rheumatoid lesion. *Ann Rheum Dis* 54: 549–555

23  Buckley MG, Gallagher PJ, Walls AF (1998) Mast cell subpopulations in the synovial tissue of patients with osteoarthritis. Selective increase in numbers of tryptase-positive, chymase negative mast cells. *J Pathol* 186: 67–74

24  Schwartz LB, Lewis RA, Austen KF (1981) Tryptase from human pulmonary mast cells. Purification and characterisation. *J Biol Chem* 256: 11939–11943

25  Glenner GG, and Cohen LA (1960) Histochemical demonstration of a species-specific trypsin-like enzyme in mast cells. *Nature* 185: 846–847

26  Tanaka T, McRae BJ, Cho K, Cook R, Fraki JE, Johnson DA, Powers JC (1983) Mammalian tissue trypsin-like enzymes. Comparative reactivities of human skin tryptase, human lung tryptase, and bovine trypsin with peptide 4 nitroanilide and thioester substrates. *J Biol Chem* 258: 3552–3557

27  Smith TJ, Hougland MW, Johnson DA (1984) Human lung tryptase. Purification and characterisation. *J Biol Chem* 259: 11046–11051

28  Caughey GH (1990) Tryptase and chymase in dog mast cells. In: Schwartz LB (ed): Neutral proteases of mast cells. *Monogr Allergy* 27: 67–89

29  Braganza VJ, Simmons WH (1991) Tryptase from rat skin: Purification and properties. *Biochem* 30: 4997–5007

30    Fiorucci L, Erba F, Ascoli F (1992) Bovine tryptase: purification and characterisation. *Biol Chem Hoppe Seyler* 373: 483–490

31    McEuen AR, He S, Brander ML, Walls AF (1996) Guinea pig lung tryptase: localisation to mast cells and characterisation of the partially purified enzyme. *Biochem Pharmacol* 52: 331–340

32    Robinson TL, Muller DK (1997) Purification and characterisation of cynomolgus monkey tryptase. *Comp Biochem Physiol* 118B: 783–792

33    Pereira PJB, Bergner A, Macedo-Ribeiro S, Huber R, Matschiner G, Fritz H, Sommerhoff CP, Bode W (1998) Human β-tryptase is a ring like tetramer with active sites facing a central pore. *Nature* 392: 306–311

34    Miller JS, Westin EH, Schwartz LB (1989) Cloning and characterisation of complementary DNA for human tryptase. *J Clin Invest* 84: 1188–1195

35    Miller JS, Moxley G, Schwartz LB (1990) Cloning and characterisation of a second complementary DNA for human tryptase. *J Clin Invest* 86: 864–870

36    Vanderslice P, Ballinger SM, Tam EK, Goldstein SM, Craik CS, Caughey GH (1990) Human mast cell tryptase: multiple cDNAs and genes reveal a multigene serine protease family. *Proc Natl Acad Sci USA* 87: 3811–3815

37    Schwartz LB, Sakai K, Bradford TR, Ren S, Zweiman B, Worobec A, Metcalfe DD (1995) The α form of tryptase is the predominant type present in blood at baseline in normal subjects and is elevated in those with systemic mastocytosis. *J Clin Invest* 96: 2702–2710

38    Sakai K, Ren S, Schwartz LB (1996) A novel heparin-dependent processing pathway for human tryptase: autocatalysis followed by activation with dipeptidyl peptidase I. *J Clin Invest* 97: 988–995

39    Buckley MG, Walters C, Wong WM, Cawley, MID, Ren S, Schwartz LB, Walls AF (1997) Mast cell activation in arthritis: detection of α and β tryptase, histamine and eosinophil cationic protein in synovial fluid. *Clin Sci* 93: 363–370

40    Schwartz LB, Bradford TR (1986) Regulation of tryptase from human lung mast cells by heparin. *J Biol Chem* 261: 7372–7379

41    Alter SC, Metcalfe DD, Bradford TR, Schwartz LB (1987) Stabilisation of human mast cell tryptase: effects of enzyme concentration, ionic strength and the structure and negative charge of polysaccharides. *Biochem J* 247: 821–827

42    Deyoung MB, Nemeth EF, Scarpa A (1987) Measurement of the internal pH of mast cell granules using microvolumetric fluorescence and isotopic techniques. *Arch Biochem Biophys* 254: 222–233

43    Lagunoff D, Rickard A (1983) Evidence for control of mast cell granule protease in situ by low pH. *Exp Cell Res* 144: 353–360

44    Alter SC, Schwartz LB (1989) Effect of histamine and divalent cations on the activity and stability of tryptase from human mast cells. *Biochem Biophys Acta* 991: 426–430

45    Ren S, Lawson AE, Carr M, Baumgarten CM, and Schwartz LB (1997) Human tryptase fibrinogenolysis is optimal at acidic pH and generates anticoagulant fragments in the presence of the anti-tryptase monoclonal antibody B12. *J Immunol* 159: 3540–3548

46    Sommerhoff CP, Sollner C, Mentele R, Piechottka GP, Auerswald EA, Fritz H (1994) A Kazal-type inhibitor of human mast cell tryptase: Isolation from the medicinal leech Hirudo medicinalis, characterisation, and sequence analysis. *Biol Chem Hoppe-Seyler* 375: 685–694

47    Alter SC, Kramps JA, Janoff A, Shwartz LB (1990) Interactions of human mast cell tryptase with biological protease inhibitors. *Arch Biochem Biophys* 276: 26–31

48    Robinson T, Delaria K, Harris P, Lindell D, Gundell D, Muller D (1986) Secretory leukocyte protease inhibitor as an inhibitor of mast cell tryptase. *Am J Respir Crit Care Med* 153: 455

49    Elrod KC, Moore WR, Abraham WM, Tanaka RD (1997) Lactoferrin, a potent tryptase inhibitor, abolishes late-phase airway responses in allergic sheep. *Am J Respir Crit Care Med* 156: 375–381

50    Goldstein SM, Leong J, Schwartz LB, Cooke D (1992) Protease composition of exocytosed human skin mast cell protease-proteoglycan complexes: tryptase resides in a complex distinct from chymase and carboxypeptidase. *J Immunol* 148: 2475–2482

51    Tam EK, Caughey GH (1990) Degradation of airway neuropeptides by human lung tryptase. *Am Rev Respir Cell Mol Biol* 3: 27–32

52    Walls AF, Brain SD, Desai A, Jose PJ, Hawkings E, Church MK, Williams TJ (1992) Human mast cell tryptase attenuates the vasodilator activity of calcitonin gene related peptide. *Biochem Pharmacol* 43: 1243–1248

53    Palmer JBD, Cuss FMC, Barnes PJ (1987) VIP and PHM and their role in noradrenergic inhibitory responses in isolated human airways. *J Appl Physiol* 61: 1322–1328

54    Brain SD, Williams TJ, Tippins JR, Morris HR, MacIntyre I (1985) Calcitonin gene related peptide is a potent vasodilator. *Nature* 313: 54–56

55    Schwartz LB, Maier M, Spragg J (1986) Interaction of low molecular weight kininogen with human mast cell tryptase. *Adv Exp Med Biol* 198A: 105–111

56    Maier M, Spragg J, Schwartz LB (1983) Inactivation of human high molecular weight kininogen by human mast cell tryptase. *J Immunol* 130: 2353–2356

57    Walls AF, Bennett AR, Suieras-Diaz J, Olsson H (1992) The kininogenase activity of human mast cell tryptase. *Biochem Soc Trans* 20: 260S

58    Proud D, Siekierski ES, Bailey GS (1988) Identification of human lung mast cell kininogenase as tryptase and relevance of tryptase kininogenase activity. *Biochem Pharmacol* 37: 1473–1480

59    Schwartz LB, Bradford TR, Littman BH, Wintroub BU (1985) The fibrinogenolytic activity of purified tryptase from human lung mast cells. *J Immunol* 135: 2762–2767

60    Gruber BL, Schwartz LB (1990) The mast cell as an effector of connective tissue degradation: a study of matrix susceptibility to human mast cells. *Biochem Biophys Res Commun* 171: 1272–1278

61    Lohi J, Harvima I, Keski-Oja J (1992) Pericellular substrates of human mast cell tryptase: 72,000 dalton gelatinase and fibronectin. *J Cell Biochem* 50: 337–349

62    Gruber BL, Marchese MJ, Suziki K, Schwartz LB, Okada Y, Nagase H, Ramamurthy NS

(1989) Synovial procollagenase activation by human mast cell tryptase. Dependence upon matrix metalloproteinase 3 activation. *J Clin Invest* 84: 1657–1662

63  Gruber BL, Schwartz LB, Ramamurthy NS, Irani AA, Marchese MJ (1988) Activation of latent rheumatoid synovial collagenase by human mast cell tryptase. *J Immunol* 140: 3936–3942

64  Stack MS, Johnson DA (1994) Human mast cell tryptase activates single-chain urinary-type plasminogen activator (pro-urokinase). *J Biol Chem* 269: 9416–9419

65  Ruoss SJ, Hartmann T, and Caughey GH (1991) Mast cell tryptase is a mitogen for cultured fibroblasts. *J Clin Invest* 88: 493–499

66  Hartmann T, Ruoss SJ, Raymond WW, Seuwen K, Caughey GH (1992) Human tryptase is a potent, cell-specific mitogen: role of signalling pathways in synergistic responses. *Am J Physiol (Lung Cell Mol Physiol 6)* 262: L528

67  Cairns, JA, Walls AF (1997) Mast cell tryptase stimulates the synthesis of type I collagen in human lung fibroblasts. *J Clin Invest* 99: 1313–1321

68  Cairns JA, Walls AF (1996) Mast cell tryptase is a mitogen for epithelial cells. Stimulation of IL-8 production and intercellular adhesion molecule-1 expression. *J Immunol* 156: 275–283

69  Thabrew H, Cairns JA, Walls AF (1996) Mast cell tryptase is a growth factor for human airway smooth muscle. J Allergy Clin Immunol 97: 969

70  Brown JK, Tyler CL, Jones CA, Ruoss SJ, Hartmann T, and Caughey GH (1995) Tryptase, the dominant secretory granular protein in human mast cells, is a potent mitogen for cultured dog tracheal smooth muscle cells. *Am J Respir Cell Mol Biol* 13: 227–236

71  Blair RJ, Meng H, Marchese MJ, Ren S, Schwartz LB, and Tonnesen MG (1997) Human mast cells stimulate vascular tube formation: tryptase is a novel potent angiogenic factor. *J Clin Invest* 99: 2691–2700

72  Compton SJ, Cairns JA, Holgate ST, Walls AF (1998) The role of mast cell tryptase in regulating endothelial cell proliferation, cytokine release and adhesion molecule expression: Tryptase induces expression of mRNA for IL-1β and IL-8 and stimulates the selective release of IL-8 from human umbilical vein endothelial cells. *J Immunol* 161: 1939–1946

73  Gruber BL, Kew RR, Jelaska A, Marchese MJ, Garlick J, Ren S, Schwartz LB, Korn JH (1997) Human mast cells activate fibroblasts. *J Immunol* 158: 2310–2317

74  He S, Walls AF (1997) Human mast cell tryptase: A stimulus of microvascular leakage and mast cell activation. *Eur J Pharmacol* 328: 89–97

75  He S, Peng Q, Walls AF (1997) Potent induction of a neutrophil and eosinophil-rich infiltrate *in vivo* by human mast cell tryptase: Selective enhancement of eosinophil recruitment by histamine. *J Immunol* 159: 6216–6225

76  He S, Gaca MDA, Walls AF (1998) A role for tryptase in the activation of human mast cells: modulation of histamine release by tryptase and inhibitors of tryptase. *J Pharmacol Exp Ther* 286: 289–297

77 Compton SJ, Cairns JA, Holgate ST, Walls AF (1999) Interaction of human mast cell tryptase to stimulate endothelial cell recruitment. *Int Arch Allergy Immunol; in press*

78 Ohkuni Y, Illig M, Numerof R, Takigawa K, Rennard SI (1997) Tryptase synergistically augments cytokine release from human lung fibroblasts in the presence of TGF-β or IL-4 driven cytokine. *Am J Respir Crit Care Med* 155: A182

79 Jung K-S, Cairns JA, Church MK, Shute JK, Walls AF (1994) Human mast cell tryptase can induce eosinophil chemotaxis and secretion. *Clin Exp Allergy* 24: 988A

80 Vu T-K, Hung DT, Wheaton VI, and Coughlin SR (1991) Molecular cloning of a functional thrombin receptor reveals a novel proteolytic mechanism of receptor activation. *Cell* 64: 1057–1068

81 Molino M, Barnathan ES, Numero R, Clark J, Dreyer M, Cumashi A, Hoxie JA, Schechter N, Woolkalis M, Brass LF (1997) Interactions of mast cell tryptase with thrombin receptors and PAR-2. *J Biol Chem* 272: 4043–4049

82 Mirza H, Yatsula V, Bahou WF (1996) The proteinase activated receptor 2 (PAR-2) mediates mitogenic responses in human vascular endothelial cells. *J Clin Invest* 97: 1705–1714

83 Molino M, Raghunath PN, Kuo A, Ahuja M, Hoxie JA, Brass LF, Barnathan ES (1998) Differential expression of functional protease-activated receptor-2 (PAR-2) in human vascular smooth muscle cells. *Arterioscler Tromb Vasc Biol* 18: 825–832

84 Santulli RJ, Derian CK, Darrow AL, Tomko KA, Eckardt AJ, Seiberg M, Scarborough RM, Andrade-Gorden P (1995) Evidence for the presence of a protease-activated receptor distinct from the thrombin receptor in human keratinocytes. *Proc Natl Acad Sci USA* 92: 9151–9155

85 Corvera CU, Dery O, McConalogue K, Bohm SK, Khitin LM, Caughey GH, Payan DG, Bunnett NW (1997) Mast cell tryptase regulates rat colonic myocytes through proteinase-activated receptor 2. *J Clin Invest* 100: 1383–1393

86 Howells GL, Macey MG, Chinni C, Hou L, Fox MT, Harriott P, Stone SR (1997) Proteinase-activated receptor-2: expression by human neutrophils. *J Cell Sci* 110: 881–887

87 Kong W, McConalogue, Khitin LM, Hollenberg MD, Payan DG, Bohmm SK, Bunnett NG (1997) Luminal trypsin may regulate enterocytes through proteinase-activated receptor 2. *Proc Natl Acad Sci* 94: 8884–8889

88 Ishihara H, Connolly AJ, Zeng D, Kahn ML, Zheng YW, Timmons C, Tram T, Coughlin SR (1997) Protease-activated receptor 3 is a second thrombin receptor in humans. *Nature* 386: 502–506

89 Schechter NM, Fraki JE, Geesin JC, Lazarus GC (1983) Human skin chymotryptic protease. Isolation and relation to cathepsin G and rat mast cell proteinase I. *J Biol Chem* 258: 2973–2978

90 Urata H, Knoshita A, Misono KS, Bumpus FM, Husain A (1990) Identification of a highly specific chymase as the major angiotensin II forming enzyme in the human heart. *J Biol Chem* 265: 22348–22357

91 Sukenaga Y, Kido H, Neki, Enomoto M, Ishida K, Takagi K, Katunuma N (1993)

Purification and molecular cloning of chymase from human tonsils. *FEBS Lett* 323: 119–122

92    Lutzelschwab C, Pejler G, Aveskogh M, Hellman L (1997) Secretory granule proteases in rat mast cells. Cloning of 10 different serine proteases and a carboxypeptidase A from various rat mast cell populations. *J Exp Med* 185: 13–29

93    Urata H, Kinoshita A, Perez DM, Misono KS, Bumpus FM, Graham RM, Huain A (1991) Cloning of the gene and cDNA for human heart chymase. *J Biol Chem* 266: 17173–17179

94    Schechter NM, Wang ZM, Blacher RW, Lessin SR, Lazarus GS, Rubin H (1994) Determination of the primary structures of human skin chymase and cathepsin G from cutaneous mast cells of urticaria pigmentosa lesions. *J Immunol* 152: 4062–4069

95    McEuen AR, Gaca MDA, Buckley MG, He S, Gore MG, Walls AF (1998) Two distinct forms of human mast cell chymase. Differences in affinity for heparin and in distribution in skin, heart, and other tissues. *Eur J Biochem* 256: 461–470

96    Heidtmann HH, Tavis J (1993) A novel chymotrypsin-like serine protease from human lung. *Biol Chem Hoppe-Seyler* 374: 871–875

97    McEuen AR, Sharma B, Walls AF (1995) Regulation of the activity of human chymase during storage and release from mast cells: the contributions of inorganic cations, pH, heparin and histamine. *Biochim Biophys Acta* 1267: 115–121

98    McEuen AR, Ashworth DM, Walls AF (1998) The conversion of recombinant human mast cell prochymase to enzymatically active chymase by dipeptidyl peptidase I is inhibited by heparin and histamine. *Eur J Biochem* 253: 300–308

99    Goldstein SM, Leong J, Schwartz LB, Cooke D (1992) Protease composition of exocytosed human skin mast cell protease-proteoglycan complexes. Tryptase resides in a complex distinct from chymase and carboxypeptidase. *J Immunol* 148: 2475–2482

100   Schechter NM, Sprows J L, Schoenberger OL, Lazarus GS, Cooperman BS, Rubin H (1989) Reaction of human skin chymotrypsin-like proteinase chymase with plasma proteinase inhibitors. *J Biol Chem* 264: 21308–21315

101   Walter M, Plotnick M, Schechter NM (1996) Inhibition of human mast cell chymase by secretory leukocyte proteinase inhibitor: enhancement of the interaction by heparin. *Arch Biochem Biophys* 327: 568–571

102   Powers JC, Takumi T, Harper JW, Minematsu Y, Barker L, Lincoln D, Crumley KV (1985) Mammalian chymotrypsin-like enzymes: comparative reactivities of rat mast cell proteases, human and dog skin proteases and human cathepsin G with peptide-4-nitroanilide substrates and with peptide chloromethyl ketone and sulphonyl fluoride inhibitors. *Biochem* 24: 2048–2058

103   Urata H, Kinoshita A, Misono KS, Bumpus FM, Husain A (1990) Identification of a highly specific chymase as the major angiotensin II-forming enzyme in the human heart. *J Biol Chem* 265: 22348–22357

104   Briggamon RA, Schechter NM, Fraki J, Lazarus GS (1984) Degradation of the epidermal-dermal junction by proteolytic enzymes from human skin and polymorphonuclear leukocytes. *J Exp Med* 160: 1027–1042

105  Kofford MW, Schwartz LB, Schechter NM, Yager DR, Diegehnan RF, Graham MF (1997) Cleavage of type I procollagen by human mast cell chymase initiates collagen fibril formation and generates a unique carboxyl terminal propeptide. *J Biol Chem* 272: 7127–7131

106  Saarinen J, Kalkkinen N, Welgus HG, Kovanen PT (1994) Activation of human interstitial procollagenase through direct cleavage of the Leu 83-Thr 84 bond by mast cell chymase. *J Biol Chem* 269: 18134–18140

107  Tunon De Lara JM, Okayama Y, McEuen AR, Heusser CH, Church MK, Walls AF (1994) Release and inactivation of interleukin 4 by mast cells. *Ann NY Acad Sci* 725: 50–58

108  Mizutani H, Schechter N, Lazarus G, Black RA, Kupper TS (1991) Rapid and specific conversion of precursor interleukin 1β (IL-β) to an active IL-I species by human mast cell chymase. *J Exp Med* 174: 821–825

109  Longley BJ, Tyrrell L, Ma YS, Williams DA, Halaban R, Langley K, Lu HS, Schechter NM (1997) Chymase cleavage of stem cell factor yields a bioactive, soluble product. *Proc Natl Acad Sci USA* 94: 9017-9021

110  He S, Walls AF (1998) The induction of a prolonged increase in microvascular permeability by human mast cell chymase. *Eur J Pharmacol* 352: 91–98

111  He S, Garca MDA, Walls AF (1997) The regulation of mast cell histamine release by human mast cell chymase and chymase inhibitors. *J Allergy Clin Immunol* 99: 588

112  He S, Walls AF (1998) Human mast cell chymase induces the accumulation of neutrophils and eosinophils and other inflammatory cells *in vivo*. *Br J Pharmacol* 125: 1491–1500

113  Sommerhoff CP, Caughey GH, Finkbeiner WE, Lazarus SC, Basbaum CB, Nadel JA (1989) Mast cell chymase. A potent secretagogue for airway gland serous cells. *J Immunol* 142: 2450–2456

114  Goldstein SM, Kaempfer CE, Proud D, Schwartz LB, Irani AA, and Wintroub BU (1987) Detection and partial characterisation of a human mast cell carboxypeptidase. *J Immunol* 139: 2724–2729

115  Goldstein SM, Kaempfer CE, Kealey JT, Wintroub BU (1989) Human mast cell carboxypeptidase: purification and characterisation. *J Clin Invest* 83: 1630–1636

116  Reynolds DS, Gurley DS, Stevens RL, Sugarbaker DJ, Austen KF, Serafin WE (1989) Cloning of cDNAs that encode human mast-cell carboxypeptidase-A, and comparison of the protein with mouse mast-cell carboxypeptidase-A and rat pancreatic carboxypeptidase. *Proc Natl Acad Sci USA* 86: 9480–9484

117  Natsuaki M, Stewart CB, Vanderslice P, Schwartz LB, Natsuaki M, Wintroub BU, Rutter WJ, Goldstein SM (1992) Human skin mast-cell carboxypeptidase: functional-characterization, cDNA cloning, and genealogy. *J Invest Dermatol* 99: 138–145

118  Goldstein SM, Leong J, Bunnett NW (1991) Human mast cell proteases hydrolyse neurotensin, kinetensin and Leu[5]-enkephalin. *Peptides* 12: 995–1000

119  Clark JM, Abraham WM, Fishman CE, Forteza R, Ahmed A, Cortes A, Warne RL,

Moore WR, Tanaka RD (1995) Tryptase inhibitors block allergen induced airway and inflammatory responses in allergic sheep. *Am J Respir Crit Care Med* 152: 2076–2083

120 Elrod KC, Moore WR, Abraham WM, Tanaka RD (1997) Lactoferrin, a potent tryptase inhibitor, abolishes late-phase airway responses in allergic sheep. *Am J Respir Crit Care Med* 156: 375–381

121 Krishna MT, Chauhan AJ, Little L, Sampson K, Mant TGK, Hawksworth R, Djukanovic R, Lee TH, Holgate ST (1998) Effect of inhaled APC-366 on allergen-induced bronchoconstriction and airway hyperresponsiveness to histamine in atopic asthmatics. *Am J Respir Crit Care Med* 157: A456

122 Holloway L, Beasley R, Roche W (1995) The pathology of fatal asthma. In: Busse WW, Holgate ST (eds): *Asthma and rhinitis*. Blackwell Scientific Publications, Boston 109–117

# Cytokine and adhesion molecule antagonists

*Paul S. Foster and Simon P. Hogan*

Division of Biochemistry and Molecular Biology, John Curtin School of Medical Research, Australian National University, ACTON ACT 0200

## Introduction

The proposed central role of specific leukocyte subsets in the pathophysiology of asthma has focused attention on the development of agents that will selectively inhibit the migration of these inflammatory cells into the lung. In asthma, airway CD4+ Th2 type lymphocytes, mast cells and eosinophils appear to be primarily effector cells that underlie the clinical manifestations of disease [1]. The cellular and molecular mechanisms involved in the regulation of the recruitment of these inflammatory cells from the blood to sites of inflammation are complex, however, cellular migration appears to be modulated by two fundamental processes; cell-adhesion systems located in the vascular endothelium and signals elicited through cytokine and chemokine (chemoattractant cytokines) receptors. Cell-adhesion and cytokine signalling systems form networks that are elegantly coordinated to promote cellular extravasation and localisation to the site of inflammation [2, 3]. At the initiation of inflammation, cytokines and chemokines play key roles in propagating the inflammatory response by eliciting signals that activate adhesion-systems, induce the secretion of other cytokines/chemokines from the vascular bed and promote chemotaxis. The type of cytokines produced in response to a particular inflammatory stimulus are intimately involved in directing the immune response by promoting the selective mobilization, attachment and recruitment of specific leukocyte sub-sets to the site of provocation [2–4].

In asthma the inflammatory response appears to be predominantly driven by the Th2 type cytokines, in particularly interleukin-(IL)-4 and IL-5 secreted from allergen-specific CD4+ T cells [1, 5]. Th2 cytokines may also be derived from activated mast cells and eosinophils. These cytokines, in association with specific adhesion molecules and other inflammatory molecules (chemokines, leukotrienes, prostaglandins, and platelet activating factor) provide the basis of the molecular network that regulates the trafficking of leukocytes to the asthmatic lung.

In this chapter we provide an overview of the molecular and cellular mechanisms that regulate the recruitment of leukocytes to sites of allergic inflammation. We also

Anti-Inflammatory Drugs in Asthma, edited by A.P. Sampson and M.K. Church
© 1999 Birkhäuser Verlag Basel/Switzerland

identify the cytokines and adhesion molecules that are currently thought to be the key molecular targets for the inhibition of leukocyte trafficking to the lung and describe their potential for future anti-inflammatory therapy of asthma. Mecha-nisms for the antagonism of cytokine and adhesion molecule function will also be discussed.

## Potential roles of cytokines and adhesion molecules in asthma

### Key cytokines involved in regulating allergic inflammation

The accumulation and/or activation of inflammatory cells during an asthmatic response may be initiated and partially sustained by cytokines released at sites of antigen provocation (such as the airway epithelium and from antigen presenting cells) and from T cells and mast cells after activation by specific antigens [1, 4]. B lymphocytes, basophils, monocytes and neutrophils may act in concert with T cells, mast cells and eosinophils in the lung to modulate the inflammatory responses. Cytokines in conjunction with chemokines are thought to play an integral role in orchestrating the molecular events that initially stimulate the inflammatory response and regulate leukocyte endothelium interactions, extravasation, chemotaxis and localization of inflammatory cells at the site of allergen provocation. Each of the events involved in the regulation of leukocyte migration provides an opportunity for therapeutic intervention and subsequent attention of the inflammatory response.

Characterisation of the immunopathogenesis of asthma suggests that Th2 type cytokines (IL-3, -4, -5, -10, -13) and granulocyte macrophage colony stimulating factor (GM-CSF) play central roles in the asthmatic response by regulating the pro-duction of IgE, the effector function of mast cells and eosinophils, and by promot-ing transendothelial cell migration [1, 4, 5]. In particular, IL-4 is thought to be a crit-ical factor for the regulation of T cell commitment to the $CD4^+$ Th2 phenotype and is known to regulate IgE production by B cells and mast cell function [6]. In addi-tion, IL-4 also has potential roles in regulating the inflammatory response to recall antigens and in the production of the eosinophil-specific chemoattractant, eotaxin [6, 7]. In conjunction with other Th2 type cytokines as well as IL-1$\beta$ and tumor necrosis factor, IL-4 may also regulate leukocyte trafficking in asthma by activating adhesion systems in the vascular endothelium [8, 9].

IL-5 has also been identified as a key mediator in the aetiology of asthma [1, 5, 10]. IL-5 not only regulates the growth, differentiation, and activation of eosinophils, but also provides an essential signal for the induction of eosinophilia during allergic inflammation [11–13]. Furthermore, in conjunction with chemokines (RANTES, monocyte chemoattractant protein-3 (CP-3), macrophage inflammatory protein-1$\alpha$ (MIP-1$\alpha$) and eotaxin) and lipid mediators (platelet-activating factor and leukotriene B$_4$), IL-5 may promote eosinophil chemotaxis [14–16]. Notably, of the cytokines/chemokines implicated in modulating eosinophilic inflammation, only IL-5 and eotaxin have been identified to selectively regulate eosinophil trafficking. Eotaxin is a newly identified member of the C-C branch of chemokines and is highly potent and extremely rapid in inducing pulmonary and intradermal eosinophil recruitment [7, 16] (recently, eotaxin-2 has been identified). Investigations in guinea pigs and mice suggest that eotaxin and IL-5 act cooperatively to promote the recruitment of eosinophils into tissues [7, 17, 18]. Evidence is also accumulating that eotaxin may play a role in the aetiology of eosinophil-associated allergic disease in humans.

## Adhesion molecules

Adhesion molecules are glycoproteins that play intimate roles in cell assembly, cell signalling and cell-cell communication [2, 3]. The adhesion molecules that are primarily involved in regulating the migration and interaction of leukocytes during inflammation are the selectins, integrins and the cell adhesion molecules (CAMs) of the immunoglobulin superfamily. It is specific members of these families of adhesion molecules that appear to constitute the adhesion systems utilized during inflammatory responses in asthma. In particular, leukocyte endothelial-cell interactions during allergic responses are regulated through the L-, P-, and E- type selectins, vascular- and intercellular-CAMs (VCAMs and ICAMs, respectively) and the integrins, lymphocytes function-associated antigen-1 ((LFA-1), the $\beta_2$-integrin, CD11a/CD18 adhesion complex), Mac-1 (the $\beta_2$ integrin, CD11b/CD18 adhesion complex) and very-late activation antigen 4 ((VLA-4), the $\beta_1$-integrin, $\alpha_4 \beta_1$) (Tab. 1).

## Molecular basis of leukocyte adhesion

The arrest and extravasation of circulating leukocytes at the vascular bed involves activation of adhesion molecules on the surfaces of both the endothelium and inflammatory cells. Leukocyte extravasation proceeds primarily through three steps that have been well characterised [2, 3, 19] (Fig. 1). The initial phase involves weak interactions between the endothelium and the migrating cell that are regulated through selectins (E-, P- or L-selectin) and their receptors (e.g. sialoglycoproteins), which promotes leukocyte tethering and rolling of the arrested cell on the endothelium. The second phase is coordinated by signals elicited by cytokines/chemokines produced in response to inflammation that up-regulate the expression of selectins, various CAMs and β-integrin adhesion complexes (e.g. VCAM-1/VLA-4, ICAM-1/LFA-1 or ICAM-1/Mac-1 interactions). The coordinated interaction between cytokines and adhesion systems promotes stable adherence of inflammatory cells to the vascular endothelium and allows for the final phase of migration, diapedesis.

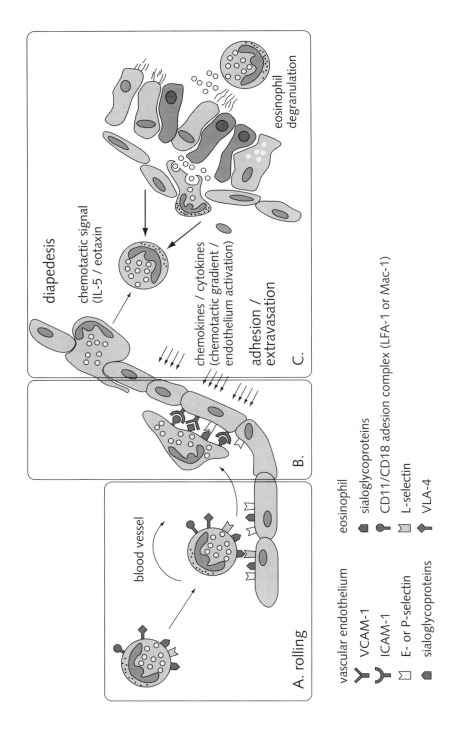

Notably, the events leading to extravasation are sequential and are mediated by distinct molecular interactions between specific adhesion-complexes that are characteristic of the immune response.

Thus, inhibition of these molecular interactions during any phase of leukocyte-endothelial cell interactions should inhibit the process of extravasation and potentially attenuate the inflammatory response within the tissue.

## Adhesion molecules and asthma

The increased expression of a number of adhesion complexes has been correlated with the clinical manifestations of asthma, which suggests a functional role for these molecules in the aetiology of disease (reviewed in [20]). Increased levels of ICAM-1 and E-selectin have been found in the blood of acute asthmatics and in the bronchial epithelium and pulmonary vascular bed of allergic and non allergic asthmatics [20–25]. The recruitment of granulocytes to the airways has also been correlated with increased levels of soluble -ICAM-1 and -E-selectin in the bronchial alveolar lavage fluid (BALF) of asthmatics after segmental antigen-challenge [26, 27]. In allergic asthmatics correlations have also been observed between elevated levels of IL-4 in BALF, eosinophil numbers in the airway wall, and increased VCAM-1 expression [28]. L-selectin has also been implicated in regulating eosinophil migration into the asthmatic lung after allergen-challenge [29].

Thus, the postulated role of leukocytes in the pathophysiology of asthma in association with evidence that suggests that cytokines and adhesion molecules are upregulated in this disease, suggests that therapeutics which target these inflammatory molecules may be effective in the relief of airways obstruction.

*Figure 1*

*Molecular regulation of eosinophil transmigration. (A) Eosinophils express L-selectin, which promotes transient interactions with the vascular endothelium through carbohydrate ligands (sialoglycoproteins). Eosinophils also express the CD11/CD18 adhesion complex and the integrin, very-late-activation-antigen 4 (VLA-4). (B) Initial activation of the endothelium occurs through interactions with chemokines and cytokines, which promote eosinophil-endothelium interactions by chemotaxis and activating adhesion pathways. Firm adhesion to the activated endothelium may be mediated by eosinophils binding to P-selectin and E-selectin, and interactions between intercellular adhesion molecule-1 (ICAM-1) and the CD11/CD18 adhesion complex. Vascular cell adhesion molecule 1 (VCAM-1) and the VLA-4 adherence pathway may promote the initial binding of activated eosinophils to the endothelium and preferentially promote eosinophil accumulation at sites of inflammation. (C) Transmigration of eosinophils across the vascular bed occurs after priming with cytokines and in response to chemotatic signals (adapted from [19]).*

*Table 1 - Key adhesion molecules involved in leukocyte trafficking in asthma*

| Adhesion molecule subtypes | | Cell localization | Ligand |
|---|---|---|---|
| *Immunoglobulin superfamily* | | | |
| VCAM-1 | | endothelial cells | VLA-4 |
| ICAM-1 | | endothelial cells | LFA-1 |
| | | leukocytes | hyaluronic acid |
| | | epithelium | Mac-1 |
| | | lymphocytes | LFA-1, Mac-1 |
| *Selectins* | | | |
| P-type | | endothelial cells | PSGL-1; SL-C |
| E-type | | endothelial cells | SL-C |
| L-type | | PMN leukocytes/lymphocytes | CD-34 |
| | | | SL-C |
| | | | GlyCAM-1 |
| | | | E-selection |
| | | | P-selection |
| *Integrins* | | | |
| $\beta_1$ | VLA-4 | lymphocytes, eosinophils monocytes, mast cells | VCAM-1, fibrinogen |
| $\beta_2$ | LFA-1 | lymphocytes, leukocytes | ICAM -1,-2,-3 |
| | Mac-1 | lymphocytes/various leukocytes | ICAM-1, fibrinogen, others |

*P-selectin glycoprotein ligand, (PSGL-1): sialyl lewis and other carbohydrate moieties, SL-C; integrin subsets, $\alpha_4\beta_1$ (VLA-4), CD11a/CD18 (LFA-1), CD11b/CD18 (Mac-1); polymorphonuclear leukocyte (PMN); other abbreviations see text. For detailed references see [2, 3, 20, 94].*

## Key cytokine targets for the inhibition of allergic airways inflammation

Glucocorticosteroids remain the current drugs of choice for the regulation of severe manifestations of asthma. These drugs may be effective, in part, because they suppress cytokine production (IL-4, IL-5 and others) by inflammatory cells and modify the participation of adhesion systems in the inflammatory response [30]. However, long-term glucocorticosteroid therapy is associated with harmful systemic effects and does not always relieve bronchial hyperreactivity. Clearly, new antagonists which target key molecules in the inflammatory cascade are required.

Clinical and experimental investigations have identified Th2-cells and -cytokines as key regulatory components of the inflammatory response associated with asthma and allergic disease. It is hoped that the delivery of specific cytokine antagonist to the airways early in an asthmatic's life will attenuate inflammatory infiltrates, the observed progressive morphological changes to the airway wall, and the development of enhanced bronchial reactivity. Specific Th2 cell suppressors may also provide a significant advance in the treatment of established disease. The immunomodulatory functions of IL-4 and IL-5 have identified these cytokines as key therapeutic targets for the relief of airways inflammation and obstruction in asthma. Furthermore, in animal models of asthma, both cytokines have been implicated in the development of airways hyperreactivity to spasmogens after antigen inhalation [13, 31–33]. Although animal models are only representative of the immunopathological process underlying asthma, they do provide important insights into the potential contribution of individual inflammatory cells and molecules to the pathogenesis of this disease which in turn allows identification of key targets for potential therapeutic intervention.

## Roles of IL-4, IL-5 and eotaxin

Currently, there are no specific antagonists of IL-4, IL-5 or eosinophil-specific-chemokines available for clinical practice. However, analysis of the literature suggests that the development of such agents will provide a significant advancement in the treatment of asthma. IL-5 plays a central role in eosinophil development and activation and has been strongly implicated in the aetiology of allergic and non-allergic asthma. In transgenic mice, the overexpression of IL-5 in the respiratory epithelium results in changes to the airways pathognomic of asthma and in enhanced bronchial reactivity [32]. Investigations in IL-5 deficient mice indicate that this cytokine is critical for regulating eosinophilia during allergic inflammation [13]. Moreover in a mouse model of asthma, IL-5 was found to be essential for the development of airways epithelial cell damage and bronchial hyperreactivity in response to inhaled allergen [13]. Recently, we have also shown that IL-5 secreted from allergen specific CD4[+] Th2 cells plays a pivotal role in the pathophysiology of allergic airways disease by regulating eosinophilia and bronchial hyperreactivity in response to allergen inhalation [34]. Notably, IL-5 deficiency does not affect the production of other cytokines or antibodies, nor significantly impair T and B cell function, suggesting that antagonism of this molecule would not significantly impair other immunological responses [35].

Interestingly, evidence is accumulating that IL-5 production can be regulated by CD4[+] T cells in the absence of IL-4. This particular sub-population of CD4[+] T cells develops into the Th2 phenotype (producing IL-4 and IL-5) independently of IL-4 and can provide enough IL-5 during allergic inflammation of the lung to induce eosinophilia, bronchial hyperreactivity and morphological changes to the airways [33, 36]. Thus, two CD4+ T cell pathways exist for the immune system to regulate IL-5 production and eosinophilia in response to inhaled allergens; one dependent on IL-4 and the other independent of this factor. The central role of IL-5 in both T cell components of allergic disease further highlights the requirements for highly specific therapeutic agents that inhibit production and/or action of this cytokine.

In conjunction with IL-5, inhibition of the function of eotaxin may markedly suppress the movement of eosinophils into tissues. Eotaxin and IL-5 may act in synergism to regulate the homing of eosinophils to sites of allergic inflammation. IL-5 mobilizes eosinophils from the bone marrow and also promotes homing to the infected organ, while eotaxin elicits signals for cell polarization and chemotaxis within the inflamed tissue [18]. It appears that "cross talk" occurs between IL-5 and eotaxin signalling systems to uniquely and selectively promote eosinophil chemotaxis/locomotion and potentially degranulation. Investigations using inhibitory mAbs in guinea pigs indicated that this chemokine may play a major role in the movement of eosinophils from the blood to the allergic lung [37]. In contrast, eosinophilia was not significantly altered in eotaxin deficient mice during the late-phase of allergic airways inflammation [38]. Recently, the eotaxin receptor has also been identified on memory Th2 cells, suggesting that eotaxin may also play a role in the recruitment of this T cell to sites of allergic inflammation [39]. The biological functions of eotaxin suggest that this molecule, in conjunction with IL-5, will provide an important new therapeutic target for the attenuation of the progression of allergic disease.

Blocking the actions of IL-4 may also provide an effective mechanism to attenuate inflammation of the airways in asthmatics. Inhibition or deletion of IL-4 during allergic airways inflammation attenuates eosinophilia, IgE production and bronchial hyperreactivity [31, 40], while overexpression of this cytokine in the lung of transgenic mice results in morphological changes to the respiratory epithelium [41]. Recently, IL-4 was also shown to play a crucial role for the homing of Th2 cells to the allergic lung [42].

Although blocking the actions of IL-4 may provide an effective mechanism for the relief of airways obstruction in asthma, evidence from animal models of Th2 dependent allergic airways inflammation indicate that targeting this cytokine alone may not be an effective therapeutic strategy. Notably, enhanced reactivity to cholinergic stimuli and eosinophilia are still features of inflammatory responses (albeit significantly reduced) in mice treated with anti-IL-4 mAbs or deficient in this factor [31, 33]. Furthermore, unlike IL-5 transgenic mice [32], over expression of IL-4 in the airway wall does not result in the induction of airways hyperreactivity, although morphological changes in the respiratory epithelium are observed [41]. Anti-IL-4 mAbs also are only effective in attenuating aeroallergen-induced airways hyperreactivity if administered during the primary sensitisation phase, but not during the period of direct provocation of the airways with allergen [31], suggesting that antagonists of the actions of IL-4 during an established asthmatic response may not attenuate bronchial hyperreactivity. Eosinophilia and bronchial hyperreactivity are also induced after allergen-inhalation in sensitised mast cell-, IgE- and CD40- (no production of IgE, IgG or IgA) deficient mice, components of the inflammatory response whose functions are intimately regulated by IL-4 [33, 40, 43, 44].

A number of other interleukins may also play important roles in regulating airways occlusion in asthma [4]. IL-13 has similar biological activities to IL-4 in the downregulation of proinflammatory cytokines and chemokine production, in the induction and expression of integrins and in the regulation of IgE synthesis [45, 46]. Thus, targeting both of these cytokines concurrently may be required to attenuate the asthmatic response. IL-1β, IL-11 and TNFα have also been implicated in various mechanisms associated with leukocyte activation and trafficking in allergic inflammation [4]. However, the role of these cytokines in a broad range of immune responses suggests that these molecules would not be suitable targets for therapeutic modulation of asthma. In contrast, the Th2 cytokine IL-10 down regulates processes associated with allergic disease, such as IL-5 and IgE synthesis. Notably, IL-10 has been shown to suppress the recruitment of leukocytes into the lung during the early-phase of allergic airways inflammation in mice [47].

Although clinical and experimental investigations indicate that IL-4 and IL-5 are primary targets for the attenuation of asthma, studies in mice also suggest that directly targeting T cell activation may be required to alleviate bronchial hyperreactivity associated with allergic inflammation of the airways [18, 48–50]. Recently, we have described a novel CD4+ T cell pathway in BALB/c mice that modulates allergen-induced airways hyperreactivity independently of the collective actions of IL-4 and IL-5 [48]. Data indicates that CD4+ T cells operate at least two pathways that can act independently to induce airways hyperreactivity. The co-existence of parallel pathways may account for the dissociation of airways eosinophilia from the development of airways hyperreactivity in some cases of asthma and in animal models of this disease [48]. Notably, the transfer of enriched naïve T cell populations from a strain of mice that displayed inherent airways hyperreactivity to methacholine to a hyporeactive strain conferred enhanced airways reactivity to this spasmogen in the absence of antigen challenge [50]. Airways hyperreactivity was directly associated with CD4+ T cells and occurred in the absence of eosinophilia and pronounced inflammation and morphological changes to the airways. Although the mechanism of T cell activation in the absence of antigen was obscure these investigations support our conclusion that factors secreted from CD4+ T cells play fundamental roles in determining the level of airways reactivity to cholinergic stimuli. Thus, while a number of molecules contribute to the mechanisms underlying the regulation of bronchial hyperreactivity in mice, only CD4+ T cells have been shown to exclusively regulate disease pathogenesis [48, 49].

# Key adhesion molecule targets for the inhibition of leukocyte-endothelium transmigration during allergic airways inflammation

The roles of various adhesion-molecules in the trafficking of leukocytes into the lung have been investigated in various animal models of asthma. Collectively, these investigations suggest that adhesion molecules play a pivotal role in controlling T cell and eosinophil trafficking into the allergic lung and in the subsequent induction of bronchial hyperreactivity in response to allergen inhalation, thus indicating the potential therapeutic value of targeting adherence pathways at the vascular endothelium for the treatment of asthma.

The potential importance of VCAM-1, ICAM-1, VLA-4, and LFA-1 on antigen-induced leukocyte recruitment to the trachea in a mouse model of allergic airways disease has been demonstrated by using inhibitory mAbs [51]. Inhibition of the VCAM-1/VLA-1 pathway, but not of ICAM-1 or of LFA-1, suppressed eosinophilia. In this model, antigen challenge induced the expression of VCAM-1, but not of ICAM-1 on the vascular endothelium. Notably, VCAM-1 expression was suppressed (27%) by anti-IL-4 mAb treatment, without significantly affecting eosinophil accumulation into the trachea. Thus, factors other than IL-4 are important in promoting VCAM-1-regulated airways eosinophilia [51]. In contrast to eosinophil transmigration, all of the adhesion molecule mAbs reduced CD4$^+$ and CD8$^+$ T cell infiltration into the trachea, indicating the importance of both LFA-1/ICAM-1 and VLA-4/VCAM-1 adhesion pathways for lymphocyte extravasation during allergic airways inflammation [51].

In similar studies, CD18 and VLA-4 were shown to play key roles in eosinophil extravasation in the lung and blockade of these integrins also suppressed the influx of mononuclear cells and neutrophils [52, 53].

A number of studies have attempted to correlate the effects of inhibiting adhesion molecules during allergic inflammation not only with the selective reduction in the trafficking of leukocyte subsets, but also with in the level of bronchial reactivity to spasmogens. In primate, rat and guinea pig models of asthma, administration of anti-ICAM-1 or anti-VLA-4 mAbs attenuated the development of inflammation and bronchial hyperreactivity [53–55]. Inhibition of integrin signalling through Mac-1 or LFA-1 also attenuated enhanced airways reactivity in models of allergic asthma [56–59].

The mechanisms whereby adhesion molecules regulate airways hyperreactivity are not clear. Observations in a sheep model of asthma suggest a key role for $\alpha_4$ integrins in the development of allergen-induced late-phase airways dysfunction independently of leukocyte recruitment [57, 60]. Systemic and airway administration of anti-$\alpha_4$ mAb (MP1/2) did not alter the composition of leukocyte subsets recovered in BALF, while significantly reducing an increase in late-phase lung resistance and bronchial hyperreactivity [60]. Inhibition of ICAM-1 signalling or of integrin function (with mAbs against VLA-4, both LFA-1 and Mac-1 or with mAbs which recognise different epitopes on the CD18 molecule) have also shown that adhesion molecules can regulate bronchial hyperreactivity in the presence of inflammatory cell influx into the airways [55–59]. Thus, adhesion systems may not only play an important role in inflammatory cell extravasation but also in their state of activation and ability to communicate directly with other inflammatory cells and pathways. This concept is supported by recent investigations which show that integrins control cell adhesion to extracellular ligands and also transduce biochemical signals both into and out of cells [61].

Mice carrying a targeted disruption of a gene encoding a particular adhesion molecule have been employed to investigate the role of the factors in leukocyte trafficking to sites of inflammation. Lymphocytes from L-selectin deficient mice do not bind to high endothelial venules of peripheral lymph nodes and total numbers of lymphocytes are decreased at these sites [62]. A central role for L-selectin in leukocyte homing to non-lymphoid tissues during contact and delayed-type hypersensitivity responses was also observed [63]. Leukocyte rolling was also significantly impaired in P- and L- selectin deficient mice [62, 64]. In P-selectin-deficient mice the accumulation of CD4+ T lymphocytes, monocytes and neutrophils, and the degranulation of mast cells were significantly reduced during contact hypersensitivity reactions [65]. Recently, endothelial selectins were also shown to be critical for $\alpha_4$-integrin dependent leukocyte rolling in chronically inflamed venules in mice deficient in P- and E- selectin [68]. P-selectin deficiency has also been associated with the attenuation of leukocyte recruitment to the lung and of airways hyperreactivity in a mouse model of asthma [66]. In ICAM-1-deficient mice, IL-5 and eosinophil peroxidase levels were significantly lower in BALF in comparison to wild type after sensitisation and exposure to aeroallergen [67]. Furthermore, aeroallergen-induced airways hyperreactivity was significantly attenuated in the absence of ICAM-1. Thus, ICAM-1 was considered to be an important molecule for regulating eosinophilia and enhanced bronchial reactivity during allergic responses of the airways [67]. Recent investigations suggest that adhesion mechanisms may also be able to distinguish between Th1 and Th2 subsets and mediate differential trafficking of these T cells [69]. Collectively, these investigations indicate that targeting specific adhesion-molecule complexes may be an efficient means of controlling leukocyte infiltration during late-phase asthmatic responses.

## Cellular and molecular approaches to antagonise adhesion pathways and cytokine signalling

Th2 type cytokines and adhesion systems activated by these factors have become a major focus of research directed at developing novel anti-inflammatory agents for the treatment of asthma. Several cellular and molecular approaches are currently being pioneered with the view to providing new insights and principles for the development of highly specific therapeutics. Experimental strategies currently are aimed at inhibiting cytokine, chemokine or adhesion molecule signalling processes by targeting molecular interactions between ligands and their receptors or by modifying specific components of signal transduction pathways or of mechanisms of transcription.

The molecular components (transcription factors and promoter elements) regulating cytokine-induced expression of specific adhesion molecules in endothelial cells and of cytokine expression by Th2 cells are being increasingly characterized. In particular, the transcription factor NF-κB plays a critical role in immune and inflammatory responses. NF-κB is regulated by the cytokine-responsive I-κB complex (IKK α and β subunits) and a catalytically inactive form of IKK-β has been shown to block cytokine-induced NF-κB activation [70]. Nitric oxide, by inhibiting the action of NF-κB has also be shown to suppress cytokine induced expression of adhesion molecules and cytokine production within endothelial cells. The signal transducers and activators of transcription (STATS) provide another target for the inhibition of cytokine gene expression [71]. In particular, IL-4 signals through STAT-6 to regulate T helper development, IgE production, expression of CD23, and presentation of MHC class II antigen on B cells [71, 72]. Importantly, IL-13 also activates the STAT-6 pathway [73]. Thus, the inhibition of STAT-6 signal transduction and/or other transcription factors involved in cytokine and adhesion molecule signalling may provide a mechanism for attenuating allergic inflammation in asthma.

Cytokine or adhesion molecule function may also be antagonised by targeting specific components of their signal transduction pathways. The intracellular domains of integrins communicate with several structural and signal transduction proteins to regulate a wide variety of cellular functions associated with leukocyte activation and recruitment [61]. Recently, the Rho subfamily of small guanosine triphosphate (GTP)-binding proteins was identified as a potential pharmacological target for the uncoupling of G-protein-linked chemoattractant receptors from integrin-mediated adhesion of leukocytes [74]. Inactivation of Rho by C3 transferase exoenzyme blocked chemokine induced lymphocyte $\alpha_4\beta_1$ adhesion to VCAM-1 [74]. Calreticulin has also been shown to be an essential modulator of both integrin adhesion functions and intercellular signalling [75]. Thus, disruption of calreticulin-integrin interactions may not only inhibit cell adhesion but also activation of other mechanisms associated with the inflammatory stimulus, perhaps providing a mechanism to attenuate bronchial hyperreactivity. However, the redundancy in the actions of cytokines and chemokines and the pleotropic actions of many of the transcription factors and intracellular transducing elements involved in both cytokine and adhesion molecule signalling suggests that modulation of specific components of the inflammatory response by targeting intracellular compartments will be very difficult and such approaches currently are far removed from clinical applications.

Animal studies with monoclonal antibodies (see above) suggest that targeting specific inflammatory molecules with humanised antibodies may provide an effective therapeutic approach to the treatment of asthma. The recent success at blocking chemokine receptors with low molecular weight compounds also indicates that the use of small molecules, peptide antagonists and perhaps non-signalling receptor binding analogues of specific cytokines/chemokines and adhesion molecules may also provide a more direct modality to attenuate inflammatory responses. Heterocyclic bicyclams, an 18 residue peptide and a highly cationic oligopeptide containing nine arginines were found to inhibit HIV entry of cells by interacting with the CXCR-4 (receptor 4 for CXC chemokines) (see [76] for review). The repeated delivery of truncated analogues of chemokines (MCP-1) has also been shown *in vivo* to inhibit chronic inflammatory arthritis that develops spontaneously in MRL-lpr mice [77]. Collectively, these investigations identify the potential for chemokine/cytokine receptor antagonists as anti-inflammatories (76).

Structural analysis of inflammatory molecules and their receptors is also allowing for the identification of specific motifs that can be targeted with small molecules/peptides to inhibit downstream activation of signal transduction pathways. For example, antagonists of the QIDSPL motif within domain one of VCAM indicate that this site is critical for VLA-4 binding [78, 79]. The EILDVPST sequence within the connecting segment-1 (CS-1) region of fibronectin is also recognised by VLA-4 [80]. Recently, the cyclic hexapeptide CWLDVS (TBC 772) has been shown to be a potent antagonist of $\alpha_4$ integrin function; inhibiting lymphocyte interactions with fibronectin, VCAM-1 and mucosal vascular adhesion-CAM-1 (MAdCAM-1) [81, 82]. This peptide is not toxic to T cells *in vitro* and is integrin selective in its suppressive activity as co-stimulation through other molecules in the presence of TBC 772 was not impaired [81]. Notably, the antagonist peptide inhibited integrin function by a mechanism independent of competitive binding [81]. Recently, a CS-1 ligand mimic was also shown to inhibit VLA-4 mediated mast cell binding to fibronectin and attenuate degranulation [83]. These *in vitro* investigations with peptide antagonists have been extended in a sheep asthma model [84]. Aerosol administration of the CS-1 ligand mimic (phenylacetyl-L-leucyl-L-aspartyl-L-phenylalanyl-D-prolineamide) before aeroallergen-challenge significantly attenuated (40%) the early-phase and almost ablated the late-phase airways response (88%). Moreover, the VLA-4 antagonist inhibited the development of airways hyperreactivity to cholinergic stimuli. Inhibition of antigen-induced changes in airways function were directly correlated with a reduction of VLA-4 positive leukocytes (eosinophils, lymphocytes and metachromatic-staining cells) in airway biopsies taken 24 h after the challenge [84]. These investigations also provide evidence that small molecules which target specific inflammatory molecule interactions can be delivered directly to the airways to potentially inhibit asthmatic like responses. These results also support investigations with anti-$\alpha_4$-integrin mAbs and studies with other small molecule VLA-4 antagonists and suggest that inhibition of CS-1 as well as VCAM-1 binding may be important for suppression of allergic airways inflammation [85]. The potential of intravenous or perhaps subcutaneous administration of specific carbohydrate antagonists as therapeutics for blocking leukocyte trafficking in asthma has also been demonstrated. Intravenous administration of fucoidin, a selectin-binding carbohydrate (blocking of selectin-carbohydrate interactions), markedly inhibited (> 98%) leukocyte rolling flux [68].

Recently, a mutant of human IL-5, E12K was shown *in vitro* to act as a potent and specific antagonist of IL-5 dependent cell proliferation and eosinophil adhesion, and of the events inducing downstream tyrosine phosphorylation [86]. Although this mutant did not inhibit all of the actions mediated by IL-5, it demonstrated the potential for inhibiting IL-5 function with engineered structural analogues. The recent demonstration that insertion mutants of IL-5 can be expressed as monomers with biological activity similar to that of native IL-5 provides a platform for the development of non-signalling receptor binding antagonists of this cytokine [87].

## Th2 cell and cytokine suppression by opposing cytokines

The molecular complexity, high receptor affinity, pleotrophic actions, and redundancy of cytokines has to date made it difficult to design pharmacological antagonists that will specifically modify the actions of an individual cytokine and/or attenuate inflammatory responses. Furthermore, once the inflammatory cascade is initiated mechanisms may operate in parallel and independently to regulate leukocyte trafficking and the induction of bronchial hyperreactivity in asthma, suggesting that strategies targeting one factor may not be sufficient to relieve airways obstruction.

Alternatively, over all suppression of a specific inflammatory response may be achieved by molecules that are normally involved in the downregulation of the particular immune response *in vivo*. The ability of cytokines to cross-regulate immune responses driven by T cells suggests a possible role for cytokine-directed therapy of the inflammatory response underlying asthma. In particular, the cytokines IFNγ IFNα and IL-12 have been shown to potentially suppress immunological responses driven by Th2 cells [88–93]. These cytokines may act by inhibiting the proliferation of Th2-cells, by suppressing IgE and IL-4 production and by downregulating adhesion pathways. IFNα and IL-12 may exert their inhibitory effects by enhancing the production of IFNγ and also independently of this cytokine. IFNα inhibits antigen-induced eosinophil and CD4+ T cell recruitment into airway tissue [93]. Furthermore, both IL-12 and IFNγ are potent inhibitors of antigen-induced airways hyperreactivity and Th2 driven inflammation [90–92]. Recently, we have demonstrated the potential of cytokine directed gene therapy for the suppression of airway inflammatory responses in asthma. The delivery of viral constructs encoding IL-12 to the lung before the onset and during an established allergic response, selectively inhibited airways eosinophilia and hyperreactivity to cholinergic stimuli [93]. This effect was accompanied by a shift to Th1 type cytokine expression in lung T cells. The protective effects of IL-12 were almost completely abolished when experiments were performed in mice with disruption of the gene encoding the IFNγ receptor. Interestingly, this strategy may promote the clearance of respiratory tract viral infections (by stimulating the proliferation of IFNγ producing CD8[+] T cells) which are thought to play key roles in inducing and exacerbating asthmatic responses.

## Summary

The proposed central role of airways inflammation in the induction and maintenance of the asthmatic responses has identified molecules that specifically regulate the migration and activation leukocytes as key therapeutic targets for the relief of airways obstruction. In asthma, leukocyte trafficking to the lung appears to be predominantly regulated by Th2 cytokines (in particularly IL-4 and IL-5) secreted from allergen-specific CD4[+] T cells in association with specific adhesion molecules (VCAM-1, ICAM-1, VLA-4, LFA-1, Mac-1 and P-, E- and L-selectin). Clinical and experimental investigations suggest that the delivery of specific antagonists of these molecules to the airways may provide a significant advance in the treatment of asthma. Currently, a range of cellular and molecular approaches are being employed with the view to identifying novel anti inflammatory targets and agents. The complexity of the inflammatory response in asthma suggests that Th2 cell suppressers may be more efficient at attenuating the inflammatory response than targeting individual inflammatory molecules.

The immunoregulatory effects of IFNγ, IFNα and IL-12 suggest that these molecules have the potential to inhibit the activation of CD4[+] Th2 cells and mast cells and suppress airways eosinophilia in asthma. The delivery of inhibitory cytokines or antagonists of cytokine and adhesion molecule signalling networks directly to the airways may provide a rapid, potent and convenient method for the treatment of developing and ongoing asthmatic responses.

*Acknowledgement*
We would like to thank Hans Matthaei for criticial reading of the manuscript.

## References

1    Bochner B, Undem B, Lichtenstein L (1994) Immunological aspects of allergic asthma. *Annu Rev Immunol* 12: 295–335
2    Springer T (1990) Adhesion receptors of the immune system. *Nature* 346: 425–434
3    Carlos T, Harlan J (1994) Leukocyte-endothelial adhesion molecules. *Blood* 84: 2068–2101

4    Hogan S, Foster P (1997) Cytokines as targets for the inhibition of eosinophilic inflammation. *Pharmacol Ther* 74: 259–283

5    Robinson D, Hamid Q, Ying S, Tsicopoulos A, Barkans J, Bentley A, Corrigan C, Durham S, Kay A (1992) Predominant TH2-like bronchoalveolar T-lymphocyte population in atopic asthma. *New Eng Med J Med* 326: 298–304

6    Finkelman F, Katona I, Urban J, Holmes J, Ohara J, Tung A, Sample J, Paul W (1988) IL-4 is required to generate and sustain *in vivo* IgE responses. *J Immunol* 141: 2335–2341

7    Rothenberg M, Luster A, Leder P (1995) Murine eotaxin: an eosinophil chemoattractant inducible in endothelial cells and in interleukin 4-induced tumor suppression. *Proc Natl Acad Sci USA* 92: 8960–8964

8    Pober J, Gimbrone M Jr, Lapierre L, Mendrick D, Fiers W, Rothlein R, Springer T (1986) Overlapping patterns of activation of human endothelial cells by interleukin-1, tumor necrosis factor, and gamma interferon. *J Immunol* 137: 1893–1896

9    Walsh G, Hartnell A, Wardlaw A, Kurihara K, Sanderson C, Kay A (1990) IL-5 enhances the *in vitro* adhesion of human eosinophils, but not neutrophils, in a leucocyte integrin (CD11/18)-dependent manner. *Immunology* 71: 258–265

10   Hamid Q, Azzawi M, Ying S, Moqbel R, Wardlaw A, Corrigan C, Bradley B, Durham S, Collins J, Jeffery P et al (1991) Interleukin-5 in the pathogenesis of asthma. *J Clin Invest* 87: 1541–1546

11   Yamaguchi Y, Hayashi Y, Sugama Y, Miura Y, Kasahara T, Kitamura S, Torisu M, Mita S, Tominaga A, Takatsu K (1988) Highly purified murine interleukin 5 (IL-5) stimulates eosinophil function and prolongs *in vitro* survival. IL-5 as an eosinophil chemotactic factor. *J Exp Med* 167: 1737–1742

12   Wang J, Rambaldi A, Biondi A, Chen Z, Sanderson C, Mantovani A (1989) Recombinant human interleukin-5 is a selective eosinophil chemoattractant. *Eur J Immunol* 19: 701–705

13   Foster P, Hogan S, Ramsay A, Matthaei K, Young I (1996) Interleukin 5 deficiency abolishes eosinophilia, airways hyperreactivity, and lung damage in a mouse asthma model. *J Exp Med* 183: 195–201

14   Dahinden C, Geiser T, Brunner T, von Tscharner V, Caput D, Ferrara P, Minty A, Baggiolini M (1994) Monocyte chemotactic protein 3 is a most effective basophil- and eosinophil-activating chemokine. *J Exp Med* 179: 751–756

15   Rot A, Krieger M, Brunner T, Bischoff S, Schall T, Dahinden C (1992) RANTES and macrophage inflammatory protein-1 alpha induce the migration and activation of normal human eosinophil granulocytes. *J Exp Med* 176: 1489–1495

16   Jose P, Griffiths Johnson D, Collins P, Walsh D, Moqbel R, Totty N, Truong O, Hsuan J, Williams T (1994) Eotaxin: a potent eosinophil chemoattractant cytokine detected in a guinea pig model of allergic airways inflammation. *J Exp Med* 179: 881–887

17   Collins P, Marleau S, Griffiths-Johnson D, Jose P, Williams T (1995) Cooperation between interleukin-5 and the chemokine eotaxin to induce eosinophil accumulation *in vivo*. *J Exp Med* 182: 1169–1174

18 Mould A, Matthaei K, Young I, Foster P (1997) Relationship between interleukin-5 and eotaxin in regulating blood and tissue eosinophilia in mice. *J Clin Invest* 99: 1064–1071

19 Hogan S, Foster P (1996) Cellular and molecular mechanisms involved in the regulation of eosinophil trafficking *in vivo. Med Res Reviews* 16: 407–432

20 Bloemen P, Henricks P, Nijkamp F (1997) Cell adhesion molecules and asthma. *Clin Exper Allergy* 21: 128–141

21 Montefort S, Lai C, Kapahi P, Leung J, Lai K, Chan H, Haskard D, Howarth P, Holgate S (1994) Circulating adhesion molecules in asthma. *Am J Respir Crit Care Med* 149: 1149–1152

22 Gosset P, Tillie-Leblond I, Janin A, Marquette C, Copin M, Wallaert B, Tonnel A (1995) Expression of E-selectin, ICAM-1 and VCAM-1 on bronchial biopsies from allergic and non-allergic asthmatic patients. *Int Arch Allergy Immunol* 106: 69–77

23 Pilewski J, Albelda S (1995) Cell adhesion molecules in asthma: homing, activation, and airway remodeling. *Am J Respir Cell Mol Biol* 12: 1–3

24 Bentley A, Durham S, Robinson D, Menz G, Storz C, Cromwell O, Kay A, Wardlaw A (1993) Expression of endothelial and leukocyte adhesion molecules intercellular adhesion molecule-1, E-selectin, and vascular cell adhesion molecule-1 in the bronchial mucosa in steady-state and allergen-induced asthma. *J Allergy Clin Immunol* 92: 857–868

25 Montefort S, Gratziou C, Goulding D, Polosa R (1994) Bronchial biopsy evidence for leukocyte infiltration and upregulation of leukocyte-endothelial cell adhesion molecules 6 hours after local allergen challenge of sensitized asthmatic airways. *J Clin Invest* 93: 1411–1421

26 Takahashi N, Liu M, Proud D, Yu X, Hasegawa S, Spannhake E (1994) Soluble intracellular adhesion molecule 1 in bronchoalveolar lavage fluid of allergic subjects following segmental antigen challenge. *Am J Respir Crit Care Med* 150: 704–709

27 Georas S, Liu M, Newman W, Beall L, Stealey B, Bochner B (1992) Altered adhesion molecule expression and endothelial cell activation accompany the recruitment of human granulocytes to the lung after segmental antigen challenge. *Am J Respir Cell Mol Biol* 7: 261–269

28 Fukuda T, Kukushima Y, Maruyama N et al (1995) Role of interleukin-4 and vascular cell adhesion molecule-1 in selective eosinophil migration into the airways in allergic asthma. *Am J Respir Cell Mol Biol* 14: 84–94

29 Mengelers H, Maikoe T, Hooibrink B, Kuypers T, Kreukniet J, Lammers J, Koenderman L (1993) Down modulation of L-Selectin expression on eosinophils recovered from bronchoalveolar lavage fluid after allergen provocation. *Clin Exp Allergy* 23: 196–204

30 Robinson D, Hamid Q, Ying S, Bentley A, Assoufi B, Durham S, Kay A (1993) Prednisolone treatment in asthma is associated with modulation of bronchoalveolar lavage cell interleukin-4, interleukin-5, and interferon-gamma cytokine gene expression. *Am Rev Respir Dis* 148 (2): 401–406

31 Corry D, Folkesson H, Warnock M, Erle D, Matthay M, Wiener-Kronish J, Locksley R

(1996) Interleukin 4, but not interleukin 5 or eosinophils, is required in a murine model of acute airway hyperreactivity [see comments]. *J Exp Med* 183: 109–117

32    Lee J, McGarry M, Farmer S, Denzler K, Larson K, Carrigan P, Brenneise I, Horton M, Hackzu A, Gelfand E et al (1997) Interleukin-5 expression in the lung epithelium of transgenic mice leads to pulmonary changes pathognomic of asthma. *J Exp Med* 185: 2143–2156

33    Hogan S, Mould A, Kikutani H, Ramsay A, Foster P (1997) Aeroallergen-induced eosinophilic inflammation, lung damage, and airways hyperreactivity in mice can occur independently of IL-4 and allergen-specific immunoglobulins. *J Clin Invest* 99: 1329–1339

34    Hogan S, Koskinen A, Matthaei K, Young I, Foster P (1998) Interleukin-5 producing CD4+ T cells play a pivotal role in aerollergen-induced eosinophilia, bronchial hyperreactivity, and lung damage in mice. *Am J Respir Crit Care Med* 157: 210–218

35    Kopf M, Brombacher F, Hodgkin P, Ramsay A, Milbourne E, Dai W, Ovington K, Behm C, Kohler G, Young I et al (1996) IL-5-deficient mice have a developmental defect in CD5+ B-1 cells and lack eosinophilia but have normal antibody and cytotoxic T cell responses. *Immunity* 4: 15–24

36    Noben-Trauth N, Shultz L, Brombacher F, Urban Jr. J, Gu H, Paul W (1997) An interleukin 4 (IL-4)-independent pathway for CD4+ T cell IL-4 production is revealed in IL-4 receptor-deficient mice. *Proc Natl Acad Sci* 94: 10838–10843

37    Humbles A, Conroy D, Marleau S, Rankin S, Palframan R, Proudfoot A, Wells T, Li D, Jeffery P, Griffiths-Johnson D et al (1997) Kinetics of eotaxin generation and its relationship to eosinophil accumulation in allergic airways disease: analysis in a guinea pig model *in vivo*. *J Exp Med* 186: 601–612

38    Rothenberg M, MacLean J, Pearlman E, Luster A, Leder P (1997) Targeted disruption of the chemokine eotaxin partially reduces antigen-induced tissue eosinophilia. *J Exp Med* 185: 785–790

39    Sallusto F, Mackay C, Lanzavecchia A (1997) Selective expression of the eotaxin receptor CCR3 by human T helper 2 cells. *Science* 277: 2005–2007

40    Brusselle G, Kips J, Joos G, Bluethmann H, Pauwells P (1995) Allergen-induced airway inflammation and bronchial responsiveness in wild-type and interleukin-4-deficient mice. *Am J Respir Cell Mol Biol* 12: 254–259

41    Rankin J, Picarella D, Geba G, Temann U, Prasad B, Dicosmo B, Tarallo A, Stripp E, Whitsett J, Flavell R (1996) Phenotypic and physiologic characterisation of transgenic mice expressing interleukin 4 in the lung: Lymphocytic and eosinophilic inflammation with airway hyperreactivity. *Proc Natl Acad Sci USA* 93: 7821–7825

42    Cohn L, Homer R, Marinov A, Rankin J, Bottomly K (1997) Induction of airways mucus production by T helper 2 (Th2) cells: A critical role for interleukin 4 in cell recruitment but not mucus production. *J Exp Med* 186: 1737–1747

43    Mehlhop P, van de Rijn M, Goldberg A, Brewer J, Kurup V, Martin T, Oettgen H (1997) Allergen-induced bronchial hyperreactivity and eosinophilic inflammation occur in the absence of IgE in a mouse model of asthma. *Proc Natl Acad Sci* 94: 1344–1349

44  Takeda K, Hamelmann E, Joetham A, Shultz L, Larsen G, Irvin C, Gelfand E (1997) Development of eosinophilic airway inflammation and airway responsiveness in mast cell deficient mice. *J Exp Med* 186: 449–454

45  Zurawski G, de Vries J (1994) Interleukin 13, an interleukin 4-like cytokine that acts on monocytes and B cells, but not on T cells. *Immunol Today* 15: 19–26

46  Punnonen J, Aversa G, Cocks B, McKenzie A, Menon S, Zurawski G, de Waal-Malefyt R, de Vries J (1993) Interleukin 13 induces interleukin 4-independent IgG4 and IgE synthesis and CD23 expression by human B cells. *Proc Natl Acad Sci USA* 90: 3730–3734

47  Zuany-Amorim C, Haile S, Leduc D, Dumarey C, Huerre M, Vargaftig B, Pretolani M (1995) Interleukin-10 inhibits antigen-induced cellular recruitment into the airways of sensitized mice. *J Clin Invest* 95: 2644–2651

48  Hogan S, Matthaei K, Young J, Koskinen A, Young I, Foster P (1998) A novel T-cell regulated mechanism modulating allergen-induced airways hyperreactivity in BALB/c mice independently of interleukin -4 and -5. *J Immunol* 161: 1501–1509

49  Gavett S, Chen X, Finkelman F, Wills-Karp M (1994) Depletion of murine CD4+ T lymphocytes prevents antigen-induced airway hyperreactivity and pulmonary eosinophilia. *Am J Respir Cell Mol Biol* 10: 587–593

50  De Sanctis G, Itoh A, Green F, Qin S, Kimura T, Grobholz J, Martin T, Maki T, Drazen J (1997) T-lymphocytes regulate genetically determined airway hyperresponsiveness in mice. *Nat Med* 3: 460–462

51  Nakajima H, Samo H, Nishimura T, Yoshida S, Iwamoto I (1994) Role of vascular cell adhesion molecule 1/very late activation antigen 4 and intercellular adhesion molecule in antigen-induced eosinophil and T cell recruitment into the tissue. *J Exp Med* 179: 1145–1154

52  Weg V, Williams T, Lobb R, Nourshargh S (1993) A monoclonal antibody recognizing very late activation antigen-4 inhibits eosinophil accumulation *in vivo*. *J Exp Med* 177: 561–566

53  Pretolani M, Ruffie C, Lapa e Silva J, Joseph D, Lobb R, Vargaftig B (1994) Antibody to very late activation antigen 4 prevents antigen-induced bronchial hyperreactivity and cellular infiltration in the guinea pig airways. *J Exp Med* 180: 795–805

54  Wegner C, Gundel R, Reilly P, Haynes N, Letts L, Rothlein R (1990) Intercellular adhesion molecule-1 (ICAM-1) in the pathogenesis of asthma. *Science* 247: 456–459

55  Sun J, Elwood W, Haczku A, Barnes P, Hellewell P, Chung K (1994) Contribution of intercellular-adhesion molecule-1 in allergen-induced airway hyperresponsiveness and inflammation in sensitised brown-Norway rats. *Int Arch Allergy Immunol* 104: 291–295

56  Rabb H, Olivenstein R, Issekutz T, Renzi P, Martin J (1994) The role of the leukocyte adhesion molecules VLA-4, LFA-1, and Mac-1 in allergic airway responses in the rat. *Am J Respir Crit Care Med* 149: 1186–1191

57  Abraham W, Sielczak M, Ahmed A, Cortes A, Lauredo I, Kim J, Pepinsky B, Benjamin C, Leone D, Lobb R et al (1994) Alpha 4-integrins mediate antigen-induced late

bronchial responses and prolonged airway hyperresponsiveness in sheep. *J Clin Invest* 93: 776–787

58    Van Oosterhout A, Hessel E, Van Esch B et al (1996) Modulation of IgE, eosinophil migration and airway hyperresponsiveness by antibodies to LFA-1, Mac-1 or VLA-4 in a murine model of allergic asthma. *Am J Respir Crit Care Med* 153: 149–A754

59    Milne A, Piper P (1994) The effects of two anti-CD18 antibodies on antigen-induced air-way hyperresponsiveness and leukocyte accumulation in the guinea pig. *Am J Respir Cell Mol Biol* 11: 337–343

60    Abraham W, Sielczak M, Ahmed A, Cortes A, Lauredo I, Kim J, Pepinsky B, Benjamin C, Leone D, Lobb R, Weller P (1994) Alpha-4 intergrin mediates antigen-induced late bronchial responses and prolonged airway hyperresponsiveness in sheep. *J Clin Invest* 93: 776–787

61    Dedhar S, Hannigan G (1996) Integrin cytoplasmic interaction and bidirectional tran-membrane signalling. *Curr Opin Cell Biol* 8: 657–669

62    Arbones M, Ord D, Ley K, Ratech H, Maynard-Curry C, Otten G, Capon D, Tedder T (1994) Lymphocyte homing and leukocyte rolling and migration are impaired in L-selectin-deficient mice. *Immunity* 1: 247–260

63    Tedder T, Steeber D, Pizcueta P (1995) L-selectin-deficient mice have impaired leukocyte recruitment into inflammatory sites. *J Exp Med* 181: 2259–2264

64    Mayadas T, Johnson R, Rayburn H, Hynes R, Wagner D (1993) Leukocyte rolling and extravasation are severely compromised in P selectin-deficient mice. *Cell* 74: 541–554

65    Subramaniam M, Saffaripour S, Watson S, Mayadas T, Hynes R, Wagner D (1995) Reduced recruitment of inflammatory cells in a contact hypersensitivity response in P-selectin-deficient mice. *J Exp Med* 181: 2277–2282

66    DeSanctis G, Wolyniec W, Green F, Qin S, Jiao A, Finn P, Noonan T, Jeotham A, Gelfand E, Doerschuk C et al (1997) Reduction of allergic airways responses in P-selectin-defi-cent mice. *Am J Physiol* 6: 681–687

67    Wolyniec W, DeSanctis G, Haynes N, Jaio A, Drazen J, Noonan T (1997) Intercellular adhesion molecule-1 (ICAM-1) mediates airway hyperresponsiveness in ovalbumin cha-lenged mice. *Proc Am Thoracic Soc*: A876

68    Kanwar S, Bullard D, Hickey M, Smith C, Beaudet A, Wolitzky B, Kubes P (1997) The association between alpha 4-integrin, P-selectin, and E-selectin in an allergic model of inflammation. *J Exp Med* 185: 1077–1087

69    Austrup F, Vestweber D, Borges E, Löhning M, Bräuers R, Herz U, Renz H, Hallmann R, Scheffold A, Radbruch A et al (1997) P- and E-selectin mediate recruitment of T-helper-1 but not T-helper-2-cells into inflamed tissues. *Nature* 385: 81–83

70    Woronicz J, Goa X, Cao Z, Rothe M, Goeddel D (1997) IκB Kinase-β: NF-κB activa-tion and complex formation with IκB kinase-α and NIK. *Science* 866–869

71    Ihle J (1995) Cytokine receptor signalling. *Nature* 377: 591–594

72    Takeda K, Tanaka T, Shi W, Matsumoto M, Minami M, Kashiwamura S, Nakanishi K, Yoshida N, Kishimoto T, Akira S (1996) Essential role for STAT-6 in IL-4 signalling. *Nature* 380: 627–631

73    Callard R, Matthews D, Hibbert L (1996) IL-4 and IL-13 receptors: are they one and the same? *Immunol Today* 17: 108–110

74    Laudanna C, Campbell J, Butcher E (1996) Role of Rho in chemoattractant-activated leukocyte adhesion through integrins. *Science* 271: 981–983

75    Coppolino M, Woodside M, Demaurex N, Grinstein S, St-Arnuad R, Dedhar S (1997) Calreticulin is essential for integrin-mediated calcium signalling and cell adhesion. *Nature* 386: 843–846

76    Baggiolini M, Moser B (1997) Blocking chemokine receptors. *J Exp Med* 186: 1189–1191

77    Gong J, Ratkey K, Waterfield J, Clarklewis I (1997) An antagonist of monocyte chemoattractant protein 1 (MCP-1) inhibits arthritis in the MRL-lpr mouse model. *J Exp Med* 186: 131–137

78    Vonderheide R, Tedder T, Springer T, Staunton D (1994) Residues within a conserved amino acid motif of domains 1 and 4 of VCAM-1 are required for binding to VLA-4. *J Cell Biol* 125: 215–222

79    Osborn L, Vassallo C, Browning B, Tizard R, Haskard D, Benjamin C, Dougas I, Kirchhausen T (1994) Arrangement of domains, and amino acid residues required for binding of vascular cell adhesion molecule-1 to its counter-receptor VLA-4 (alpha 4 beta 1). *J Cell Biol* 124: 601–608

80    Komoriya A, Green L, Mervic M, Yamada S, Yamada K, Humphries M (1991) The minimal essential sequence for a major cell type-specific adhesion site (CS1) within the alternatively spliced type III connecting segment domain of fibronectin is leucine-aspartic acid-valine. *J Biol Chem* 266: 15075–15079

81    Vanderslice P, Ren K, Revelle J, Kim D, Scott D, Bjercke R, Yeh E, Beck P, Kogan T (1997) A cyclic hexapeptide is a potent antagonist of alpha 4 integrins. *J Immunol* 158: 1710–1718

82    McIntyre B, Woodside D, Caruso D, Wooten D, Simon S, Neelamegham S. Revelle J, Vanderslice P (1997) Regulation of human T lymphocyte coactivation with an alpha 4 integrin antagonist peptide. *J Immunol* 158: 4180–4186

83    Ra C, Yasuda M, Yagita H, Okumura K (1994) Fibronectin receptor integrins are involved in mast cell activation. *J Allergy Clin Immunol* 94: 625–628

84    Abraham W, Ahmed A, Sielczak M, Narita M, Arrhenius T, Elices M (1997) Blockade of late-phase airway responses and airway hyperresponsiveness in allergic sheep with a small-molecule peptide inhibitor of VLA-4. *Am J Respir Crit Care Med* 156: 696–703

85    Abraham W, Ahmed A, Cortes A, Sielczak M (1996) Effect of TYB-2285 on antigen-induced airway responses in sheep. *Pharmacol* 9: 49–58

86    McKinnon M, Page K, Uings I, Banks M, Fattah D, Proudfoot A, Graber P, Arod C, Fish R et al (1997) Interleukin 5 mutant distinguishes between two functional responses in human eosinophilis. *J Exp Med* 186: 121–129

87    Dickason R, Huston D (1996) Creation of a biologically active interleukin-5 monomer. *Nature* 379: 652–655

88    Finkelman F, Katona I, Mosmann T, Coffman R (1988) IFN-gamma regulates the iso-

types of Ig secreted during *in vivo* humoral immune responses. *J Immunol* 140: 1022–1027

89   Parronchi P, De Carli M, Manetti R, Simonelli C, Sampognaro S, Piccinni M, Macchia D, Maggi E, Del-Prete G, Romagnani S (1992) IL-4 and IFN (alpha and gamma) exert opposite regulatory effects on the development of cytolytic potential by Th1 or Th2 human T cell clones. *J Immunol* 149: 2977–2983

90   Gavett S, O'Hearn D, Li X, Huang S, Finkelman F, Wills-Karp M (1995) Interleukin-12 inhibits antigen-induced airway hyperresponsiveness, inflammation, and Th2 cytokine expression in mice. *J Exp Med* 182: 1527–1536

91   Kips J, Brusselle G, Joos G, Peleman R, Tavernier J, Devos R, Pauwels R (1996) Interleukin-12 inhibits antigen-induced airway hyperresponsiveness in mice. *Am J Respir Crit Care Med* 153 (2): 535–539

92   Nakajima H, Nakao A, Watanabe Y, Yoshida S, Iwamoto I (1994) IFN-alpha inhibits antigen-induced eosinophil and CD4+ T cell recruitment into tissue. *J Immunol* 153: 1264–1270

93   Hogan S, Foster P, Tan X, Ramsay A (1998) Mucosal interleukin-12 gene delivery inhibits allergic airways disease and restores local antiviral immunity. *Eur J Immunol* 28: 413–423

94   Albelda S, Smith C, Ward P (1994) Adhesion molecules and inflammatory injury. *FASEB J* 8: 504–512

# Index